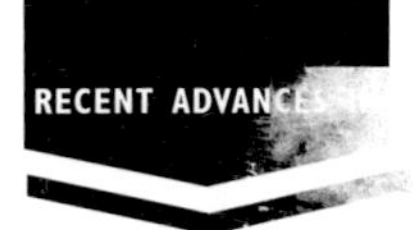




# Paediatrics

RECENT ADVANCES IN PAEDIATRICS

***Contents of Number 13***
*Edited by T. J. David*



ISBN 0443 051003

You can place you order by contacting your local medical bookseller or the Sales Promotion Department, Churchill Livingtone, Robert Stevenson House, 1-3 Baxter's Place, Leith Walk, Edinburgh EH1 3AF, UK

Tel: (0131) 556 2424; Telex: 727511 LONGMN G; Fax: (0131) 558 1278

Look out for *Recent Advances in Paediatrics* 15 in November 1996

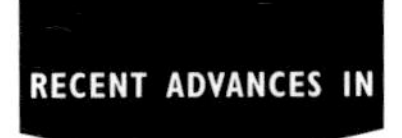


# Paediatrics

Edited by

**T. J. David** MD PhD FRCP DCH

Professor and Head,
Department of Child Health,
University of Manchester;
Honorary Consultant Paediatrician,
Booth Hall Children's Hospital,
Royal Manchester Children's Hospital and
St Mary's Hospital,
Manchester, UK

NUMBER FOURTEEN

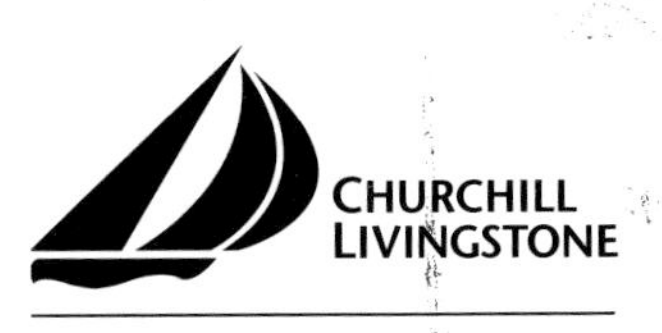


NEW YORK, EDINBURGH, LONDON, MADRID, MELBOURNE, SAN FRANCISCO AND TOKYO 1995

CHURCHILL LIVINGSTONE
Medical Division of Pearson Professional Ltd

Distributed in the United States of America by Churchill Livingstone Inc., 650 Avenue of the Americas, New York, N.Y. 10011, and by associated companies branches and representatives throughout the world.



First published 1995

ISBN 0-443-053081
ISSN 0-309-0140

**British Library Cataloguing in Publication Data**
A catalogue record for this book is available from the British Library

**Library of Congress Cataloguing in Publication Data**
A catalogue record for this book is available from the Library of Congress

Page layout: Janet Smith

Produced by Longman Singapore Publishers Pte Ltd
Printed in Singapore

The publisher's policy is to use **paper manufactured from sustainable forests**

# Contents

# Preface

The aim of Recent Advances in Paediatrics is to provide a review of important topics and help doctors keep abreast of developments in the subject. The book is intended for the practising clinician and the postgraduate student. There are 12 chapters which cover a variety of general paediatric and neonatal areas. Six chapters have a community orientation, and there are two chapters on the important tropical paediatric subjects of vitamin A deficiency and trachoma. The selection of topics has veered towards those of general rather than special interest.

The final chapter, an annotated literature review, is a personal selection of key articles and useful reviews published in 1994. As with the choice of subjects for the main chapters, the selection of articles has inclined towards those of general rather than special interest. There is, however, special emphasis on community paediatrics and tropical paediatrics, as these two important areas tend to be less well covered in general paediatric journals. Trying to reduce to an acceptable size the short-list of particularly interesting articles is an especially difficult task.

Annual publication of this book provides the opportunity to respond to the wishes of readers, and any suggestions for topics to be included in future issues would always be welcome. Please write to me at the address below.

I am indebted to the authors for their hard work, prompt delivery of manuscripts and patience in dealing with my queries and requests. I would also like to thank my secretaries Angela Smithies and Val Smith, Yvonne O'Leary and Gill Haddock of Churchill Livingstone for all their help, and my wife and sons for all their support.

Professor T. J. David
University Department of Child Health
Booth Hall Children's Hospital
Manchester M9 7AA,
UK

1995

# Contributors

**Peter S. Baxter** MA MBBS MD MRCP DCH
Consultant Paediatrician/Paediatric Neurologist, Northern General Hospital NHS Trust, Sheffield, UK

**Howard M. Berger** MRCP BSc PhD
Professor in Neonatal Medicine, Neonatal Unit, Department of Paediatrics, University Hospital, Leiden, The Netherlands

**Linda Bobo** PhD
Assistant Professor, Department of Pediatric Infectious Diseases, Dana Center for Preventive Ophthalmology, Baltimore, Maryland, USA

**T. J. David** MD PhD FRCP DCH
Professor and Head, Department of Child Health, University of Manchester; Honorary Consultant Paediatrician, Booth Hall Children's Hospital, Royal Manchester Children's Hospital and St Mary's Hospital, Manchester, UK

**Máire Messenger Davies** BA PhD
Principal Lecturer, Media Studies, School of Media, London Institute, London, UK

**S. N. Jarvis**
Donald Court Professor of Community Child Health, Department of Child Health, University of Newcastle upon Tyne, Gateshead, UK

**Harriet L. MacMillan** MD
Assistant Professor, Departments of Psychiatry and Pediatrics, Centre for Studies of Children at Risk, McMaster University, Hamilton, Ontario, Canada

**Ralf M. W. Moison** MSc
Analytical Chemist, Neonatal Unit, Department of Paediatrics, University Hospital, Leiden, The Netherlands

**Colin Morley** MA DCH FRCP MD
Honorary Consultant Paediatrician, Addenbrookes Hospital and University of Cambridge, Cambridge, UK

**Anne C. Niec** MD
Assistant Professor, Departments of Pediatrics and Psychiatry, McMaster University, Hamilton, Ontario, Canada

**David R. Offord** MD
Professor, Department of Psychiatry, Director, Centre for Studies of Children at Risk, McMaster University, Hamilton, Ontario, Canada

**Bosco Paes** MD FRCP(I) FRCP(C)
Professor, Department of Pediatrics (Neonatal Division), Children's Hospital at Chedoke-McMaster and Director of Nurseries, St Joseph's Hospital, Hamilton, Ontario, Canada

**Janet Pinelli** RN MScN DNS(Cand)
Associate Professor and Clinical Nurse Specialist/Neonatal Practitioner, Children's Hospital at Chedoke-McMaster, Hamilton, Ontario, Canada

**C. D. Rittey** MB ChB MRCP
Consultant Paediatric Neurologist, Ryegate Childrens Centre, Sheffield, UK

**Martin P. Samuels** BSc MD MRCP
Senior Lecturer in Paediatrics, Professor of Paediatrics, Academic Department of Paediatrics, North Staffordshire Hospital, Stoke on Trent, UK

**S. M. Shalet** MD FRCP
Professor, Department of Endocrinology, Christie Hospital, Manchester, UK

**David P. Southall** MD FRCP
Professor of Paediatrics, Academic Department of Paediatrics, North Staffordshire Hospital, Stoke on Trent, UK

**Peter G. F. Swift** MA FRCP DCH
Consultant Paediatrician, Leicester Royal Infirmary Children's Hospital, Leicester, UK

**E. M. L. Towner**
Senior Lecturer in Community Child Health, Department of Child Health, University of Newcastle upon Tyne, Gateshead, UK

**Keith P. West** Jr DrPH RD
Associate Professor of International Health and Ophthalmology, The Johns Hopkins School of Public Health and Medicine, Baltimore, Maryland, USA

**Sheila West** PhD
Associate Professor, Wilmer Eye Institute, Dana Center for Preventive Ophthalmology, Baltimore, Maryland, USA

**Diny van Zoeren-Grobben** MB
Neonatologist, Neonatal Unit, Department of Paediatrics, University Hospital, Leiden, The Netherlands

# 1

# The continuing enigma of cot death

*C. J. Morley*

The most remarkable change in cot death (sudden infant death syndrome) over the last few years has been the dramatic reduction in the incidence. This seems to be related to sleeping position but the enigma is that there is no satisfactory explanation why prone sleeping should be involved in sudden unexpected infant deaths and how this fits in with all the pathological abnormalities which have been found in the infants who die.

## REDUCE THE RISK CAMPAIGNS

The data for the change in cot deaths in England and Wales for the last six years are shown in Figure 1.1.[1] There has been a similar reduction in Australia, New Zealand and Holland. This appears to be related to the 'Reduce the Risk Campaigns' in each country where mothers were advised in words similar to: 'do not lie your baby on the front, do not smoke in the presence of the baby and do not to let the baby get too warm'. Interestingly, the UK campaign was not launched until the end of 1991 and, as can be seen from Figure 1.1, the incidence of cot death had started to fall several years before this, although the rate of fall increased from 1991 to 1992. The decline from 1988 is still probably related to a change in infant sleeping position. Christine Hiley (personal communication) has found that information relating sleeping

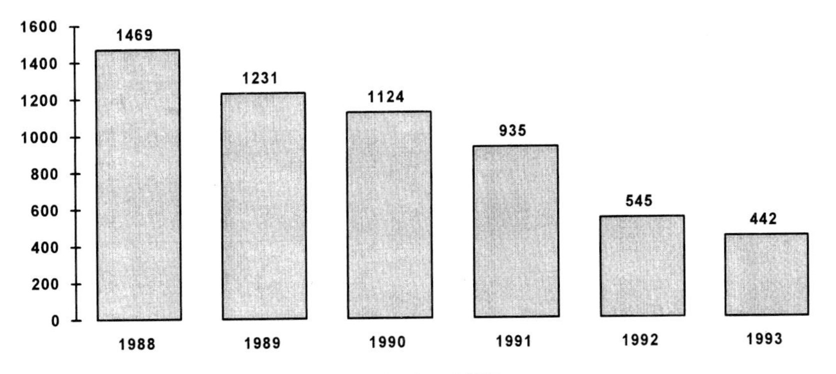


**Fig. 1.1** Number of cot deaths in England and Wales.

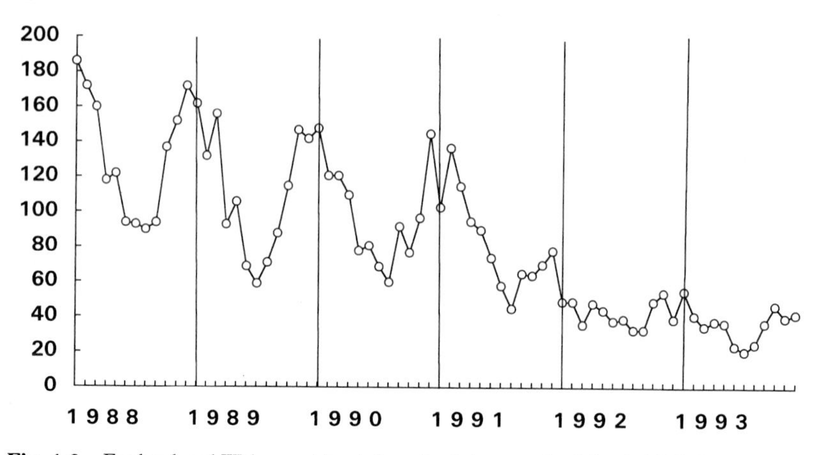


**Fig. 1.2** England and Wales: sudden infant death by month of death 1988-93.

position to cot death was being published in magazines and papers from the end of 1988 with an explosion of information about sleeping position from 1989. Mothers were changing the sleeping position of their babies from front to side from 1988.

With the reduction in the incidence of cot death there has also been a change in season of death. There used to be a peak in the winter but this has now almost disappeared (Fig. 1.2). The peak age for cot death used to be two to four months and this has also become less obvious (Fig. 1.3).

There are many other aspects of child care which have changed over the last few years and may also be related to the reduction in cot deaths (infra vide).

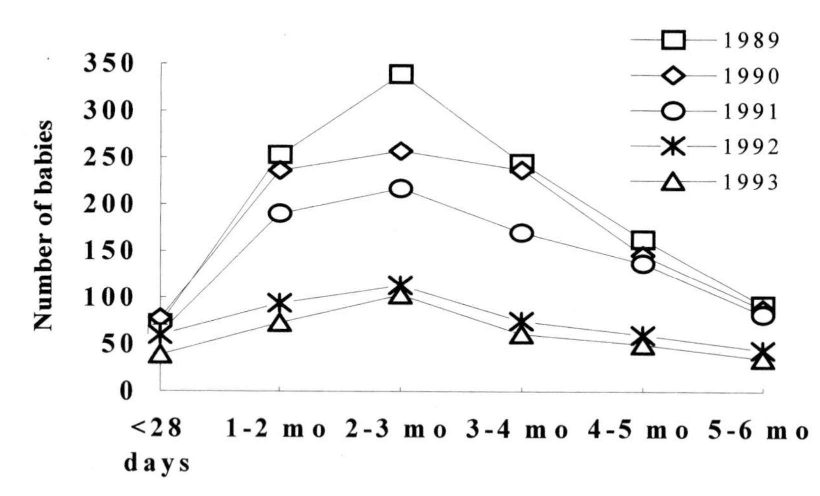


**Fig. 1.3** Age at death 1989-93.

## RISK FACTORS FOR COT DEATH

There is now extremely good data to show that prone sleeping position is a very important risk factor for cot death. The main UK study, undertaken in the district of Avon,[2] compared 72 infants dying suddenly and unexpectedly with two controls matched for age and date. Parents were interviewed and information was collected on bedding, sleeping position, heating and recent signs of illness for index and control infants. Compared with the controls the infants who had died from cot death were more likely to have been sleeping prone (relative risk 8.8), to have been more heavily wrapped (relative risk 1.14 per tog above 8 togs), and to have had the heating on all night (relative risk 2.7). The infants older than 70 days with these factors were at higher risk than the younger infants.

In 1993, Mitchell[3] reviewed all the evidence about sleeping position and cot death, analysing the 17 best case-control studies. He points out that there are difficulties with comparing the studies, such as: different case and control definitions, the bias introduced by case selection and matching, definitions of sleeping position, recall bias of the carers, and confounders such as age, birthweight, social class, rank, ethnicity, geography and sex. Despite these problems, a meta-analysis showed the pooled relative risk associated with the prone sleeping position was 2.8 (95% CI from 2.1 to 3.6) and none of the studies suggested the converse. Mitchell cogently argues, using the nine criteria of Hill (Table 1.1),[4] that prone sleeping is not just associated with cot but that it should be considered to be a cause.

**Table 1.1** The criteria of Hill used to prove that prone sleeping is a cause of cot death

| | |
|---|---|
| Strength | The stronger the association the more likely it is to be causal. The odds ratio for a baby dying from cot death if he is lying prone is moderately strong. |
| Consistency | All studies have shown an odds ratio greater than 1 for cot death in a prone sleeping baby, even where it did not reach statistical significance. |
| Specificity | Prone sleeping would appear to be a risk factor across the world although so far the risk appears to be greatest in Australasia and Europe. |
| Temporal sequence | In this, the factor thought to be causative must precede the event and not be a consequence of it. Babies who are put down to sleep prone are at greatest risk of subsequent cot death. |
| Biological gradient | There is a gradient in the risk for cot death with different sleeping positions, with prone sleeping being a greater risk than side sleeping, which is greater than supine. |
| Biological plausibility | At the moment this is not fulfilled because so far there is no known reason why prone sleeping causes cot death. |
| Coherence | The assumption of a causal relationship between prone sleeping and cot death does not conflict with what is known about the disease. |
| Experiment | The most striking experiments are the effect of the 'Reduce the Risk Campaigns' on the incidence of prone sleeping and cot death. |
| Analogy | There are other environmental factors which affect health, such as smoking and lung cancer or pollution and asthma. |

**Table 1.2**

| | Before the campaign n = 385 | After the campaign n = 399 | Event rate difference and 95% CI | *P* |
|---|---|---|---|---|
| Sleeping on their front | | | | |
| Newborn | 81 (21%) | 16 (4%) | –17 (–13 to –22) | < 0.0001 |
| 3 months old | 105 (27%) | 29 (7%) | –20 (–15 to –25) | < 0.0001 |
| 6 months old | 94 (25%) | 32 (8%) | –17 (–11 to –21) | < 0.0001 |
| Sleeping on their back | | | | |
| Newborn | 36 (10%) | 158 (40%) | 30 (25 to 36) | < 0.0001 |
| 3 months old | 55 (14%) | 215 (54%) | 40 (34 to 46) | < 0.0001 |
| 6 months old | 117 (31%) | 257 (65%) | 34 (28 to 41) | < 0.0001 |
| Sleeping on their side | | | | |
| Newborn | 262 (68%) | 224 (56%) | –12 (–5 to –19) | < 0.0001 |
| 3 months old | 225 (58%) | 154 (39%) | –20 (–13 to –27) | < 0.0001 |
| 6 months old | 169 (45%) | 108 (27%) | –17 (–10 to –23) | < 0.0001 |
| Duvets or quilts used | | | | |
| Newborn | 139 (36%) | 104 (26%) | –10 (–4 to –17) | 0.011 |
| 3 months old | 196 (51%) | 152 (38%) | –13 (–6 to –20) | 0.0003 |
| 6 months old | 258 (67%) | 223 (56%) | –11 (–18 to –44) | 0.006 |
| Babies covered with three blankets or more | | | | |
| Newborn | 58 (15%) | 92 (23%) | 8 (3 to 14) | 0.0045 |
| 3 months old | 50 (13%) | 76 (19%) | 6 (2 to 11) | 0.016 |
| 6 months old | 27 (7%) | 64 (16%) | 9 (5 to 13) | 0.0005 |
| Mothers' worries about their babies' temperature | | | | |
| Baby too cold | 119 (31%) | 76 (19%) | –12 (–6 to –18) | 0.0001 |
| Baby too hot | 91 (24%) | 149 (37%) | 13 (7 to 20) | 0.0003 |
| Used a wall thermometer | 40 (10%) | 87 (22%) | 12 (6 to 17) | 0.0013 |
| Babies sleeping in the parents' room | | | | |
| Newborn | 300 (78%) | 315 (79%) | 1 (–5 to 6) | NS |
| 3 months old | 150 (39%) | 188 (47%) | 8 (1 to 15) | 0.028 |
| 6 months old | 77 (20%) | 120 (30%) | 10 (4 to 16) | 0.004 |
| Babies in the parents' bed | | | | |
| At any time in first six months | 193 (50%) | 243 (61%) | 11 (4 to 18) | 0.002 |
| Usually | 15 (4%) | 24 (6%) | 2 (–1 to 5) | NS |
| Smoking | | | | |
| Mothers smoking in pregnancy | 72 (19%) | 87 (22%) | 3 (–3 to 9) | NS |
| Other members of the household | 109 (28%) | 104 (26%) | -2 (–4 to 9) | NS |
| Not smoking near the baby | 242 (63%) | 286 (72%) | -9 (2 to –15) | 0.022 |
| Breast feeding | | | | |
| Breast fed in the first month | 226 (58%) | 242 (60%) | 2 (–5 to 9) | NS |

The 'Reduce the Risk Campaigns' were associated with a fall in the incidence of cot death. However, it was not clear whether this was coincidence or whether the mothers had followed the advice of the campaigns. Hiley[5] showed that several aspects of baby care were changed by the campaign. These are shown in Table 1.2. During this time the incidence of cot death in the region fell. The numbers of babies dying were 40 in 1989, 56 in 1990, 33 in 1991, 12 in 1992, 14 in 1994.

These data showed that the campaign had a very significant influence on babies' sleeping position and mothers were also more aware of not letting their babies get too hot, although overall they seemed to clothe them appropriately. Sadly, it had no effect on the incidence of smoking, probably one of the highest risk factors for cot death. However, it is possible that families are being more careful about not smoking near their babies. There was also no change in the incidence of breast feeding, a factor considered in some studies to be a preventative factor.

In a study published in 1994,[6] comparing different factors before and during the 'Reduce the Risk Campaign' in Avon, Wigfield et al showed there was a significant reduction in cot death from 3.5 to 1.7 per 1000 live births. This was associated with a reduction in prone sleeping from 60% to 28%. The seasonal variation in incidence also changed and a higher proportion of deaths in the second study occurred to ex-premature babies than in the first and the male predominance was accentuated. Prone sleeping still carried a highly significant risk in the second study but the relative importance of other risk factors had apparently changed: maternal smoking in pregnancy and the use of bottle feeding from birth had higher odds ratios in the second study whereas the odds ratio for heavy wrapping and overnight heating no longer reached significance.

In The Netherlands,[7] the incidence of cot death has fallen from 1.04/1000 live births in 1986 to 0.44 in 1991. This was closely related to national advice in 1987 that babies should not sleep prone. At that time, about 60% were sleeping prone but by 1990 this had fallen to 16%. This reduction in cot death was accompanied by a reduction in all respiratory deaths. The fall in cot death in The Netherlands has paralleled the continuing decrease in the prone sleeping position.

## CLOTHING AND BEDDING

The large New Zealand case control study, set up to investigate risk factors that contribute to cot death, identified prone sleeping position, smoking by adults, lack of breast feeding and sharing a bed with an adult who smoked as prime modifiable risk factors. They also showed that infants dying of cot death were more likely to be male, with young unmarried parents, of Maori race and more likely to die during the winter months. A paper on these data, by Wilson et al,[8] describes the infants' clothing and bedding and their relationship with the risk of cot death. There was little difference in the clothing worn by the two groups of infants. Their most interesting findings are shown in Table 1.3.

In a longitudinal study by Wigfield et al,[9] overnight recordings were made in the bedrooms of 152 babies aged 3–18 weeks, the insulation provided by their bedclothes was assessed and the outside temperature measured. The

**Table 1.3** Data from the New Zealand cot death case control study

| | Cot deaths n = 393 | Controls n = 1592 |
|---|---|---|
| In a cot at death (or index night) | 28% | 40% |
| In a parent's bed at death (or index night) | 21% | 10% |
| No waterproof layer over mattress | 68% | 52% |
| Sheepskin under baby | 32% | 32% |
| Only a sheet under the baby | 40% | 28% |
| Woven woollen waterproof under blanket `drycot' | 16% | 32% |
| Adult pillow | 13% | 8% |
| Layers over the baby | 3 | 3 |
| Use of duvets | 58% | 46% |
| Firm tucking of covers | 62% | 74% |
| Bonnet worn | 8% | 5% |

amount of clothing and bedding varied widely from 0.1 tog to 23 tog. Very few babies slept with their heads covered. There was little correlation between age and insulation and no correlation between age and bedroom temperature. The amount of insulation did not vary with sleeping position. There was an inverse relationship between the level of insulation and the minimum bedroom temperature. The babies were, on average, covered with an extra 2 tog in the winter compared with the summer, for the same room temperatures. The levels of thermal insulation to achieve thermoneutrality were calculated from measurements on infants over a range of air temperatures for each age group of babies. Broadly based thermal guidelines for night-time covers for babies up to 4 months derived from the studies are shown in Table 1.4. These calculations all include one sheet (0.2 tog) over the baby. In this study, they found there was a close similarity between the average amount of clothing and bedding that parents chose for their babies and values calculated from their laboratory studies. Obviously the clothing may need to be varied depending on the exact nature of the covers and the type of mattress and the environmental conditions. Covering a baby's head may profoundly affect the thermal balance of the baby.

**Table 1.4** Levels of insulation calculated for babies in the first few months of life

| Season | Usual range of night time temperature (°C) | Total tog of covering required | Clothing (0.8 tog) | Layers of blanket (1.2 tog/layer) |
|---|---|---|---|---|
| Winter (cool) | 14–17 | 6–9 | Babygro, vest | 4–7 |
| Winter (average) | 16–19 | 5–8 | Babygro, vest | 4–6 |
| Summer (average) | 20–22 | 4–6 | Babygro, vest | 3–4 |
| Summer (warm) | 23–25 | 3–4 | Babygro, vest | 2–3 |

## ETHNIC AND CULTURAL DIFFERENCES IN COT DEATH RATES

In 1985, Davies,[10] commenting on the low incidence of cot death in Hong Kong, speculated 'that the possible influence of lifestyle and care taking practices such as posture and babies never being left alone were being underestimated in preference to more exotic and esoteric explanations for the aetiology of cot death'. In 1994,[11] he reviewed the background to ethnic differences in the incidence of cot death. In the USA, the incidence is higher in blacks than whites and Hispanics with the lowest incidence in the oriental Americans. In New Zealand, the Maori population has a higher incidence than the Europeans. In the UK, despite a higher post-neonatal mortality among Asian people (India, Pakistan and Bangladesh), the cot death rate was lower in these groups than among the infants born to mothers born in Britain or Ireland with higher rates among Afro-Caribbean people. The paradox was that Asian mothers were often poorer, had more children and less satisfactory housing than Caucasian mothers, all factors that might be expected to increase cot death. In a Chicago study, the Hispanics shared many of the adverse social and environmental factors of black families and yet their incidence of cot death was four times less. A study by Grether et al,[12] showed that the longer oriental families lived in the USA the greater became the risk of cot death, implying local social and environmental influences. In Hong Kong with a low incidence of cot death, overcrowding, lack of breast feeding and a high incidence of respiratory infections could also have been considered risk factors. We are left with the provoking thought, 'could culturally associated infant care practices provide an important clue to sudden infant death?'

Mitchell and Scragg[13] have shown that the ethnic differences in New Zealand are largely due to the differences in known risk factors between the Maori and non-Maori populations.

Petersen and Wailoo[14] found differences in the maturation of night time body temperature patterns in infants and correlated this with an increased risk of cot death. They have now shown that there is no difference in the maturation of body temperature patterns between Asian and European infants. If anything, the Asian infants were slightly less mature, the opposite of what would have been expected if the racial differences in cot death rate were due to physiological differences. Interestingly, the Asian infants slept in warmer bedrooms than the white infants.

Farooqi,[15] in a study of 374 multiparous women in Birmingham, conducted before the 'Reduce the Risk Campaign', showed that 94% of Asian infants slept in their parents' bedroom during the first year at night compared with 61% of whites and 36% slept in their parents' bed compared with 11% of whites. Only 4% of Asian infants slept prone, compared with 33% of white infants. The majority of Asian and white mothers placed their infants on the side, 46% and 58% respectively, and only 6% of white mothers placed their infant supine, compared with 34% of Asian mothers.

Studies have shown that infant-parent co-sleeping alters the infant's sleep experience as, for example, the characteristics of arousals, the frequency and duration of nursing, infant sleep position and the number of maternal inspections. For example, while sleeping in the same bed mothers nursed their infants three times more frequently than they do while their infants are sleeping in an adjacent room. Preliminary data from McKenna et al[16] demonstrate significant differences between routine co-sleeping and solitary sleeping environments.

## DO PRONE SLEEPING BABIES GET CARBON DIOXIDE NARCOSIS?

Bolton et al[17] explored the idea that the reported association between cot death and sleeping prone could be due to rebreathing expired carbon dioxide. They constructed a model to investigate this and suggested that with the head face down in the mattress, particularly if it was soft, an infant would rapidly accumulate a dangerous level of carbon dioxide. Kemp et al[18] also investigated this with sedated rabbits breathing through a tracheostomy attached to the nares of an infant mannequin head placed on a child's bedding in the same position as a child who had died while face down. The bedding had low resistance to air flow and caused considerable rebreathing that was lethal in five of the seven rabbits studied. Their conclusion was that infants who were face down in the bedding could rebreath exhaled gases and that this might be lethal.

Chiodini et al[19] investigated 11 infants aged 0.2 to 6 months while sleeping in different positions. Before the study all infants had predominantly slept prone. They were studied on soft and firm mattresses. Their face was passively placed in the face down position. All infants were observed to sleep in this position at some time during the study. Spontaneous turning of the head to the face down position during sleep occurred in 10/11 infants. Once in this position the infants stayed for a range of 0.1–19.2 min before turning their face to the side. All infants, regardless of age, were capable of turning the head out of the face down position. Sometimes they lifted it up and sometimes they slip it round. There was an increase in end tidal partial pressure of carbon dioxide in infants sleeping face down on soft bedding which corresponded to an increase from 36 mmHg to 40 mmHg. There was no significant change in the end tidal partial pressure of carbon dioxide in infants face down in firm bedding. There was no significant change in heart rate or respiratory rate during face down breathing, nor was there any change in oxygen saturation. One infant did drop his oxygen level to 85% but he showed no signs of arousal. This study suggests that infants can easily sleep face down without any apparent difficulty. However, these were all healthy children and it gives no indication of how they would behave if they were ill with an upper respiratory tract infection or fever.

In a review of this area of research, Johnson[20] dismisses the idea of carbon dioxide rebreathing as a cause of death, commenting that the studies were unphysiological and clinical studies realistically conducted show that the inspired carbon dioxide did not rise above 2–3% and only increased expired carbon dioxide from 36 Torr to 40 Torr in the worst situation with unchanged oxygen levels.

## PATHOLOGICAL FINDINGS AND COT DEATH

In spite of the encouraging decline in the incidence of sudden infant deaths, it is still the single commonest cause of death between 1 and 12 months. It was thought, and still is by some, that the infants who died of cot death are not entirely normal. They 'exhibit structural and functional abnormalities during life and at post mortem, which serve to indicate in some way, not as yet defined, that they are physiologically defective'. The enigma is that if this is true why has the cot death rate fallen so dramatically with the 'Reduce the Risk Campaign'?

One of the problems with discussing cot death incidences is that there is a disagreement about the percentage of cases presenting as cot deaths that eventually were found to be due to other causes. Byard et al[21] examined all cases presenting in Adelaide over 10 years from 1983 to 1992. There were 361 cases of unexpected death in infants who had been considered well by their parents with only minimal symptoms and signs. Of these, 329 (91%) were identified as cot death. Of the others, 9 (2.5%) were due to accidental asphyxia based on death scene investigation and 23 (6.4%) were due to a variety of other diseases. This paper emphasises the importance of high class paediatric pathology with routine microbiological testing – bacteriology of lung, faeces, spleen, CSF and blood with the option of the middle ear, and virological testing of lung, faeces, liver and CSF with the option of nasopharyngeal, blood and spleen. It also emphasises the importance of a careful death scene examination and careful sympathetic questioning of the parents. This is something long overdue in the UK, where it is done sporadically and rarely so completely. With fewer babies dying of cot death there is even more reason why paediatric pathologists must undertake all post-mortem examinations on these infants to determine whether the causes of death are changing.

### Abnormalities of the diaphragm

A study by Lamont et al[22] examined the type 1 and type 2 fibres in the diaphragm, external intercostal and psoas muscles of 37 cot death cases and 20 controls. Type 1 are fatigue resistant fibres. The fatiguability of a muscle can be related to its proportion of type 1 to type 2 fibres. There were fewer type 1 fibres in cot death cases (median 30%) compared with control infants (median 40%) ($P < 0.02$) whereas the diameter of type 1 fibres in the cot deaths was larger (median 33.9 μm) than in control (median 30.3 μm) infants ($P < 0.007$). The total cross-sectional area occupied by type 1 and type 2 fibres was similar in both groups. There were no differences in the external intercostal or psoas muscles. The percentage of type 1 fibres correlated poorly with post conceptional age, sex, body weight, length and postmortem delay. The finding suggests these infants may be predisposed to diaphragmatic fatigue. The hypertrophy of type 1 fibres could be explained by increased resistive loads on the muscle but it does not explain why the children have fewer type 1 fibres. This could be congenital, either genetic or due to intrauterine factors. An upper respiratory tract infection might be the final insult if the child had an abnormal diaphragm liable to fatigue.

## Endotoxins

Bacterial toxins have been proposed as one cause of sudden unexpected death. Bettelheim et al[23] examined gut segments from 46 cot death cases of which 37 (80%) grew *Escherichia coli* and 21 (46%) were carrying toxigenic strains. Stools were obtained from live infants admitted to hospital and selected on the basis of age, socio-economic status, race, gestational age, feeding and having a condition unrelated to the gastrointestinal tract and had not taken antibiotics in the preceding month. *E. coli* strains were isolated from 20/24 (83%) but none were toxigenic. No toxigenic strains were isolated from infants dying of other conditions. There was a trend towards the babies with toxigenic strains of *E. coli* being bottle fed but this did not reach statistical significance. This extremely high isolation rate of toxigenic *E. coli* from infants dying of cot death suggests a possible causal relationship.

## Abnormal immune responses

It has been hypothesized that cot death may be an abnormal immune response to common respiratory pathogens in the lungs of vulnerable infants. Howat et al[24] studied the lungs of 48 infants who had died of cot death and compared them with 30 who had died of non-pulmonary causes with no lung inflammation. They examined the lungs for eosinophil and neutrophil leucocytes, mast cells, and T and B lymphocytes. There were three times more eosinophils in the lungs of infants who had died of cot death both for the parenchyma (28 vs 8 cells/mm$^2$) and the peribronchial region (19 vs 5 cells/mm$^2$). This was independent of the age and sex of the child. There was an increase in CD3 positive T lymphocytes and B CD20 positive lymphocytes in both the parenchyma and peribronchial tissues. There were more peribronchial mast cells in the cot death group (22 vs 15 cells/mm$^2$). There were insignificant differences in the neutrophils and parenchymal mast cells at both sites in either group. This finding suggests that an abnormal or inappropriate inflammatory response had occurred in association with cot death. This inflammatory reaction is similar to that seen in an allergic inflammation. However, it may be that the immature immune system lacks the fine control necessary to produce appropriate immune responses to common pathogens. An aberrant response to viral infection is a possible explanation for these findings. Compared with controls, cot death infants had higher blood levels of CD19 (B cells), higher levels of CD29 and CD38 (lymphocyte activation markers). In the thymus, CD38 and CD58 (lymphocyte activation markers) were higher in cot death. In the tonsils, CD45RA (immature T cells) were at lower levels and the activated counterpart

CD45RO (activated mature T cells) at higher levels in cot death. This lends support to the view that there is immunological activation occurring in cot death. There is some limited evidence suggestive of B cell activation (involved in humoral activity) and more striking evidence of T cell activation.

Platt et al[25] analysed the blood tryptase levels in 50 cot death infants and 15 controls and also investigated sections of lung for mast cells. They showed the tryptase in serum was significantly higher in the cot death group (median 6.2 ng/ml) compared with the controls (1.1 ng/ml) ($P = 0.0004$). Tryptase levels in 20 (40%) of the cot death cases were greater than 10 ng/ml, a value recommended for adults to indicate mast cell activation premortem. Living infants under 1 year of age without active allergic disease or mastocytosis typically have tryptase levels below 1 to 1.7 ng/ml. The level of tryptase was not influenced by death to postmortem interval or whether resuscitation had been attempted or not. To investigate whether mite or milk allergens could be involved in the pathogenesis of cot death, IgE-specific antibodies to bovine β-lactalbumin, α-lactalbumin, κ-casein and mite extracts were analysed. There were no differences between the groups for α-lactalbumin, κ-casein and mite extracts. For the β-lactalbumin, 15/38 of the cot death subjects had detectable antibody compared with 1/9 of the controls. Lung sections showed no significant differences in the number or type of mast cells in the entire lung or in the peribronchiolar, perivascular or interstitial areas between the cot death and the controls. This was not related to different levels of tryptase.

This study provides further evidence that mast cell activation is involved in some cot death cases and indicates that one cause of cot death may be anaphylaxis caused by mast cell activation. The findings suggest that cow's milk may be an offending allergen and induce an IgE mediated anaphylaxis in some cases. However, milk allergy involvement in the mast cell activation remains uncertain.

Forsyth et al[26] showed increased levels of immunoglobulins in pulmonary lavage specimens taken from infants dying of cot death. Raised IgG, IgM, and IgA concentrations were found to be associated with sudden unexpected deaths. It is not certain whether this is local secretion or just passive diffusion as part of the pulmonary oedema, but it again suggests an immunological reaction in the lungs.

## Cot death and organ size

In a comprehensive study of organ weights in 500 cot death cases over 15 years at the University of Washington, Seattle, Siebert et al[27] compared their data with norms published by Coppoletta and Wolbach,[28] Schulz et al,[29] TÑhkÑ[30,31] and Shankle.[32] All dissections were performed by one individual. The mean body weights for females and males were generally between the 10th and 50th centiles for normal living infants. For the infants more than 8 months old, the mean weight was well below the 10th centile. Organ weights for thymus, lungs, liver and brain were significantly above those expected for published norms in the majority of cases, the adrenal gland being a prominent exception. The heart weight was borderline elevated.

The weight of the thymus was high, but possibly because published norms are too low, being derived from infants who were ill prior to death. Increase in lung weight is because they were congested and oedematous. It remains unclear whether cot death brains have normal weights and the published standards are low or whether they are disproportionately heavy.

Hinchcliffe et al[33]<D> investigated the total number of nephrons in the kidneys of 24 cot death cases with those of 16 controls of the same age who were born at more than 36 weeks' gestation and weighed between the 10th and 90th centiles. They were estimated blind to the origin of the specimen using a new technique. The number in both the cot death groups was significantly less (P <0.001) than the number in the controls: cot death birth weight <10th centile (n = 9) 635 000 (range 327 000–1 010 000); cot death normal birth weight (n = 15) 690 000 (range 361 000–1 040 000); controls (n = 16) 903 000 (range 740 000–1 060 000).

This renal developmental arrest may be only one manifestation of a general, somatic developmental defect, reflecting adverse intrauterine conditions. The mean (range) for renal weight of the cot death group was 19.5 g (12.5 to 26.9 g). This was significantly different from the controls 23.2 g (13.3 to 32.8 g). This was considered to be due to the presence of proportionally more cases of greater postnatal age in the control group than a real difference in mean weight. None of the renal weight fell outside the 95% for age. There was no relationship between birthweight and nephron number. The cot death infants tended to be light for their postnatal age.

What we do not know is whether the reduction in cot death rate in the last few years has altered the known risk factors of: young maternal age, high parity, winter deaths, peak at 2 to 4 months, low birth weight, multiple birth, low social class, smoking or the typical postmortem findings of: frothy blood-tinged fluid around the nose, thymus with petechial haemorrhages, petechial haemorrhages below the visceral pleura, epicardial petechiae, liquid heart blood (80%), prominent lymph nodes and Peyer's patches, pulmonary congestion and oedema, mild inflammation of the upper respiratory tract, focal fibrinoid necrosis of the vocal cords, persistent haematopoiesis in the liver.

What is not clear is how these factors can be related to the profound influence of sleeping position on cot deaths. Unless prone sleeping is just the final common pathway that stresses a vulnerable infected infant. Nevertheless it is not clear why these otherwise healthy infants should have such profound pulmonary congestion and oedema. Is this primary or secondary? Will these change with the changing incidence? With a fall in the incidence of pure cot death the proportion of sudden and unexpected deaths that are due to explicable causes should increase.

Fortunately, the incidence of cot deaths has fallen but frustratingly we still do not have a satisfactory explanation for this, particularly in the face of all the data suggesting these babies have pathological abnormalities. It is possible that the babies who are now dying of cot death may have different problems and risk factors. We are beholden not only to maintain the momentum of the campaign but also to carefully investigate and tabulate each new death to try to determine which factors are now responsible for increasing the risk of cot death.

## KEY POINTS FOR CLINICAL PRACTICE

- Cot death is causally related to prone sleeping with a relative risk of at least 2.8. Wherever babies' sleeping positions have changed from prone to supine or side, the incidence of cot death has fallen.
- The incidence of maternal smoking and bottle feeding, known risk factors for cot death, has not changed with the campaigns. There is good statistical evidence that if the incidence of these were reduced there would be a further reduction in cot deaths.
- Over-wrapping babies is a risk factor for cot death but most mothers cover their babies with appropriate layers, although more layers are used in the winter for the same room temperature.
- There are large ethnic differences in the incidence of cot death with some of the poorest and over crowded Asian families having the lowest incidence. Together with McKenna's studies of the sleeping patterns of infants sleeping with their mothers, this suggests that hitherto unsuspected cultural aspects of infant care may be very important.
- Despite studies to suggest carbon dioxide narcosis may be a factor in cot death among prone sleeping babies they are so far unconvincing.
- There are many new pathological findings in cot death babies: abnormal diaphragm muscle cells; a high incidence of colonisation with toxigenic bacteria; abnormal immune responses; and abnormally small organs. All these suggest that the babies who died a cot death were not normal healthy babies at the time of death.

## REFERENCES

1 Office of Population Census and Surveys. OPCS Monitor 1993; DH3 93/2.
2 Fleming PJ, Gilbert R, Azaz Y et al. Interaction between bedding and sleeping position in the sudden infant death syndrome: a population based case-control study. BMJ 1990; 301: 85-89
3 Mitchell EA. Sleeping position of infants and the sudden infant death syndrome. Acta Paediatrica 1993; 389 Suppl: 26-30
4 Hill AB. The environment and disease: association or causation? Proc R Soc Med 1965; 58: 295-300

5 Hiley CMH, Morley CJ. Evaluation of government's campaign to reduce the risk of cot death. BMJ 1994; 309: 703-704
6 Wigfield R, Gilbert R, Fleming PJ. SIDS: risk reduction measures. Early Hum Dev 1994; 38: 161-164
7 de Jonge GA, Burgmeijer RJF, Engleberts AC et al. Sleeping position for infants and cot death in the Netherlands 1985-91. Arch Dis Child 1993; 69: 660-663
8 Wilson CA, Taylor BJ, Williams SM et al. Clothing and bedding and its relevance to sudden infant death syndrome: further results from the New Zealand cot death study. J Paediatr Child Health 1994; 30: 506-512
9 Wigfield RE, Fleming PJ, Azar YEZ et al. How much wrapping do babies need at night? Arch Dis Child 1993; 69: 181-186
10 Davies DP. Cot death in Hong Kong: a rare problem? Lancet 1985; 2: 1346-1349
11 Davies DP. Ethnicity and sudden infant death syndrome: an introduction. Early Hum Dev 1994; 38: 139-141
12 Grether JK, Schulman J, Croen LA. Sudden infant death syndrome among Asians. J Pediatr 1990; 116: 525-528
13 Mitchell EA, Scragg R. Observations on ethnic differences in SIDS mortality in New Zealand. Early Hum Dev 1994; 38: 151-157
14 Petersen SA, Wailoo MP. Interactions between infant care practices and physiological development in Asian infants. Early Hum Dev 1994; 38: 181-186
15 Farooqi S. Ethnic differences in infant care practices and in the incidence of sudden infant death syndrome in Birmingham. Early Hum Dev 1994; 38: 209-213
16 McKenna JJ, Mosko S. Evolution and infant sleep: experimental studies of infant-parent co-sleeping and its implication for SIDS. Acta Paediatr 1994; 389 Suppl: 31-36
17 Bolton DPG, Taylor BJ, Campbell AJ, Galland BC, Cresswell C. Rebreathing expired gases from bedding: a cause of cot death? Arch Dis Child 1993; 69: 178-190
18 Kemp JS, Kowalski RM, Burch PM, Graham MA, Thach BT. Unintentional suffocation by rebreathing: a death scene and physiologic investigation of a possible cause of sudden death. J Pediatr 1993; 122: 874-880
19 Chiodini BA, Thach BT. Impaired ventilation in infants sleeping facedown: potential significance for sudden infant death syndrome. J Pediatr 1993; 123: 686-692
20 Johnson P. Infant care practices and the investigation of physiological mechanisms. Early Hum Dev 1994; 38: 165-179
21 Byard RW, Carmichael E, Beal S. How useful is post-mortem examination in sudden infant death syndrome? Pediatr Pathol 1994; 14: 817-822
22 Lamont P, Chow C, Hilton J, Pamphlett R. Differences in diaphragm fibre types in SIDS infants. J Neuropathol Exp Neurol 1995; 54: 32-37
23 Bettelheim KA, Goldwater PN, Dwyer BW, Bourne AJ, Smith DL. Toxigenic Escherichia coli associated with sudden infant death syndrome. Scan J Infect Dis 1990; 22: 467-476.
24 Howat WJ. Moore IE, Judd M, Roche W. Pulmonary immunopathology of sudden infant death syndrome. Lancet 1994; 343: 1390-1392
25 Platt MS, Yunginger JW, Sekula-Perlman et al. Involvement of mast cells in sudden infant death syndrome. J Allergy Clin Immunol 1994: 94; 250-256
26 Forsyth KD, Weeks SC, Koh L, Skinner J, Bradley J. Lung immunoglobulins in the sudden infant death syndrome. BMJ 1989; 289: 23-26
27 Siebert JR, Haas JE. Organ weights in sudden infant death syndrome. Pediatr Pathol 1994; 14: 973-985
28 Coppoletta JM, Wolbach SB. Body length and organ weights in infants and children: study of body lengths and normal weights of more important vital organs of body between birth and 12 years of age. Am J Pathol 1933; 9: 55-70
29 Schulz DM, Giordano DA, Schulz DH. Weights of organs of fetuses and infants. Arch Pathol 1962; 74: 244-250
30 Tähkä H. The weight of the thymus in children of 0-2 years of age. Acta Paediatr 1951; 40: 469-485
31 Tähkä H. The weight of the adrenal glands. Acta Paediatr Scand 1951; 40 (Suppl 1): 1
32 Shankle WR, Landing BH, Gregg J. Normal organ weights of infants and children: graphs of values by age, with confidence intervals. Pediatr Pathol 1983; 1: 399-408
33 Hinchcliffe SA, Howard CV, Lynch MRJ et al. Renal developmental arrest in sudden infant death syndrome. Pediatr Pathol 1993; 13: 333-343

# 2

# Childhood diabetes in the community

*P. G. F. Swift*

*Much that we now accept as mainstream practice for the person with diabetes was being pioneered by Dr Joan Walker in Leicester 40 years ago. The invaluable role of the nurse specially trained in diabetes, the dietitian and the broader team, the recognition of the patient's emotional response to diabetes, the impact of social factors, the expanded role of day-care facilities were being incorporated into the ethos of diabetes care. Starting treatment for diabetic children in their homes, an almost heretical notion in its time and still not universally accepted, was initiated because of the conviction that it was in the home that lifelong therapeutic fashions should be set.* [1]
Harry Keen

The paediatrician with expertise in diabetes should help to set lifelong therapeutic 'fashions'. This is no easy task. Successful management of diabetes is often thwarted by a combination of uniquely difficult features (see Table 2.1). In the UK, it is only recently that childhood diabetes has been accorded the intellectual energy and practical commitment that it deserves. The paediatrician's excuse has been that 'the ravages of diabetic (microvascular) complications are not seen in the children's diabetic clinic'.[2] The important message in the above quotation should be that the organisation of preventative care to delay adult complications is a central task for paediatricians.

Despite these difficulties, when diabetes is well managed it is possible for a child and adolescent to develop self confidence and a feeling of achievement by maintaining acceptable metabolic control over many years and be able to live an active, healthy life without major social, intellectual or physical restrictions. As a consequence of better understanding of diabetes and its requirements the prognosis of childhood diabetes has improved significantly over the past three decades.[3] It is clear that many children and their families are managing diabetes with extraordinary skill, determination and success. To achieve consistent success within a community it must be recognised by purchasers of health-care that children with diabetes need specialist expertise and special facilities. Latterly, advice to purchasers in the UK has come through local planning groups, now commonly known as Local Diabetes Services Advisory Groups, which should include paediatric members (BDA Communication 1994). In the UK, the NHS has been ideally placed to provide not only the essential medication and equipment, free at the point of

**Table 2.1**

| | |
|---|---|
| **Diagnosis:** | is usually sudden and unexpected in a previously healthy child ('like a bereavement') |
| **Aetiology:** | remains elusive ('who is to blame') |
| **Hereditary components:** | are proposed ('family guilt') |
| **Life long disorder** | |
| **Life-endangering crises:** | punctuate its progress (hypoglycaemia and ketoacidosis) |
| **Unremitting:** | invasion of attention and thought every day and night during all types of activity including sleep and leisure |
| **Sudden unexplained fluctuations:** | in metabolic control occur |
| **Treatment:** | requires regular daily self-injection which nevertheless provides imperfect control because of extreme variability of insulin absorption |
| **Monitoring:** | demands frequent biochemical self-assessment of blood and/or urine, interpretation and action |
| **Dietary management:** | (including restriction of sweets) is important but inexact and variable in effect |
| **Chronic anxiety:** | pervades the situation because of potential long-term vascular complications when optimal control is not achieved |
| **Optimal metabolic control:** | requires self-discipline, high motivation, attention to detail and a degree of perfectionism |

contact, but also to develop comprehensive care plans. It is one of the major achievements of the NHS that diabetes has been the front runner in the development of shared-care arrangements,[4] patient centred education,[5] seeing patients in an holistic or 3-dimensional (physical, social and psychological) terms[6] (Waine, Chapter 35) and moving management away from the hospital towards the home.[1]

## THE COMMUNITY

In the context of diabetes the much used and abused word 'community' may have a variety of meanings. This review will focus on community management in the context of a UK District Health Authority having the characteristics of:

1. Primary care – family doctor services immediately accessible for:
   (a) prompt diagnosis
   (b) immediate referral to secondary care services
   (c) rapid management of intercurrent health problems which might otherwise provoke decompensation in a child with diabetes

2. Secondary care – specialised hospital-centred services based on recommendations[7] that each District should have a Children's Diabetes Team available for the care of children with diabetes working in specialist diabetes clinics. Members of the Children's Diabetes Team should be able to work both in hospital and in the community and should have close links with the adult diabetes services.

3. The child's geographically identifiable community including within it child health and education services.

The 'diabetic community' will also be considered – often organised around voluntary self-help groups where the people involved have a commonality of interest, namely diabetes. In order to avoid a parochial view, diabetes in the wider context of national and global communities will also be discussed.

## DIABETES MANAGEMENT IMPERATIVES

A modern perspective on diabetes has been covered in a previous chapter in this series.[7a] Treatment protocols and imperatives should be part of a chronic disease management programme, the characteristics and demands of which have been described by several authors.[8, 9] Etzwiler[10] has recently emphasised that although health care delivery in the USA is inordinately costly, it has had little success in managing chronic diseases like diabetes because the medical model is still physician-dominated and hospital-based instead of being patient-centred and community-orientated. The latter is essential because professional responsibility for people with diabetes amounts to only 1–10% of a patient's life experience, whereas patient responsibility is 90–99% of the time. Recognition has been made of the crucial importance of patient-centred education[5] and attempts to change attitudes and motivation rather than a knowledge-based educational programme.[11] Further progress is needed in training for the management teams not only in diabetes management, but in educational theory and communication skills.

Even when well organised expert services are available, young people from disorganised or distressed families will sabotage attempts at achieving good metabolic control. Compromises have to be made when individual and family circumstances adversely affect self control, motivation and adherence to the management regimens. Nevertheless a sensitive, consistent and integrated multi-disciplinary community team is in the best position to recognise family problems and crises at an early stage[12] and to diminish their effect by applying counselling skills in a non-authoritarian environment. Some children and parents will still regard the hospital clinic as a hostile place where it is difficult to express emotions and describe personal problems.

## MODERN EXPECTATIONS OF METABOLIC CONTROL

In the past, paediatricians have taken the soft option of not attempting tight control of diabetes for two reasons: (1) the potential for provoking damaging hypoglycaemia; and (2) the lack of evidence for a direct link with vascular complications.

Although recurrent hypoglycaemia particularly in the pre-school age group has been associated with cognitive and learning difficulties, recent evidence paints a more optimistic picture.[13] Modern management – including high carbohydrate, high fibre dietary recommendations, blood glucose monitoring and a clearer understanding of glucose variability – enable many children of all ages to control their diabetes within acceptable limits without frequent or damaging hypoglycaemia.

Despite persuasive studies in animal models and increasing evidence in human populations, including children, that better metabolic control decreases the rate of microvascular complications, the control:complications controversy has persisted. The controversy is over – the results of the Diabetes Control and Complications Trial (DCCT) have been published.[14] The DCCT, costing $168 million, was terminated after 9 years because the result had become significantly impressive. The study involved 1441 highly selected and motivated individuals (14% were aged 13 to 17 years) who were randomised to follow one of two treatment regimens.

1. An intensive therapy (IT) regimen with strictly defined goals of preprandial blood glucose (BG) <7 mmol/l postprandial BG <10 mmol and $HbA1_c$ within the normal range (<6%). This was to be accomplished by multiple daily insulin injections or by continuous subcutaneous infusion of insulin, BG monitoring at least 4 times per day, weekly discussion with the professional team members, monthly clinic visits for check-ups, dietary instruction,[15] support and $HbA1_c$ measurements.

2. A conventional treatment (CT) group in contrast gave themselves one or two injections per day, daily self monitoring with much less stringent goals, three-monthly clinic attendance when $HbA1_c$ was measured.

The report[16] on the sub-group of 13 to 17 year olds (n = 195) shows that the IT cohort attained a mean $HbA1_c$ of 8.1% (1% higher than the adult IT group) compared with $HbA1_c$ of 9.8% in the CT group. After an average follow-up duration of 7 years, the IT group had decreased risks of developing retinopathy by 53%, progression of existing retinopathy by 70% and microalbuminuria by 55%. There was however a 3-fold increase in severe hypoglycaemia in the IT group. The study group concluded that the benefits outweighed the risk of hypoglycaemia.

It should be noted that in the IT adolescent group (n = 92) severe hypoglycaemia (coma or seizure) occurred at a rate of 27 episodes per 100 patient years (14 hospitalisations) and did not have a significant effect on neuropsychological function nor on quality-of-life questionnaires. This incidence of hypoglycaemia would not seem to be excessive compared with rates described in children's clinics elsewhere.[17,18]

The implications of this landmark trial have been widely debated.[19–21] The scientific conclusion is clear – a 2% reduction in glycated haemoglobin sustained over a decade is associated with a reduction of microvascular complications of 60%. Unfortunately, most paediatricians faced with a child from an unhappy broken home, failing at school, and other problems will realise the impossibility of attempting to achieve normoglycaemia. Fortunately, the trial results show that a reduction of $HbA1_c$ by 2% from any starting level will significantly reduce the risks of complications.

Another worrying escape from tighter glycaemic control has been encouraged by some commentators. It is believed by some that because vascular complications have been reported rarely before puberty, the contribution of the pre-pubertal years of diabetes to long-term prognosis may be minimal.[22] This extraordinary conclusion was reached from a study comparing children diagnosed pre-pubertally with those diagnosed in the pubertal years. Both these groups, however, had very high complication rates before aged 30 years, whereas a recent local study,[23] where overall control was probably more satisfactory, concluded that the pre-pubertal phase did indeed influence the subsequent development of complications.

What is clearly of major importance is that good habits, skills, techniques and understanding of good control must be instilled in young children and their parents from the onset of diabetes so that the best achievable BG control is maintained during the accelerated growth phase of adolescence when significant increases occur in insulin, sex steroids, growth factors and growth hormone all of which may influence the development of vascular complications.

In other words, poor control of diabetes pre-pubertally plus poor control in adolescence is a recipe for disastrous vascular complications in early adulthood. In contrast, the maintenance of acceptable glycaemic control in early childhood and during puberty will enable most adults to remain complication free for many years.[3]

## LOCAL COMMUNITY MANAGEMENT

Leicestershire is an English shire county of some 860 000 people, 23% being less than 16 years of age. Epidemiologically it is of interest because of its stable geographical boundaries, a centrally placed major city and suburbs wherein 60% of the population reside and in the surrounding rural county there are several towns with considerable populations. Leicester City and the town of Loughborough (population 55 000) are ethnically diverse.

The first diabetic incidence survey of a total community in Britain was carried out in the old mining village of Ibstock in West Leicestershire in 1957.[1,24] It was initiated from the diabetic clinic at Leicester Royal Infirmary by Dr Joan Walker and carried out by one of the health visitors based in the clinic. Dr Walker had appointed the first specialist diabetes health visitor in Britain in 1950 and in her book[1] she makes a most telling comment which is highly relevant to the discussion of community diabetes. When exploring the houses in the village she 'was certain the front doors would remain firmly closed against the survey. But the nurse did not share the same gloomy view. *There was a back door*'. There is always a back or side door through which we may try to enter the anxiety filled world of diabetes. A direct frontal approach is often the least rewarding! Lateral thinking with a sensitive indirect approach is likely to be more acceptable and successful, particularly in children.

Even before the advent of the National Health Service in 1948, Dr Walker had begun to diagnose and treat children entirely on an out-patient basis. 'The parents saw the rapid improvement in their child and realised the benefit of insulin. They brushed aside their own emotion and set themselves to organise a simple routine, eager to share their responsibility with us. The specialist nurses continued the education in the parents' own home. *The parents were in command.* These methods for caring for newly diagnosed diabetic children were not those in common practice. There was some disbelief that our method was safe and caused curiosity and much discussion'.[1]

Since that time, non-hospital initiation of treatment has been extended and refined by Dr John Hearnshaw (Diabetes Physician), who eloquently described the results of successfully managing children at home on domiciliary visits in his Nabarro lecture to the International Diabetes Federation (IDF) in 1985.[25] Since 1979, the author has had the privilege of being the first paediatrician in Leicester to carry forward these radical community management policies, details of which will be described.

## 'The diagnosis presented little difficulty with acute onset and classic symptoms'[1]

In a recent survey, 61% of parents reported that they were the first to suspect the diagnosis.[26] In the past three years, an identical proportion of local parents thought that the symptoms were due to diabetes and indeed several obtained testing equipment to confirm the diagnosis.

Even so, in our recent study,[27] 18% of children had significant acidosis (pH $<7.20$) at presentation necessitating hospital care with IV fluids. When the parents do not clearly describe the symptoms, the primary care physician must elicit the history, test the urine immediately and refer immediately to the Children's Diabetes Team. Despite heightened public awareness of diabetes, primary care staff still occasionally request a urine specimen the next day or next visit by which time ketoacidosis may supervene. Pitfalls and hazards in diagnosis include:

1. Frequent micturition (polyuria and nocturia not elicited); urinary infection suspected (bacteruria tested but glycosuria not sought)
2. Abdominal pain (liver distension and gastritis) presenting as an acute abdomen
3. Impaired consciousness (mimicking meningo-encephalitis)
4. Persistent vomiting (suspected gastroenteritis)
5. Dyspnoea (suspected pneumonia) due to severe acidosis.

Diabetes in a child presents to a general practitioner very infrequently, so it is not surprising that the diagnosis is occasionally delayed. The crucial thought process is to turn 'frequency' of micturition or thirstiness into an immediate test for glycosuria.

### 'General practitioners were notified that young diabetics be *referred immediately*'[1]

If the child has not vomited and is not seriously dehydrated or acidotic there is no obvious need to admit the child to a hospital bed. Local GPs are encouraged to phone the children's admissions unit or the consultant directly who will then arrange to see the child at home, nearly always the same evening. If there is some doubt about the degree of dehydration the child will be assessed initially in the hospital and, if appropriate, given the first insulin injection before being allowed home.

In Leicestershire, between 15–40 children under 15 years are diagnosed each year. In the decade 1979–1988, 62% of children did not come into hospital at diagnosis. We remain unable to keep 25–35% out of hospital because of delays in diagnosis or non-availability of staff.

At the first contact with the Children's Diabetes Team, the diagnosis must be unequivocally confirmed. This always includes heavy glycosuria (± ketonuria) and a diagnostically raised capillary or venous blood glucose (>11 mmol/l). In the past 12 months, two very young children have been referred with a history of polydipsia, no urine test had been performed but apparently had a raised capillary BG. When tested at home, having washed chocolate or sweet biscuits from the fingers, they were both normoglycaemic and the polydipsia was due to excessive habit drinking of hyposmolar fluids.

Heavy ketonuria without symptomatic acidosis or vomiting is not a contra-indication to home treatment. Having confirmed the diagnosis with the assistance and understanding of the child and parents, the significance of the findings are explained. It is useful to a child to explain that the word DIABETES means 'a fountain' just like the child has been day and night for the past days or weeks. Other explanations are helpful:

- How ill the child would become without receiving immediate treatment – but with positive encouragement that the diagnosis has been confirmed early before acidosis has supervened.
- The self destructive process within the pancreas.
- The dramatic improvements which will occur in the next 24 hours, for example the sudden reduction or disappearance of nocturia – this effect is intriguing even though the BG might not have fallen below the renal threshold.

### 'The *first injection* of insulin would be given meticulously'[1]

The first injection is the most important in the child's life. It carries with it enormous psychological and physical significance. A criticism that one consultant paediatrician made about not admitting a child to hospital was that

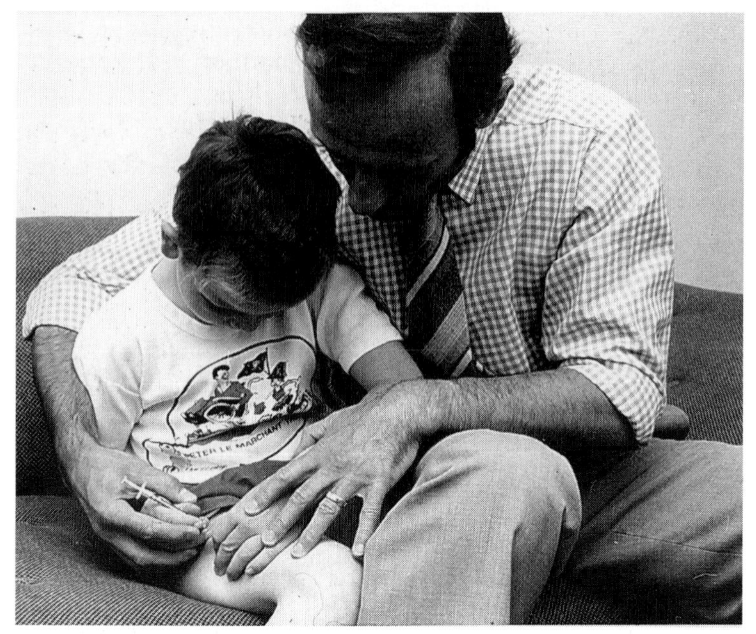

**Fig. 2.1** The cuddling technique for the first injection.

it devalued the serious nature of the disorder; that a significant 'initiation process' was lost. This criticism carries no weight. Helping to give the first insulin injection to a child, with the family watching in their own home is one of the most powerful initiation ceremonies that a doctor can experience.

The injection is best given by approaching a young child from the side (Fig. 2.1) not allowing a prolonged sight of the needle and asking the child either to hold the syringe or one's own hand to help the insertion of the needle. The pain of the first injection, when well performed, is much less than expected enabling a rapid dissolution of fear encouraging the child to help with or even give subsequent injections.

## 'Estimating the first dose of insulin can only be done by experience'[1]

If soluble insulin is given as the first dose, there is no doubt that the BG level falls more quickly and symptoms disappear promptly. The use of soluble insulin also teaches the parents that it can be used in the context of marked hyperglycaemia in the future. A safe dose to use, avoiding hypoglycaemia, is approximately 0.25–0.3 units/kg but, as the weight is not known at the first home visit, we usually give approximately the same number of units as the child's age in years.

After the insulin has been injected, a brief description of how insulin works and its positive effects can be given as well as demonstrating fully the drawing up and injection technique. The analogy of insulin being like the ignition key in a car seems a useful one for young children (and therefore parents).

Subsequent insulin injections will usually be a medium acting isophane insulin for the under fives or a pre-mixed 30/70 insulin for older children.

### 'The diet pattern employed was one which could be used for the rest of the family'[1]

After the first visit, it is extremely important to avoid hypoglycaemia by emphasising the basic carbohydrate requirements for the next 24 hours, particularly at supper time before bed. The paediatric dietitian arranges to see the family the following day to give a further explanation of a modern diabetic healthy eating plan,[28] without the regular counting or calculation of grams or exchanges which have been favoured by dietitians and yet found to be impractical by patients.[29,30] The huge appetite of the first two weeks of insulin therapy should be explained and accepted as a normal process of anabolic recovery.

### 'The value of testing and recording was explained'[1]

Having already demonstrated that urine and blood glucose measurements are required to confirm the diagnosis, these techniques can be demonstrated again so that self monitoring can begin and be recorded in a monitoring diary. The diagnostic results on this first visit are entered into the diary and a note is written that the child has helped with or given the first injection. The diary is used as an immediate educational and informational tool:

- The rapid changes and improvements in BG can be documented immediately.

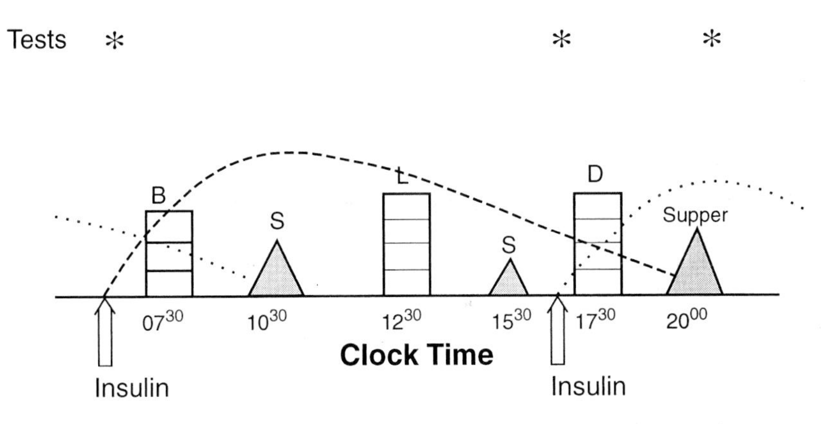


**Fig. 2.2** Chronological cartoon to illustrate a day with diabetes. B = breakfast; S = snack; D–dinner; L = lunch; * = useful monitoring times.

- Telephone contact numbers can be given to ensure 24-hour support during the next days/weeks.
- A chronological cartoon of a day with diabetes (see Fig. 2.2) can be constructed illustrating a basic guide to the requirements of a normal (school) day.
- A personal hand-held record of achievement – a teaching aid enabling the parent or child to make adjustments in treatment (not an excuse for ritual inspection and judgement by the didactic doctor).

A clearly stated aim of reducing blood glucose levels to less than 9 or 10 mmol/l is explained linking this to:

1. The balance between insulin, food and exercise
2. Frequent contact with the team to discuss alterations in insulin dose to achieve near normoglycaemia
3. The avoidance of low sugar reactions by regular carbohydrate intake
4. The successful prevention of older age complications by our modern knowledge of good BG control and healthy living.

A strong positive message is emphasised that, although diabetes is a serious disorder, with good care and attention the great majority of children with diabetes are extremely healthy, rarely missing time off school and can continue to pursue all their usual hobbies and activities with vigour and success. The naming of top sports and show business personalities with diabetes is another helpful positive message.

This 'initiation ceremony' lasting about 1.5 hours accomplishes several important and perhaps crucial functions:

1. Unequivocal demonstration of *diagnosis*
2. *Simple description* of the serious nature of diabetes and outcome without insulin
3. The *first injection* given by experienced professional but helped by child or parent
4. *Positive educational messages* and practical management skills transmitted in an unhurried manner to the whole family
5. Giving immediate *practical* responsibility to the people who want it and need it (the child and parents)
6. Establishment of a close *professional relationship* based on mutual trust including a secure 24-hour contact support service and an immediate contact with the other key members of the diabetes team.

Such an immediate practical approach is more likely to be educationally successful as emphasised by Coles[5] – practice should come before theory, particularly at a time of heightened anxiety. Nevertheless, the usual professional response to this type of home-management programme is to say that parents need hospital admission to give them time to cope with the shock and distress. This is at total variance with our experience of community care. The parents learn by instant practical experience, they are not overloaded with information, anxieties are reduced by seeing their child improve rapidly with their own help and the child is not inhibited by inevitable hospital boundaries.

### 'Continuity of care is indeed the key to good health of the diabetic'[1]

There is little doubt that parents and children appreciate the opportunity of building up strong bonds of trust in their professional carers, particularly if the trust is based on the knowledge that their advisors are experienced in practical diabetes management, consistent in their views and allow a two-way interaction. Parents object strongly and children rebel if they see different professional staff with different prejudices on successive ward rounds or clinic visits. Inconsistency and inexperience in managing diabetes are recipes for rejection, rebellion and metabolic chaos.

For domiciliary care of diabetes to be successful there must be a small consistent team available to carry forward the messages of the initial visit. In Leicestershire we have 5.5 full-time equivalent Diabetes Specialist Health Visitors working in both the children's and adult services. Each is allocated to a particular geographical sector and one will always be able to visit a newly diagnosed child the next day to:

1. Supervise further injections
2. Consolidate the education
3. Advise on equipment and skills and joining the British Diabetic Association
4. Provide psychological support
5. Liaise with the family doctor
6. Discuss immediate return to nursery or school
7. Initiate the long-term continuity of care
8. Advise on benefits, such as Disability Living Allowance.

The third member of the team who visits is the paediatric specialist diabetes dietitian. At this stage, therefore, only three professional advisors are involved. Compare this with the large number of contacts when a child is admitted to hospital all able to offer words of 'kindly advice' to the stressed but impressionable parents; but all liable to add elements of conflict and confusion to the picture. Experience shows that at home the initial injections and blood tests in most cases are more likely to become an acceptable part of the regime when consistently performed by the parents rather than a number of alien professionals.

During the first week there will be at least five personal or telephone contacts with the parents and child. One of these might be the first visit to the hospital clinic.

## THE CHILDREN'S SPECIALIST DIABETIC CLINIC

Specialist diabetes clinics in the UK have taken some time to be accepted and developed. They provide a concentration of expertise[9] and special facilities, such as on site capillary glycated haemoglobin measurements, educational and play services,[7a] voluntary stalls for diabetic provisions and the launching pad for group activities outside the clinic.

In a relatively small district, all the children with diabetes should be accommodated within one consultant-led clinic. In Leicestershire we have developed a variety of children's diabetic clinics to suit differing groups and localities:

1. Midweek clinic within the Children's Hospital
2. Monthly Saturday morning clinics jointly with the adult diabetologist
3. Bimonthly outreach clinics in county towns.

This flexible range of clinics allows:

1. An attempt at age-banding
2. A service (on Saturdays) for families (particularly fathers) who find midweek clinics difficult
3. Realistic hand-over of older adolescents to the adult services
4. Consultant-led clinics close to the child's home. The outreach clinics are held in the smaller community hospitals and in one case in a GP health centre (Latham House, Melton Mowbray) in a county town with the UK's largest single practice population of 33 000.

One of the drawbacks to such a specialist consultant/nurse/dietitian service with very few hospital admissions or re-admissions is the lack of experience gained by junior doctors and medical students. This can only be remedied by practical teaching within the clinic and on the ward, enabling students to discuss diabetes with parents and children, sitting-in with nurses or the dietitian and, whenever possible, allowing staff and students to accompany the consultant or nurses on home visits.

Psychological problems encountered in children with diabetes usually reflect the family milieu and individual personality rather than diabetes itself. Any chronic disease highlights or exaggerates pre-existing psychosocial difficulties. Psychological disturbance then promotes secondary metabolic instability which may be of an extreme severity. A clinic with a regularly attending psychologist or child psychiatrist with a special interest in diabetes is in a fortunate position because incipient and fully evolved emotional disturbances may be more successfully managed. Unfortunately, specialist psychological skills in childhood diabetes are unusual in the UK. Most clinic teams attempt to prevent behavioural problems by consistent support and advice in patient-centred discussions in the clinic and during community activities. The severe psychological disturbances which inevitably affect a proportion of the diabetic population may precipitate referral to psychiatric colleagues who, in some instances, have remarkable success in altering family and personal dynamics. Unfortunately, all clinics have a small number of children and particularly adolescents who remain totally resistant to even the most comprehensive hospital and community support services. In the words of the late Oman Craig 'One's attitude to the "Impossible Case" should be to stick with it even if it makes one feel useless for years on end'.[31] Many of these recidivists some years down the line express appreciation for the ongoing commitment of their professional friends and advisors, even though they have rejected it during the difficult adolescent years.

## COMMUNITY SUPPORT AND ACTIVITIES OUTSIDE THE CLINIC

### School

Children with diabetes spend at most 3 or 4 hours per year in direct contact with hospital-based clinic staff, i.e. 0.8% of waking hours! In contrast, something like 25% of their daytime life is spent in school. It is unfortunate, therefore, that the teaching profession, school doctors, school nurses and paediatricians in many districts do not provide a successful integrated diabetes service within schools, see Strang (Chpt 33) in Kelnar.[6] Children with diabetes may still occasionally be restricted by schools in activities such as swimming, educational trips or even statutory physical education. Moreover, parents frequently criticise teachers' lack of knowledge and information about diabetes.[26,32] These difficulties can often be alleviated by the provision of immediate information from the hospital and parents to schools at diagnosis, visits to school by members of the diabetes team, the proper utilisation of the British Diabetic Association (BDA) School Pack (recently revised) and subsequent direct contact with teachers and other staff. The children themselves must be encouraged to be completely open with their friends and teachers about diabetes so that there is a healthy understanding of the skills and demands required to look after the condition effectively.

### Educational holidays and other activities

The BDA has been organising diabetes 'camps' or educational holidays since 1936, initially for children from underprivileged homes. In succeeding decades, the holiday concept has broadened to provide important educational experiences for children who learn more about diabetes away from their home routine, gain independence, take part in unfamiliar or novel activities, meet new friends and learn the social skills of living with others who are 'in the same boat' – a sharing of experience. The national BDA holidays provide each year, 800 or so children with a diverse range of activities. Parents also benefit from these holidays, which provide a period of relief whilst their children are supervised in a safe environment. The holiday staff benefit by living alongside children with diabetes which is equivalent to a life time behind a hospital desk.

Two criticisms have been levelled at nationally organised holidays. First, that the standards of care and methodology may differ from local policies causing conflict and confusion in the children. Secondly, that medical officers who help the children on holiday never see them again causing a disappointing lack of continuity of care. There is, therefore, an increasing movement towards the organisation of locally-based holidays, weekends away and a variety of innovative activities. These are usually organised by clinic staff but may involve the leadership qualities of parents. Parental involvement can be of great educational potential and may enhance the confidence of a local parent support group.[33] Locally-based holidays enable staff to get to know their clinic children better, recognise their habits and difficulties and develop more practical and realistic strategies. The key issue in organisation is meticulous planning, careful choice of skilled supervision and close attention to detail in providing a safe holiday. The BDA have guidelines to help those wishing to plan holidays for children and the Association hopes to regionalise their holidays more in the future. The organisation of camps has recently been described in some detail by Thompson et al (Chpt 36) in Kelnar[6] as have the conceptual background and practical benefits of self-help organisations by Swift (Chpt 37) in Kelnar.[6] The extensive national and international travel undertaken by families nowadays generates much discussion in clinics and we have designed a travel advice booklet *Have Diabetes – Will Travel* to complement those obtainable from the BDA.

## Evaluation of a modern comprehensive community diabetes service

The development of community-based or non-hospital management of children with diabetes has not gone unchallenged. Although, in the UK, 60% of children now stay in hospital for less than 8 days,[26] in many countries, even those with sophisticated health care systems such as Sweden, Switzerland and Germany, children are routinely kept in hospital for 2 or 3 weeks; in Finland 4 weeks and in Eastern Europe 6 weeks.[34] In comparison with units where community services allow children to be managed out of hospital such as in Israel,[12] the USA,[35] Australia or the UK[27] this prolonged incarceration seems particularly harsh and extraordinarily costly in both financial and personal terms.[36]

Proponents of strict hospitalisation regimens criticise the community approach with the accusation of "not taking diabetes seriously, of creating the impression that diabetes is nothing remarkable and that it is easy for patients to live a so-called 'normal' life. This is hypocritical. Sooner or later children will discover that diabetes is not that simple".[37] There is persuasive scientific evidence that strict metabolic control with high dose insulin on a Biostator for the first 14 days after diagnosis helps to preserve pancreatic function and may improve control for the first 12 months,[38] but it is the longer view that needs to be considered. We and others have shown that children treated out of hospital have similar indices of control over the first few years, have fewer re-admissions to hospital and in the long-term with excellent continuity of care have an extremely favourable prognosis.[3,12,27] Also, in a study where newly diagnosed children were randomised to continuous subcutaneous infusion of insulin or conventional treatment, there was no significant difference in the phase of partial remission (honeymoon period).[39]

The arguments in favour of prolonged hospital admission with intensified insulin therapy need to be looked at in the terms of potentially adverse effects on the child in hospital, the doctors need to maintain authoritative control over the situation, the requirements of research and a reluctance to empower parents in assuming long-term expert management of their child. It is gratifying to record that several units in the UK are now managing children with newly diagnosed diabetes outside the hospital.

## ANATOMY OF A DISTRICT SERVICE

To help paediatricians discuss the size and scope of childhood diabetes with purchasers and adult colleagues, it may be useful to describe a District demography.

One of the few community surveys of diabetes showed that 46% of all true insulin dependent diabetes mellitus (IDDM) is diagnosed before age 15 years and 63% before age 19 years.[40] The Department of Public Health and Epidemiology, Leicester University, has compiled a Register of all insulin-taking diabetics since 1987 (J.L. Botha, N. Raymond, personal communication). From these data it can be seen that only 3% of all people taking insulin in December 1994 were under the age of 16 years of age (Fig. 2.3). However, 22% of all people taking insulin were diagnosed before this age (Fig 2.4). If one estimates that about 80% of all people with diabetes under the age of 45 years have true IDDM, then 50% of IDDM was diagnosed before age

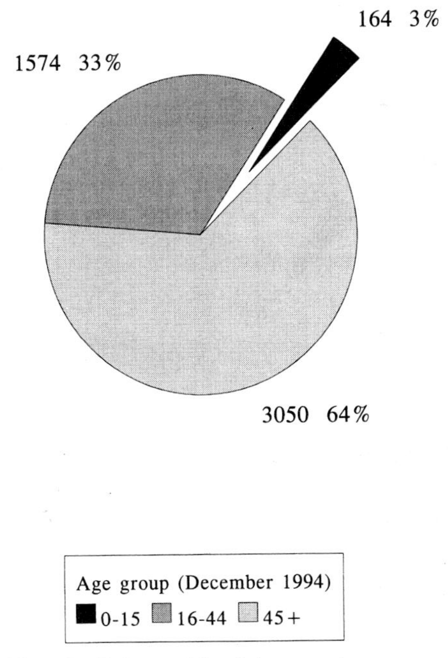


**Fig 2.3** Leicestershire diabetes register. People treated with insulin, ages in December 1994.

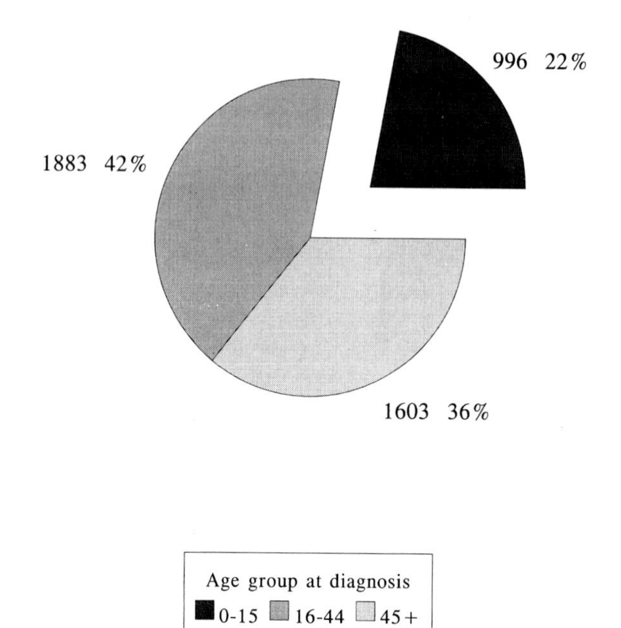


**Fig 2.4** Leicestershire diabetes register. People treated with insulin, age at diagnosis.

16 years, almost identical to the Finnish study.[40] The incidence of diabetes varies across the country and has increased in recent decades. Recent audits in Scotland, Wessex and Leicestershire have given prevalence figures for children under 15 years of 1.4, 0.8 and 0.8 per 1000, respectively.

It is important, therefore, that purchasers of health care should understand that childhood diabetes:

- carries a potentially serious long-term morbidity when inappropriately managed
- is increasing in prevalence
- 50% of people with true life long IDDM are diagnosed before the age of 16 years
- requires specialist care and community facilities.

## THE NATIONAL PERSPECTIVE

In 1988, the BPA Working Party found that the services provided by paediatricians for children with diabetes were patchy, inconsistent and in places inadequate.[7] The national survey was repeated in 1994 and shows some gratifying improvements in services. Specialist care is now provided by a smaller cohort of consultants, running larger specialist clinics with improved services (see Table 2.2).

Despite these improvements, 10% of paediatricians do not regularly measure glycated haemoglobin and 32% of districts still have 3 or more consultants caring for small numbers of children with diabetes often in general paediatric clinics.

A recent national survey of dietitians caring for children with diabetes confirmed the general improvement in availability of dietetic advice but uncovered a continuing alarming lack of uniformity in dietetic educational messages.[41]

Parents find the lack of consistency in standards and policies very difficult to understand, particularly when they move from district to district. Those involved in paediatric diabetes care must continue to work towards more unified standards of care. The establishment of Regional Diabetes Interest Groups may help this process.

**Table 2.2**

| | 1988 | 1994 |
|---|---|---|
| Consultants seeing children in specialist diabetes clinics | 63% | 88% |
| Diabetes nurse specialist (DNS) attending clinics | 61% | 87% |
| Dietitian attending clinic | 72% | 91% |
| Psychologist/psychiatrist attending clinic | 9% | 20% |
| DNS regularly visit schools | 54% | 82% |
| Facilities for adolescents/young adults | 57% | 68% |

## THE INTERNATIONAL COMMUNITY OF CHILDHOOD DIABETES

The incidence and presentation of childhood diabetes has been extensively studied in many countries by organisations with intriguing acronyms such as DERI, DIAMOND and EURODIAB. The incidence (number per 100 000 children) varies enormously from minimal in the Far East (Japan 2, China 1) to high and increasing figures in Scandinavia (Sweden 32, Finland 40) and Scotland (10 in 1968; 18 in 1976; 24 in 1990).

The extreme inequalities in social circumstances and child health mean that in the majority of countries around the world, insulin is either unavailable or only erratically available. Many children worldwide die with untreated diabetes or when given small intermittent doses of insulin rapidly begin to suffer the severe complications of diabetes, such as cataracts, which are rarely seen in more privileged societies. It remains a health priority to provide not only adequate insulin and monitoring equipment for children but also experienced health workers who are accepted by the community to manage diabetes effectively. Specialist nurses have had an enormous impact in improving diabetes management in this country, but in many parts of the world nurses have such a low social status that they are not accepted as experts in diabetes care.

Cultural differences across the world influence the acceptance of western style medicines including insulin and different countries adopt their favourite insulin regimens; the USA using self-mixing Reg/NPH mixtures; the Scandinavians using 3–6 multiple pen injections per day; the UK moving towards fixed-mixtures of insulin which although despised by some paediatric endocrinologists in other countries, have been shown to be more acceptable to people with diabetes[42] and equally efficacious.[43]

Cultural dietary differences may have a considerable impact on diabetes management worldwide. In the UK, it is difficult to persuade children to eat a diet containing 50% of total energy from carbohydrate and less fat, whereas the traditional Japanese diet may contain 70% carbohydrate with very low fat levels and in Italy children regularly consume 60% carbohydrate diets. More work needs to be done on how to change dietary patterns and whether changes affect outcome.

In Europe, The St Vincent Declaration[44] has attempted to define standards of diabetes care and to promote improvements which may benefit the whole diabetic community. Similar Declarations of commitment towards improving worldwide care of children with diabetes have been made by the IDF and more recently by the International Society For Paediatric and Adolescent Diabetes (ISPAD) making a pledge to work towards the following:

1. Making insulin and self-monitoring equipment available for all children and adolescents with diabetes.
2. Reducing morbidity and mortality of acute metabolic complications or missed diagnosis of IDDM.
3. Making age appropriate care and education accessible to all children and adolescents and their families.
4. Encouraging research on childhood diabetes.
5. Preparing and disseminating guidelines and written standards of care for realistic management of childhood diabetes.

In the worldwide context, the development of community care depends not only on the commitment of diabetes teams but also on geographical characteristics. In Leicestershire we travel only 20 miles to outreach clinics, whereas in Scotland the paediatric team fly to the Shetlands to see diabetic children and in Australia they fly hundreds of miles from Sydney or Perth to outreach clinics. Similarly, the scope of educational holidays continues to widen. In November 1994, the third International Conference on Camping was held in Osaka, Japan, representing perhaps 400 camps worldwide. Vivid descriptions of a huge variety of different camping experiences from 20 different countries were presented including the third Pacific International Camp organised in Honolulu by Professors Kida (Ehime, Japan) and Court (Melbourne, Australia) with children from many countries and islands throughout the Pacific area. Such international collaboration with increasing co-ordination of services and supplies, exchange of ideas, educational interaction, must help to foster improvements in care for children worldwide.

Diabetes is an international problem. Worldwide, it kills or debilitates many thousands of children. Optimal care demands not only individualised, sensitive, home-centred local community services but also a co-operative integrated global approach.

## KEY POINTS FOR CLINICAL PRACTICE

- Childhood diabetes is potentially a highly destructive disorder.
- Primary care diagnosis must be prompt.
- Referral to specialist secondary care services must be immediate to avoid life-endangering diabetic ketoacidosis.
- Management is best performed by an integrated Specialist Children's Diabetes Team in each District.
- Home-based community management from the onset is becoming increasingly accepted in the UK and worldwide.
- Home-based management puts parents and children in control from the start.
- Specialist children's diabetes clinics and outreach clinics are now well established.
- The Diabetes Control and Complications Trial has confirmed that for every 2% improvement in $HbA_{1C}$ over 10 years there is a 60% reduction in risk of microvascular complications.
- Paediatricians should aim at the best possible glycaemic control for children in the context of the individual family circumstances.
- There is evidence of an improving prognosis for children with diabetes.
- Worldwide there remain major inequalities in acceptance and treatment of diabetes.

### REFERENCES

1 Walker JB. Chronicle of a Diabetic Service. London: The British Diabetic Association, 1989.
2 Baum JD. Children with diabetes. Every health district should have a specialist clinic for their care. BMJ 1990; 301: 502-503
3 McNally PG. Childhood-onset diabetes: is the prognosis improving? Practical Diabetes 1991; 8: 133-136

4 Orton P. Shared care. Lancet 1994; 344: 1413-1415
5 Coles C. Diabetes education: letting the patient into the picture. Practical Diabetes 1990; 7: 110-112
6 Kelnar CJH. ed. Childhood and Adolescent Diabetes. London: Chapman & Hall, 1995.
7 British Paediatric Association Working Party. The organisation of services for children with diabetes in the United Kingdom. Diabetic Med 1990; 7: 457-464
7a Court S. Diabetes mellitus: a perspective. In: David TJ. ed. Recent Advances in Paediatrics, vol 9. Edinburgh: Churchill Livingstone 1991: 75-91
8 Riddle MC. A strategy for chronic disease. Lancet 1980; 2: 734-736
9 Swift PGF. Specialist clinics for children with diabetes. Curr Paediatr 1993; 3: 147-150
10 Etzwiler DD. Diabetes translation: a blue print for the future. Diabetes Care 1994; 17: 1-4
11 Lockington TJ, Powles S, Meadows KA et al. Attitudes, knowledge and blood glucose control. Diabetic Med 1989; 6: 309-313
12 Galatzer A, Amir S, Gil R et al. Crisis intervention program in newly diagnosed diabetic children. Diabetes Care 1982; 5: 414-419
13 Rovet JF, Czuchta D, Ehrlich RM. Neuropsychological sequelae of diabetes in childhood. A three year prospective study. Diabetes 1991; 40 (suppl. 1): 430a (abstract)
14 The Diabetes Control and Complications Trial Research Group. The effect of intensive treatment of diabetes on the development and progression of long-term complications in IDDM. N Engl J Med 1993; 14: 977-986
15 Delahanty LM, Halford BN. The role of diet behaviours in achieving improved glycemic control in intensively treated patients in the DCCT. Diabetes Care 1993; 16: 1453-1458
16 Diabetes Control and Complications Trial Research Group. Effect of intensive diabetes treatment on the development and progression of long-term complication in adolescents with IDDM: DCCT. J Pediatr 1994; 125: 177-188
17 MacFarlane PJ, Walters M, Stutchfield P, Smith CS. A prospective study of symptomatic hypoglycaemia in childhood diabetes. Diabetic Med 1989; 6: 627-630
18 Bergada I, Suissa S, Dufresne J, Schiffrin A. Severe hypoglycaemia in IDDM children. Diabetes Care 1989; 12: 239-244
19 Boulton AJM. DCCT: implications for diabetes care in the UK. Diabetic Med 1993; 10: 687
20 Drash AL. The child, the adolescent and DCCT. Diabetes Care 1993; 16: 1515-1516
21 Rubin RR, Peyrot M. Implications of the DCCT: looking beyond tight control. Diabetes Care 1994; 17: 235-236
22 Kostraba JN, Dorman JS, Orchard TJ et al. Contribution of diabetes duration before puberty to development of microvascular complications in IDDM subjects. Diabetes Care 1989; 12: 686-693
23 McNally PG, Raymond NT, Swift PGF et al. Does the prepubertal duration of diabetes influence the onset of microvascular complications? Diabetic Med 1993; 10: 906-908
24 Walker JB, Brown P. Early diabetes. Five year follow-up of diabetes in an English community. Lancet 1964; 2: 248-250
25 Hearnshaw JR. Childhood and after – a review of childhood diabetes in an English community 1930-1985. In: Serrano-Rios M, Lefebre PJ, eds. Diabetes 1985. Amsterdam: Elsevier, 1986: 31-42
26 Lessing DN, Swift PGF, Metcalfe MA et al. Newly diagnosed diabetes: a study of parental satisfaction. Arch Dis Child 1992; 67: 1011-1013
27 Swift PGF, Hearnshaw JR, Botha JL et al. A decade of diabetes: keeping children out of hospital. BMJ 1993; 307: 96-98
28 Waldron S. Childhood diabetes – current dietary management. Curr Paediatr 1993; 3: 138-140
29 Hackett AF, Rugg-Gunn AJ, Appleton DR et al. Sugar eating habits of 405, 11–14 year old English children. Br J Nutr 1984; 51: 347-356
30 Price KJ, Lang JD, Eiser C, Tripp JH. Prescribed v unrestricted carbohydrate diets in children with type I diabetes. Diabetic Med 1993; 10: 962-967
31 Craig O. Childhood diabetes and its management. In: Apley J ed. London: Butterworths 1977: 108
32 Parker H, Swift PGF, Botha JL, Raymond NT. Early onset diabetes: parents' views. Diabetic Med 1994; 11: 593-596

33 Swift PGF, Waldron S. Have diabetes – will travel. Practical Diabetes 1990; 7: 101-104
34 Simell T, Kaprio EA, Maenpaa J et al. Randomised prospective study of short-term and long-term initial stay in hospital by children with diabetes mellitus. Lancet 1991; 337: 656-660
35 Schneider AJ. Starting insulin therapy in children with newly diagnosed diabetes. Am J Dis Child 1983; 137: 782-786
36 Simell T, Simell O, Sintonen H. The first two years of type I diabetes in children: length of the initial hospital stay affects costs but not effectiveness of care. Diabetic Med 1993; 10: 855-862
37 Ludvigsson J. Treatment of diabetes in children and adolescents: art and science. IDF Bull 1993; 38: 6-9
38 Shah SC, Malone JI, Simpson NE. A randomised trial of intensive insulin therapy in newly diagnosed IDDM. N Engl J Med 1989; 320: 550-554
39 de Beaufort CE, Bruining GJ. Continuous subcutaneous insulin infusion in children. Diabetic Med 1987; 4: 103-108
40 Laakso M, Pyorala K. Age of onset and type of diabetes. Diabetes Care 1985; 8: 114-117
41 Waldron S, Swift PGF. The dietetic management of children with diabetes. Diabetic Med 1994; 11 Suppl 2: A9.55
42 McEvilly EA, Eccles L, Rayner PHW. An assessment of the benefits of pre-mixed insulins in childhood diabetes. Practical Diabetes 1990; 7: 122-124
43 Roland JM. Need stable diabetics mix their insulins? Diabetic Med 1984; 1: 51-53
44. Krans HMJ, Porta M, Keen H. Diabetes care and research in Europe: the St Vincent Declaration Action Program. Giornale Italiano di Diabetologia 1992; 12 Suppl 2.

3

# Home oxygen therapy

*M. P. Samuels  D. P. Southall*

The use of additional inspired oxygen in the home for surviving preterm infants with bronchopulmonary dysplasia was first reported from the USA nearly 20 years ago.[1,2] General practitioners were able to prescribe oxygen concentrators from 1985 after their addition to the UK drug tariff. This followed the results of studies which showed the benefit of long-term oxygen therapy at home in adults with chronic obstructive airway disease.[3,4] In recent years, there has been an increase in knowledge of normal and abnormal levels of blood oxygen in infants and children. Along with an increase in the availability of non-invasive oxygen monitoring, there has been greater awareness of hypoxaemia and a recognition of the need to correct this in order to avoid potentially adverse consequences.

There is little data on how many paediatric patients are receiving oxygen at home, but a recent working group from the Royal College of Physicians estimated that there were about 200 home oxygen concentrators installed in England and Wales in 1990, compared with about 7000 in use for adults with obstructive airway disease.[5] A regional neonatal intensive care unit found that 17% of infants who were ventilated in the first 48 hours of life developed chronic lung disease, and 9% were eligible for home oxygen therapy (although, for various reasons, only 5% received it).[6] Chronic lung disease of prematurity is the single most common situation for which paediatricians prescribe oxygen at home, and current trends suggest that the numbers of such infants may continue to increase.[7]

In addition to infants with chronic lung disease of prematurity, there are a number of other clinical situations wherein oxygen therapy may be used (Table 3.1). Patients with cyanotic congenital heart disease and no lung disease have low levels of arterial oxygen saturation ($SaO_2$). In these patients, there may be less significant consequences from the hypoxaemia, because there is not airway/alveolar hypoxia present. When hypoxaemia is due to chronic respiratory failure, however, pulmonary hypertension and right heart failure result, with an associated increase in mortality and morbidity. Additional inspired oxygen may be given to prevent this, although in certain circumstances, hypoventilation may be so severe that oxygen alone is inadequate, and respiratory support is then required.

Assessment of the need for additional inspired oxygen is sometimes

**Table 3.1** Conditions for which oxygen therapy may be required in paediatric practice

- Chronic lung disease of prematurity
- Chronic hypoxaemia from other neonatal respiratory disease
  e.g. meconium aspiration, pulmonary hypoplasia
- Recurrent cyanotic-apnoeic episodes or life threatening events with documented hypoxaemia
- Parenchymal or interstitial lung disease
  e.g. fibrosing alveolitis or alveolar lipoproteinosis
- Disorders of central respiratory control*
  e.g. congenital central hypoventilation syndrome
- Respiratory failure due to neuromuscular disease*
  e.g. myopathy
- Restrictive lung disease*
  e.g. kyphoscoliosis
- Respiratory problems in association with hypoxaemia at high altitude
  e.g. severe asthma or cyanotic breathholding
- Cyanotic congenital heart disease, with pulmonary hypertension
- Idiopathic pulmonary hypertension

*May require nasal mask positive pressure ventilation or negative pressure ventilation.

straightforward, in that such patients demonstrate clear-cut desaturation ($SaO_2$ < 85%) when breathing room air. The difficulty lies in those patients in whom hypoxaemia is less severe, and this inevitably depends upon what levels of oxygen are considered acceptable. At $SaO_2$ levels of 90–97%, there is also more dependence upon the correct use and interpretation of oxygen monitoring equipment. These issues will be discussed below.

Decisions on whether long-term oxygen therapy is administered are subsequently based on such factors as whether the acute illness has resolved, whether or not care in hospital continues, and whether or not there are likely benefits from its administration. A period of observation in hospital may confirm short-term benefits, whilst the practical issues involved in the long-term administration of oxygen are organised. As most experience with home oxygen therapy has been gained from infants with chronic lung disease of prematurity, this chapter will inevitably focus on this condition.

## BENEFITS OF OXYGEN THERAPY

### Prevention of pulmonary hypertension and heart failure

Chronic or repeated hypoxaemia can lead to pulmonary vasoconstriction, an elevated pulmonary vascular resistance, pulmonary hypertension and right sided heart failure. These result in poor growth, cardiorespiratory compromise with intercurrent respiratory infections, and ultimately death. These effects of chronic airway hypoxia can be assessed by performing an ECG, chest x-ray and echocardiography. These may demonstrate right ventricular hypertrophy, cardiomegaly, large trunk pulmonary arteries with peripheral pruning, increased right ventricular muscle mass and end-diastolic volume, more rapid pulmonary valve closure and blood flow in the pulmonary artery, and mitral valve regurgitation.

The use of long-term oxygen therapy has prolonged survival and improved the quality of life in adults with chronic obstructive airway disease.[3, 4] Oxygen is the most easily used selective pulmonary vasodilator, particularly for long-term use. Ensuring adequate oxygenation can help to prevent the development of cor pulmonale in infants with chronic lung disease of prematurity. The exact level of arterial $pO_2$ or $SaO_2$ that reflects sufficient airway oxygenation to maintain pulmonary artery pressures in the normal range is unknown, and may be different in different individuals. Halliday et al suggested that the maintenance of an arterial $pO_2$ above 55 mmHg was effective, based upon an echocardiographic assessment of pulmonary vascular resistance in infants with bronchopulmonary dysplasia.[8] As transcutaneous $pO_2$ monitoring has been noted to read a mean of 14 mmHg below arterial values,[9] it would be necessary to maintain transcutaneous $pO_2$ values above 70 mmHg in order to avoid the development of right heart failure.

Abman et al measured the pulmonary vascular response to oxygen at cardiac catheterisation, and demonstrated greatest changes in pulmonary artery pressure when $SaO_2$ was below 90%, but also showed increased values when $SaO_2$ fell from levels of 96–98% to 93–94%.[10] This study concluded that there were two components to pulmonary hypertension in chronic lung disease of prematurity, one responsive and the other unresponsive to additional inspired oxygen. The latter component was thought possibly to be due to longer term fibrotic or obliterative changes in the pulmonary vasculature. It is unknown, however, whether the provision of additional inspired oxygen for a duration longer than adopted in this study may reduce this so-called second component. This is more likely to be the case in infants with chronic lung disease of prematurity who have ongoing pulmonary vascular remodelling occurring as result of growth and repair. The pulmonary vascular bed in the older child with pulmonary hypertension may be more resistant to change. However, such children may benefit from the long-term administration of additional inspired oxygen at home.[11]

## Reduction of bronchoconstriction

Whilst some studies in healthy adults have shown no significant response to a change in the inspired oxygen concentration within the peripheral airways,[12] others have shown that it can lead to airway constriction.[13] The latter is supported by the observation that supplemental oxygen is associated with a decrease in airway resistance in adults with chronic obstructive airway disease.[14] In infants with chronic lung disease of prematurity, there is a significant decrease in total pulmonary resistance, and an increase in dynamic compliance during the administration of 100% oxygen.[15] In a different study, infants who were exposed to a reduced inspired oxygen concentration showed an increase in lung resistance and lung volume, with a reduction in mid-expiratory flow and dynamic compliance.[16] There were no significant changes in tidal volume, respiratory frequency, calculated minute volume or transcutaneous $pCO_2$ to suggest that hypoxaemia was affecting ventilatory regulation, and the authors concluded that hypoxaemia or airway hypoxia was the probable mechanism for the observed airway constriction.

It is possible that changes in airway tone or patency are responsible for some of the falls in transcutaneous $pO_2$ or $SaO_2$ that are manifested by infants with chronic lung disease of prematurity during activities such as feeding, moving, crying and sleeping.[2,17,18] In turn, the hypoxaemia that develops may further exacerbate airway calibre, with the result that major hypoxaemia may arise. The use of long-term oxygen therapy may thus help reduce the tendency to episodic desaturation by stabilisation of airway tone. This also provides a theoretical basis for the administration of additional inspired oxygen, perhaps long term, in patients with cystic fibrosis or asthma, who have chronic hypoxaemia.

## Reduction in apnoeic/cyanotic episodes

It has been demonstrated that the frequency of apnoeic pauses, obstructive apnoea and periodic breathing all were significantly reduced when additional inspired oxygen was recommenced in recently weaned premature infants.[19] When supplemented, the infants' $SaO_2$ levels were 95%, as opposed to 90% in air. Thus central respiratory motor activity may be affected by lung hypoxia or hypoxaemia. In a study looking at hypoxic arousal, Garg et al demonstrated that in twelve infants with bronchopulmonary dysplasia exposed to a 3 minute hypoxic challenge (inspired oxygen tension 80 mmHg [10.7 kPa]), eight (67%) experienced prolonged apnoea with bradycardia, and four of these infants required bag and mask resuscitation to restore normal breathing.[20]

The development of hypoxaemia, with a sudden catastrophic deterioration, in infants with chronic lung disease may explain some sudden deaths in this group.[21, 22] Further support for this idea comes from the study of 92 infants who had been born prematurely and subsequently had apparent life-threatening events.[23] Abnormalities in oxygenation were demonstrated in 46% at median of 3 days after referral. Baseline hypoxaemia ($SaO_2 < 95\%$) was found in 25% and abnormal episodic desaturation in 40%.[23] Recommencement of additional inspired oxygen to produce normal baseline levels of $SaO_2$ (95–100%) resulted in episodes either stopping or reducing in frequency or severity in 94% of patients.

## Improvement in growth

Groothuis and Rosenberg followed 22 infants who had bronchopulmonary dysplasia and were receiving home oxygen therapy.[24] Apart from 7 infants in whom parents decided prematurely to discontinue oxygen therapy, growth proceeded equally well in these infants as in healthy, full term infants. In

the 7 in whom oxygen was discontinued, weight gain fell significantly. On recommencing oxygen therapy, their weight never returned to the percentiles followed whilst receiving oxygen. It was of concern that 7/22 families did not comply with home oxygen therapy. Unfortunately, the discontinuation of therapy was reinforced by private physicians in 3 of the 7 patients because the infants 'looked well'. This reiterates the need for an adequate objective assessment of oxygenation, since clinical signs or symptoms are insensitive with respect to the detection of mild to moderate degrees of hypoxaemia.

### Reductions in mortality

Infants born before 32 weeks' gestation or weighing less than 1500 g at birth are at particularly increased risk for subsequent sudden death.[25] Infants with chronic lung disease of prematurity have an even greater risk. In one study, 6 out of 53 infants (11%) died suddenly and unexpectedly at between 16 and 30 weeks postnatal age.[21] Such deaths may result from clinically undetected hypoxaemia. Airway hypoxia, as described above, may induce bronchoconstriction, small airway occlusion and sudden, severe ventilation-perfusion mismatch.[26] A rise in intrapulmonary shunting may then produce profound and catastrophic hypoxaemia.[26]

In 7 follow-up studies from the literature of 183 infants on home oxygen therapy, there were 10 deaths (6%).[1, 6, 27–31] Three infants (1.6%) died suddenly and unexpectedly, without adequate explanation at postmortem; all occurred within a few weeks of stopping home oxygen therapy. In these particular patients, there was infrequent, intermittent monitoring of oxygenation using transcutaneous $pO_2$ and it is possible that these infants may have sustained chronic hypoxaemia. There were no sudden deaths in those infants receiving oxygen, even though these are likely to have been the more severely lung damaged infants when compared with infants with chronic lung disease from other studies.[21, 25]

There is only one controlled study looking at mortality with or without long-term oxygen therapy. This is an MRC study of adults with chronic obstructive pulmonary disease, which randomised patients to receive oxygen at 2 l/min via nasal cannulae for at least 15 hours daily.[4] At the end of 5 years follow up, mortality was 30/45 in controls and 19/42 in oxygen treated patients ($P < 0.05$).

### Non-clinical benefits

When receiving oxygen at home, the infant or child is cared for by his/her family, thereby providing a more normal environment for development. In addition, nosocomial infection is a significant risk for any child who spends a long time in hospital, such infections being potentially fatal for patients with chronic respiratory disease. Parents have commented that 'having their babies at home was worth any anxiety they experienced by having the infants on oxygen'.[1] Personal circumstances may sometimes mean, however, that parents do not wish to have their child on oxygen at home. Although Greenough and colleagues considered that 15 infants fulfilled the criteria for home oxygen therapy, in 7 cases parents did not wish to take part because they were either unsupported, working or from overseas.[6]

Several studies from the US have calculated that the discharge home of preterm infants on oxygen therapy is less expensive than keeping such infants in hospital. Studies have calculated savings of $11 990, $18 000, $33 370, and $60 690 per patient treated at home.[1,27,32,33] The Royal College of Physicians working group calculated that 1 patient year's use of a special/intensive care cot would save around £150, 000 and that this would amply fund both a community neonatal nursing sister who can look after up to 10 infants on home oxygen therapy as well as the cost of the necessary equipment to give oxygen and monitor the patients.[5]

## BENEFITS IN OLDER CHILDREN

Provision of long-term oxygen therapy may provide symptomatic relief and an improved quality of life in severe chronic lung disease, such as cystic fibrosis,[34] or in congenital heart disease with pulmonary vascular disease.[11] In conditions involving neuromuscular weakness, loss of lung volume or hypoventilation, additional inspired oxygen may improve $SaO_2$ values, provide a feeling of improved wellbeing, reduce sleep disturbance and delay the development of pulmonary hypertension. In many of these conditions, however, the disturbance in respiratory function may require the use of additional respiratory support, particularly if there is carbon dioxide retention. For conditions which are inevitably terminal in the short term, this may be considered not only inappropriate, but also unethical. Nevertheless, there have been patients awaiting heart and lung transplantation who may have benefited from the provision of additional inspired oxygen and nasal mask ventilation until a donor organ has become available.

It has traditionally been considered that providing oxygen therapy to patients with respiratory failure might lead to hypercapnia, narcosis and worsening of the respiratory failure. This can readily be assessed by utilising transcutaneous carbon dioxide monitoring when commencing oxygen therapy.[35] Hazinski and colleagues found little or no rise in transcutaneous carbon dioxide levels in 10/12 patients with respiratory failure, validated against arterial measurements. Two of these 12 patients, both with cystic fibrosis, showed elevations of 18 and 24%. Similarly, oxygen therapy may be detrimental or even dangerous in children with sleep related upper airway obstruction. Measures to deal with the upper airway, such as removal of adenoids and tonsils, or use of nasal mask continuous positive airway pressure, are more appropriate, and may fully correct the abnormal hypoxaemia.

## ASSESSMENT OF OXYGENATION

The non-invasive assessment of oxygenation is best achieved using pulse oximetry. This technique may be applied for long periods of time. Only the

Nellcor N100 and N200, the Ohmeda Biox III and 3700, Criticare 501, Kontron 7840 and Radiometer OXI3 have been validated against arterial blood samples from infants and children.[36] The users of pulse oximeters should be aware of some of the problems which may lead to inaccuracies in the measurements obtained.[36] These include:

1. Too small signals as a result of improper probe placement or low pulse pressures, as may occur if non-compliant tape is used to secure the sensor. Some pulse oximeters do not ignore such signals and continue to provide a display of erroneous measurements.
2. Falsely low or high readings as a result of an optical shunt from a misplaced sensor or excess ambient light
3. Averaging times that differ between the different pulse oximeters (from 2 to 15 seconds, or 4 to 32 heart beats), resulting in difficulty in defining normal ranges for the frequency and severity of intermittent episodes of hypoxaemia: such data are valid only for the specific brand and averaging mode of the pulse oximeter which is used.
4. Underestimation of episodic or baseline hypoxaemia – this may occur in situations where the $SaO_2$ is changing rapidly as, for example, in periodic breathing. It is due to oximeters with longer averaging times failing to show that a patient might be reaching a normal baseline blood oxygen level between pauses in breathing movements.
5. Missing significant hypoxaemic episodes due to motion artefact – unfortunately a proportion of hypoxaemic episodes may be missed because the hand or foot to which the sensor is attached is moving. This is particularly likely during feeding, crying or care procedures. This may be overcome partly by simultaneous monitoring of transcutaneous $pO_2$.[2, 37]

The normal range of $SaO_2$ depends on gestational and postnatal age, the instrument used to monitor oxygenation, and the definitions used to measure baseline and episodic hypoxaemia. Using the Nellcor pulse oximeter, measurements of baseline $SaO_2$ and the frequency of episodic desaturation have been made in normal term and preterm infants, and in children 2–16 years of age [see references 26, 80, 81, 86, 90 in reference[36]]. These are shown in Table 3.2. In summary, the normal range for baseline $SaO_2$ with the Nellcor pulse oximeter is between 95 and 100%, regardless of age.

Based on these data, we would advocate that infants who have reached 37 weeks' gestational age or over are maintained within the normal range (preterm infants might also be kept at the lower end of this range). This is in keeping with the evidence that even at $SaO_2$ levels of 93–94%, pulmonary artery pressures may be elevated.[10] Similarly, there may be as yet unknown effects on airway function even at these minimally lowered $SaO_2$ levels.

**Table 3.2** Normal data for baseline SaO2 and desaturation frequency. These are based upon studies (listed in,36, as references 26, 80, 81, 86 and 90) using the Nellcor pulse oximeter. Median, range (in brackets), and 5th or 95th centile (in italics) are given for each variable and age group

| Study group | Patient numbers | Age | Birth GA | Baseline $SaO_2$* (%) | Desaturation Frequency† |
|---|---|---|---|---|---|
| Preterm infants at discharge | 160 | 20 days (3–165) | 33 (25–36) | 99.6 (88.7–100) *95.7* | 3/12 hours (0–355) *61* |
| Preterm infants 6 weeks after discharge | 110 | 70 days (26–180) | 33 (25–36) | 100.0 (95.3–100) *97.9* | 0/12 hours (0–17) *3* |
| Full term infants in the 2nd month | 67 | 39 days (29–54) | | 99.8 (97.0–100) | 0.9 /hour (0.0–15.1) |
| Full term infants in the 1st year | 16 | 191 days (171–273) | | 99.8 (97.3–100) | 0.5 /hour (0.0–7.9) |
| Children 2–16 years | 70 | 8 years (2–16) | | 99.5 (95.8–100) | 0.0 /hour (0.0–2.7) |

*Baseline $SaO_2$ is measured during breathing of a regular amplitude and frequency, away from pauses, sighs or movement artefact (see[36]).
†Desaturation is defined as a fall in $SaO_2$ to ≤ 80% for ≥ 4s in preterm infants, ≤ 80% for any duration in full term infants, and to ≤ 90% in older children.

Because of the difficulty of ensuring adequate pulse detection during motion, when hypoxaemia is likely, we would aim to give too much rather than too little inspired oxygen.

When the inspired oxygen concentration is reduced, or the patient is breathing room air and $SaO_2$ levels fall to less than 92%, it is usually possible to decide upon the need for oxygen by clinical observation. It is when levels are in the mid 90s that a physiological recording or sleep study is of particular value. We record the following signals in the child breathing air over an 8–12 hour period: (i) $SaO_2$, in the beat-to-beat mode; (ii) the pulse waveform to assess the adequacy of pulse detection; (iii) breathing movements, to assess whether episodic desaturation is related to apnoeic pauses or periodic apnoea, and hence is normal; and (iv) ECG. An activity chart kept by the nurses or parents allows any clinical changes to be related to the recording, and recording abnormalities to be related to the activity or state of the patient.

## MONITORING AFTER DISCHARGE

Prior to the availability of non-invasive methods for measuring blood oxygen levels, patients were monitored by either clinical symptoms such as cyanosis, tachypnoea, apnoea and respiratory infections, or by intermittent arterial blood gas sampling.[1] Such symptoms are not adequately sensitive for hypoxaemia, and arterial puncture is of little value in infants with chronic lung disease because of the upset and subsequent desaturation that it causes. Some studies have reported the use of an intermittent application of transcutaneous $pO_2$ sensor for the monitoring of such infants and have advocated maintenance of transcutaneous $pO_2 > 50$ or 55 mmHg.[2, 27–29] The advantage of transcutaneous $pO_2$ monitoring is that, unlike pulse oximetry, it is not sensitive to motion artifact. It can, therefore, provide a more adequate assessment of oxygenation during motion, feeding, and upset. However, the poor correlation with arterial values[9] means that transcutaneous $pO_2$ monitoring is not a satisfactory way of assessing the adequacy of oxygenation or deciding when it is appropriate to wean the patient from oxygen therapy.

More recently, pulse oximetry has been used to monitor such patients. Larger neonatal units may have a nurse specialist who attends the homes for one or more days per week, or less frequently, depending on the duration of time since discharge and the parents' confidence. Their protocol provides an effective and regular method of assessing the adequacy of oxygenation whilst under direct clinical observation in the daytime. Some units may also provide pulse oximeters for long-term use at home. In our experience, the frequency of false alarms makes this form of monitor unsuitable for continuous monitoring of oxygen levels, particularly at night.[37]

An alternative to pulse oximetry for continuous monitoring is transcutaneous $pO_2$ using an electrode temperature of 43°C, thereby allowing re-siting of the sensor every 8 hours.[37] Although transcutaneous $pO_2$ does not provide an *accurate* measurement of blood oxygen levels, parents soon learn values of transcutaneous $pO_2$ that are compatible with pulse oximeter values $\geq 95\%$, and then can maintain these $pO_2$ values thereafter at home. This form of monitoring can be used by day and by night, and has a relatively low frequency of false alarms.[37] If the nasal cannulae supplying the oxygen become blocked or fall out, or if the infant develops a respiratory infection, parents can see a fall in the levels of transcutaneous $pO_2$ and may commence or increase the oxygen flow as required. Both gradual improvements and deteriorations in oxygenation may be seen on a day-to-day basis and sudden hypoxaemic episodes will also be detected. We have used transcutaneous $pO_2$ monitoring in over 400 infants and children on home oxygen. In the future, the ideal oxygen monitor might incorporate not only transcutaneous $pO_2$ for trend and alarm purposes, but also pulse oximetry for intermittent measurements, for example when the transcutaneous $pO_2$ value is low.

The presence of an increased frequency of apnoeic pauses, periodic breathing and obstructive apnoea in infants recently weaned from oxygen compared with when they were on supplemental oxygen, or with control infants[19] might support the use of apnoea ± ECG monitors. Garg and colleagues, however, did not find that abnormal findings on a pneumogram, a long-term recording of breathing movements, ECG and heart rate, predicted the occurrence of prolonged episodes of hypoxaemia, apnoea or bradycardia.[20] Despite this, apnoea-ECG monitors are in widespread use in the US for oxygen-dependent infants. In the UK, there are reports of infants who have died suddenly and unexpectedly whilst being cared for on apnoea monitors on special care baby units.[38] Such infants may well have had clinically unrecognised hypoxaemic events.

## WEANING FROM ADDITIONAL INSPIRED OXYGEN

It is not possible to predict the duration over which oxygen therapy is likely to be needed in infants with chronic lung disease of prematurity. Average durations in follow-up studies are between 3 and 6 months, but a proportion may require oxygen therapy for between 1 and 5 years of age. With increasing age and mobility, it becomes more difficult to apply oxygen during the daytime. Toddlers are particularly prone to removing their nasal cannulae.

When $SaO_2$ levels are maintained consistently $\geq$ 95%, the inspired oxygen flow may be reduced in increments (e.g. 0.1–0.25 l/min), depending on the initial flow. For infants on home transcutaneous $pO_2$ monitoring, $pO_2$ values consistently $\geq$ 80 mmHg may indicate that the inspired oxygen flow may be reduced, but under these circumstances, pulse oximetry should be used to confirm adequate oxygenation. Sleep studies that show the majority of an overnight recording with $SaO_2$ levels $\geq$ 95%, but with some periods between 93 and 95% could indicate that oxygen therapy be discontinued in the daytime, but still administered overnight.

Following their experience of two infants dying suddenly and unexpectedly 5 weeks after stopping oxygen therapy, Campbell and colleagues recommended continuation of apnoea monitoring for a further 2 months at home.[27] As this technique fails in 90% of instances to detect the development of sudden hypoxaemia,[37] we would recommend continuing transcutaneous $pO_2$ monitoring for a similar duration. If this includes a period when the infant suffers a respiratory tract infection, this may provide further reassurance that a renewed need for oxygen therapy is unlikely.

## METHODS OF ADMINISTRATION OF OXYGEN THERAPY

### Catheter or cannulae

Two methods are mainly used for long-term administration: (i) insertion of a size 8 French gauge feeding tube, 2–4 cm into one nostril; and (ii) nasal cannulae, such as provided by DeVilbiss (Feltham, Middlesex, UK), with nasal prongs 2–4 mm long. In acutely unwell children, an 8FG catheter inserted into the pharynx may achieve higher transcutaneous values than when the tip of the catheter ends in the nose.[39] Compared with nasal cannulae, this technique may have the benefit of conserving oxygen supplies. Nasopharyngeal and intra-nasal catheters are more likely than nasal prongs to become blocked with mucus and may need to be removed and cleaned up to twice daily. This can be a particularly unpleasant procedure for some infants. We prefer to supply nasal cannulae which may be left in place for long periods of time. They may provide up to 40% inspired oxygen with flows up to 2 l/min. The main problem with any tubing that has to be taped on to the cheek is the development of sore skin. The use of a karaya gum base below the cannulae followed by tape over the top may prevent this complication.

**Oxygen source**

Oxygen may be provided from either a cylinder, a concentrator or a liquid oxygen tank. The first two are able to be prescribed by general practitioners. A recent review calculated that the provision of cylinders for continuous oxygen therapy over a 6 month period at home, cost 5–8 times more than the provision of a concentrator.[40] Concentrators with a low flow meter are supplied in the home, along with tubing outlets to different rooms, by one of three companies in the UK, dependent on area of residence: DeVilbiss, Omnicare and the Oxygen Therapy Company. All such devices are provided with a non-portable back-up cylinder (usually British Oxygen Company (BOC) cylinder sizes F or AF, see Table 3.3) in the home, in case of concentrator or electricity mains failure.

Problems still exist with the supply of equipment to allow portability. Parents may use a BOC cylinder size C or D, but empty cylinders have to be exchanged for full ones at a pharmacy and this may cause practical problems. Alternatively, a small cylinder (e.g. Sabre AAV or BOC) may be used and topped up from a cylinder at home (size F or AF). Although the larger cylinder is able to be prescribed, the small cylinders and recharging adaptors must be purchased by the hospital, parents or charities. This also applies to the low flow meters which are used with these small cylinders.

The most recent advance in conserving oxygen in small portable cylinders, thus providing prolonged use away from the home, is the use of an electronic oxygen conserver (Oxymatic, Life Support (Europe) Ltd, Dunstable, UK). This senses pressure changes in the nasal cannulae (about 0.5 cm $H_2O$), and delivers a small pulse of oxygen with inspiration. This system may extend the duration of available oxygen by up to 7 times. Although use has been made of this in older children with cystic fibrosis, it is unknown how well this would function in infants, who generally have faster respiratory rates.

**Table 3.3** Details of commonly used cylinders (British Oxygen Company)

| Cylinder size | Contents (l) | Weight of gas (kg) | Cylinder weight* (kg) | Cylinder dimensions (mm) | Main use |
|---|---|---|---|---|---|
| C | 170 | 0.23 | 2 | 430 x 89 | portable |
| D | 340 | 0.46 | 3.4 | 535 x 102 | portable |
| F | 1360 | 1.84 | 14.5 | 930 x 140 | in home |
| AF | 1360 | 1.84 | 9.9 | 670 x 175 | in home |
| G | 3400 | 4.60 | 34.5 | 1320 x 178 | in home |

*This is weight of cylinder and valve without gas. Add weight of gas to obtain weight of full cylinder.

**Table 3.4** List of people involved in planning the discharge home of a child on oxygen therapy

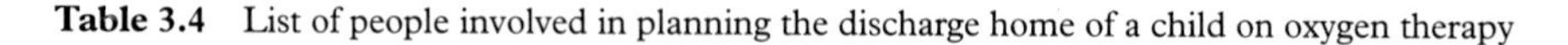

- Parents
- Paediatric medical and nursing staff
- General practitioner
- Health visitor
- Liaison nursing staff/clinical nurse specialist
- Social worker
- Business manager

**Table 3.5** Areas needing organisation prior to discharge home of a child on oxygen therapy

- Home oxygen supply
- Home oxygen monitor
- Training in resuscitation
- Training in tube feeding/changing (if relevant)
- Medications
- Immunisations
- Availability of telephone/priority telephone repair service
- Fire and electricity services
- Home and car insurance
- Identification of lines of communication
  - with nursing, medical and ambulance staff
- Discharge transport
- Respite care
- Financial issues
- Follow up

## PLANNING FOR DISCHARGE HOME

Good communication between the parents and all of those professionals listed in Table 3.4 is essential if the family are to be adequately supported at home. Most general practitioners and health visitors have little experience of infants or children on long-term oxygen therapy or home oxygen monitoring. It is optimal if a planning meeting can be held prior to discharge.

The issues that require discussion and arrangement are listed in Table 3.5. Parents and other friends or relatives who will be involved in the care of the infant or child need to be given full training in the use of all equipment. They will also be required to know how to observe changes in the child's condition, and know who to contact for help. Parents and any other carers all need to be confident in these areas. Allowing the parent(s) to look after the child undisturbed in a hospital cubicle for a day or more before discharge may help to achieve this. Standard immunisations should be given at the usual ages, and consideration should be given to influenza vaccination during the winter months.

Parents must be aware of safety issues concerning storage and usage of oxygen, including the avoidance of naked flames and secure placement of oxygen cylinders in the home and car. Electricity costs for running the concentrator are reimbursable, but parents may also be in need of other financial support to help in the provision of a telephone, child care facilities or transport to and from the hospital. Help may also be obtained from a Disability Living Allowance.

There are many practical issues relating to the assessment of oxygenation and provision of home oxygen therapy, which make it more suitable for this to be performed by paediatricians who have the relevant expertise and equipment. This particularly applies to its use in older children, as it is in this group that the benefits and outcome are less clear.

## KEY POINTS FOR CLINICAL PRACTICE

- Do not rely on clinical signs to detect hypoxaemia – it may exist in mild to moderate degrees without being clinically apparent.
- Pulse oximetry is the best method for performing long-term, non-invasive assessment of oxygenation. Be familiar with the workings of your model of oximeter, and only use those that have been well validated in children.
- Normal baseline $SaO_2$ in infants and children is 95–100%, measured with a Nellcor pulse oximeter during regular amplitude and frequency breathing. Be aware of the normal variations and pitfalls in measurement.
- In children who have suffered severe respiratory illness or an apparent life-threatening event, an assessment of oxygenation should be performed. Such illnesses may result in, or occur on a background of, hypoxaemia resulting from airway hypoxia.
- Failure to thrive may be due to chronic hypoxaemia and an assessment of oxygenation should be performed as part of the investigation – particularly in infants with a history of chronic lung disease.
- Consider prescribing additional inspired oxygen for any infant or child who is persistently hypoxaemic ($SaO_2 < 95\%$). This is not usually necessary with right to left intracardiac shunts, and may produce carbon dioxide retention in a child with upper airway obstruction.
- In hypoxaemic children, associated hypoventilation can be readily assessed by the use of transcutaneous carbon dioxide monitoring, before and after starting oxygen therapy.
- For infants under 1 year, consider home monitoring of oxygenation continuously, or at least at night, in order to detect changes in oxygenation, particularly sudden and severe hypoxaemia.

- Utilise a multi-disciplinary approach to the discharge of patients receiving long-term oxygen – this will reduce potential problems once home.

## REFERENCES


1 Pinney MA, Cotton EK. Home management of bronchopulmonary dysplasia. Pediatrics 1976; 58: 856–859
2 Philip AGS, Peabody JL, Lucey JF. Transcutaneous $PO_2$ monitoring in the home management of bronchopulmonary dysplasia. Pediatrics 1978; 61: 655–657
3 Nocturnal Oxygen Therapy Trial Group. Continuous or nocturnal therapy in hypoxemic chronic obstructive lung disease. Ann Int Med 1980; 93: 391–398
4 Medical Research Council Working Party. long-term domiciliary oxygen therapy in chronic hypoxic cor pulmonale complicating chronic bronchitis and emphysema. Lancet 1981; i: 681–686
5 Silverman M. Domiciliary oxygen therapy for children. Report of a Working Group of the Committee on Thoracic Medicine of the Royal College of Physicians. J R Coll Physicians Lond 1992; 26: 125–127
6 Greenough A, Hird MS, Gamsu HR. Home oxygen therapy following neonatal intensive care. Early Hum Dev 1991; 26: 29–35
7 Shaw N, Gill B, Weindling M, Cooke R. The changing incidence of chronic lung disease. Health Trends 1993; 25: 50–53.
8 Halliday HL, Dumpit FM, Brady JP. Effects of inspired oxygen on echocardiographic assessment of pulmonary vascular resistance and myocardial contractility in bronchopulmonary dysplasia. Pediatrics 1980; 65: 536–540
9 Ramanathan R, Durand M, Larrazabal C. Pulse oximetry in very low birthweight infants with acute and chronic lung disease. Pediatrics 1987; 79: 612–617
10 Abman SH, Wolfe RR, Accurso FJ, Koops BL, Bowman M, Wiggins JW. Pulmonary vascular response to oxygen in infants with severe bronchopulmonary dysplasia. Pediatrics 1985; 75: 80–84
11 Bowyer JJ, Busst CM, Denison DM, Shinebourne EA. Effect of long-term oxygen treatment at home in children with pulmonary vascular disease. Br Heart J 1986; 55: 385–390
12 Goldstein RS, Zamel M, Rebuck AS. Absence of effects of hypoxia on small airway functioning in humans. J Appl Physiol 1979; 47; 251–256
13 Saunders NA, Betts MF, Pengelly D, Rebuck AS. Changes in lung mechanics induced by acute isocapnic hypoxia. J Appl Physiol 1977; 42: 413–419
14 Libby DM, Briscoe WA, King TKC. Relief of hypoxia–related bronchoconstriction by breathing 30% oxygen. Am Rev Respir Dis 1981; 123: 71–75
15 Tay-Uyboco JS, Kwiatkowski K, Cates DB, Kavanagh L, Rigatto H. Hypoxic airway constriction in infants of very low birth weight, recovering from moderate to severe bronchopulmonary dysplasia. J Pediatr 1989; 115: 456–459
16 Teague WG, Pian MS, Heldt GP, Tooley WH. An acute reduction in the fraction of inspired oxygen increases airway constriction in infants with chronic lung disease. Am Rev Respir Dis 1988; 137: 861–865
17 Singer L, Martin RJ, Hawkins SW, Benson-Szekely LJ, Yamashita TS, Carlo WA. Oxygen desaturation complicates feeding in infants with bronchopulmonary dysplasia after discharge. Pediatrics 1992; 90: 380–384
18 Garg M, Kurzner SI, Bautista DB, Keans TG. Clinically unsuspected hypoxia during sleep and feeding in infants with bronchopulmonary dysplasia. Pediatrics 1988; 81: 635–642
19 Sekar AC, Duke JC. Sleep apnea and hypoxaemia in recently weaned premature infants with and without bronchopulmonary dysplasia. Pediatr Pulmonol 1991; 10: 112–116
20 Garg M, Kurzner SI, Bautista D, Keens TG. Hypoxic arousal response in infants with bronchopulmonary dysplasia. Pediatrics 1988; 82: 59–63
21 Werthammer J, Brown ER, Neff RK, Taesch HW. Sudden infant death syndrome in infants with bronchopulmonary dysplasia. Pediatrics 1982; 69: 301–304

22 Abman SH, Burchell MF, Schaffer MS, Rosenberg AA. Late sudden unexpected deaths in hospitalized infants with bronchopulmonary dysplasia. Am J Dis Child 1989; 143: 815–819

23 Samuels MP, Poets CF, Southall DP. Abnormal hypoxemia after life threatening events in infants born pre-term. J Paediatr 1994; 125: 441–446

24 Groothuis JR, Rosenberg AA. Home oxygen promotes weight gain in infants with bronchopulmonary dysplasia. Am J Dis Child 1987; 141: 992–995.

25 Yu VYH, Watkins A, Bajuk B. Neonatal and post-neonatal mortality in very low birth weight infants. Arch Dis Child 1984; 59: 987–999

26 Poets CF, Samuels MP, Southall DP. Potential role of intrapulmonary shunting in the genesis of hypoxemic episodes in infants and young children. Paediatrics 1992; 90: 385–391

27 Campbell AN, Zarfin Y, Groenveld M, Bryan MH. Low flow oxygen therapy in infants. Arch Dis Child 1983; 58: 795–798

28 Abman SH, Accurso FJ, Coops BL. Experience with home oxygen in the management of infants with bronchopulmonary dysplasia. Clin Paediatr 1984; 23: 471–476

29 Daily DK. Home oxygen therapy for infants with bronchopulmonary dysplasia. Perinatol Neonatol 1987; 11: 26–35

30 Sauve RS, McMillan DD, Mitchell I, Creighton D, Hindle NW, Young L. Home oxygen therapy: outcome of infants discharged from NICU on continuous treatment. Clin Pediatr 1989; 28: 113–118

31 Hudak BB, Allen MC, Hudak ML, Loughlin GM. Home oxygen therapy for chronic lung disease in extremely low-birth-weight infants. Am J Dis Child 1989; 143: 357–360

32 Donn S. Cost effectiveness of home management of bronchopulmonary dysplasia. Pediatrics 1982; 70: 330–331

33 Thilo EH, Comito J, McCullis D. Home oxygen therapy in the newborn. Am J Dis Child 1987; 141: 766–768

34 Zinman R, Corey M, Coates AL et al. Nocturnal home oxygen in the treatment of hypoxaemic cystic fibrosis patients. J Paediatr 1989; 114: 368–377

35 Hazinski TA, Hansen TN, Simon JA, Tooley WH. Effect of oxygen administration during sleep on skin surface oxygen and carbon dioxide tensions in patients with chronic lung disease. Pediatrics 1981; 67: 626–630

36 Poets CF, Southall DP. Non-invasive monitoring of oxygenation in infants and children: practical considerations and areas of concern. Paediatrics 1994; 93: 737–746

37 Poets CF, Samuels MP, Noyes JP, Jones KA, Southall DP. Home monitoring of transcutaneous oxygen tension in the early detection of hypoxaemia in infants and young children. Arch Dis Child 1991; 66: 676–682

38 Samuels MP, Stebbens VA, Poets CF, Southall DP. Deaths on infant ‘apnoea’ monitors. Mat Child Health 1993; 18: 262–266

39 Shann F, Gatchalian S, Hutchinson R. Nasopharyngeal oxygen in children. Lancet, 1988; ii: 1238–1240

40 McFadyen UM. Home oxygen treatment. Paediatr Respir Med 1993; 1: 10–14

# 4

# Child physical abuse: risk indicators and prevention

*H. L. MacMillan   A. C. Niec   D. R. Offord*

This chapter will review recent data on the risk indicators for and prevention of child physical abuse. It will include a discussion of screening for child physical abuse, as well as a section outlining what the clinician can do. Physical abuse is defined broadly as any physical force inflicted on a child causing harm. Child neglect is a separate category of maltreatment not included within the definition of physical abuse, although prevention strategies are often targeted at both physical abuse and neglect. It is essential that pediatricians are familiar with the diagnosis, assessment and management of child physical abuse. These topics have been reviewed in two recent publications[1,2] and are beyond the scope of this chapter.

## BURDEN OF SUFFERING

The prevalence of physical abuse is unknown, but there is evidence that official reports to child protective agencies underestimate the extent of the problem. Many episodes of child physical abuse go unreported because of failure to detect, recognize or officially report the abuse.[3] One of the difficulties in determining the magnitude of physical abuse is the lack of a common definition. In other conditions affecting children, such as infectious diseases or chronic illnesses, there is relative agreement about the definition of specific disorders. It is only in recent years that any type of child maltreatment has come to be considered a public health problem (and therefore of interest to physicians), rather than a social problem.

Much of the research to determine the prevalence of physical abuse has been carried out in the United States. A US national survey conducted in 1985 estimated the rate of physical violence against children among households with two caretakers and at least one child aged 3 to 17 years; 10.7% of the parents admitted to having carried out 'a severe violent act' against their child in the previous year.[4] A recent province-wide survey (Ontario Health Supplement, OHSUP) carried out in Canada examined the prevalence of a history of physical abuse within a community sample.[5] The definition of child physical abuse (abuse by an adult of someone growing up) included one or more of the following occurring often or sometimes: (1) being pushed, grabbed, shoved; (2) having something thrown at; and (3) being hit with something, or one or more of the following occurring often, sometimes or rarely: (1) being kicked, bitten or punched; (2) being choked, burned or scalded; and (3) being physically attacked in some other way. Within this general population sample which included residents 15 years of age and older, 31.2% of males and 21.1% of females reported a history of physical abuse by an adult during childhood.[5]

Child physical abuse is clearly a common and pervasive problem associated with a heavy burden of suffering. In evaluating the consequences of physical abuse, it can be difficult to separate the direct effects of abuse from other factors such as low socioeconomic status. Nevertheless, there is evidence that physically abused children suffer cognitive, emotional and social impairment in addition to physical disabilities.[6–8] Finkelhor emphasizes that the psychological sequelae of sexual victimization have received much more attention than non-sexual assaults involving injury,[9] yet the latter are also associated with serious psychological disturbances.[10] In addition, physical abuse is frequently underestimated as an important cause of childhood fatalities.[11]

## STRATEGIES FOR PREVENTION OF CHILD PHYSICAL ABUSE

Prevention can occur at three levels: primary, secondary and tertiary. Primary prevention includes any intervention that is provided to the general population or a sample of the general population to stop something before it ever occurs. According to a public health model of prevention, secondary prevention generally implies early detection of a condition with the aim of shortening the duration of a disorder.[12] In the child maltreatment literature, the category of secondary prevention has been applied to interventions targeted at those who are high risk for committing child maltreatment, even though abuse has not yet occurred.[13] In other fields, such interventions would be categorized as primary prevention, since there has been no onset to the condition at that point. Tertiary prevention addresses those situations in which a condition has already occurred and the aim is to prevent recurrence and impairment.

This chapter will focus on primary prevention, defined as any intervention that is provided to prevent child physical abuse from occurring. This definition includes some interventions which have been defined by others as secondary prevention. Tertiary prevention, which includes treatment, is beyond the scope of this chapter, but this topic has been reviewed elsewhere recently.[14]

## SCREENING FOR CHILD PHYSICAL ABUSE

The concept of screening individuals for increased risk of committing physical child abuse has been evaluated over the past two decades. Methods of screening include three main approaches: a staff-administered checklist, a self-administered questionnaire and a standardized interview.[15] The Family Stress Checklist[16] is an example of the first approach. Self-administered questionnaires include the Child Abuse Potential Inventory[17,18] and the Michigan Screening Profile of Parenting.[19] A standardized interview format has been used by one group of investigators.[20] In addition, Leventhal and colleagues examined whether clinicians could correctly identify infants at high risk for physical abuse without the use of specific instruments.[21]

These screening methods have been used most commonly during the newborn period to predict which individuals are at risk of physically abusing a child. Decisions about the accuracy of prediction must take into account sensitivity, specificity and misclassification rates. The main problem with the available screening methods is the high false-positive rate.[22] A sizeable number of people classified by such techniques as being at risk for committing physical abuse would never go on to abuse a child. Several authors have emphasized the potential harm associated with mislabelling people as child abusers.[23,24] The stigma may put people under increased stress and further undermine their ability to parent.[23] This may place children at greater risk than before the prediction of physical abuse.

Because there are problems with all of these screening approaches, screening individuals for potential risk of child abuse does not provide a rational basis for narrowing service delivery.[24] Kaufman and Zigler have concluded that 'accurate prediction of individual cases is not possible' and have advocated that 'efforts at predicting individual cases of child abuse should be abandoned'.[25] Nevertheless, it is still useful to evaluate risk factors for child physical abuse, since interventions can be targeted at groups of individuals or communities at increased risk while avoiding the stigma of labelling a specific individual as at risk.

## RISK INDICATORS FOR CHILD PHYSICAL ABUSE

This section briefly discusses the etiology of child physical abuse, defines the concept 'risk indicator' and summarizes what is known currently about associated features of child physical abuse. Child physical abuse is a complex, multifaceted problem; no single factor accounts for its occurrence. Several theoretical models have been developed over the years. One of the earliest approaches focused on the abusing caretaker as suffering from some form of psychiatric illness.[26] Although there continues to be uncertainty about the true prevalence of mental illness among physically abusive adults, it now appears that the majority of people who abuse their children are not mentally ill.[27]

More recent theoretical models emphasize the multicausal nature of child abuse.[28] One of the most comprehensive models describes child physical abuse as the consequence of interactions between individual characteristics of the caretaker, familial variables, factors in the environment, and cultural determinants.[28,29] In a 'developmental-ecological analysis' of the problem, Belsky underscores that what determines whether child abuse will occur is the balance of stressors and supports; therefore no single solution to child abuse exists.[29] Identification of risk factors for child physical abuse provides important information about causal pathways.

**Table 4.1** Risk indicators for child physical abuse

- low socioeconomic status
- social isolation
- young maternal age
- large family size
- single parent family
- spousal violence
- parent's childhood experience of physical abuse
- unplanned pregnancy or negative parental attitude toward pregnancy

Risk factor is a concept used extensively in the field of epidemiology. Although the term 'at risk' seems obvious, there is disagreement among experts about the definition of risk factor. For a variable to be a true risk factor for physical abuse, it must meet the following criteria: (1) the variable must be associated with an increased probability of physical abuse; (2) onset of the variable must antedate abuse; and (3) there must be evidence that the variable plays a causal role in abuse.[30] If there is an association but the temporal relationship is unclear, the variable is an indicator or correlate of physical abuse. Since much of the work assessing variables associated with physical abuse has involved cross-sectional studies, with a few exceptions it is only possible to state that the variable is an indicator of abuse. For the purpose of this chapter, a risk indicator is any factor associated with an increased likelihood of child physical abuse.

The following sections provide a summary of the variables associated with child physical abuse (see Table 4.1). It is not exhaustive; one author estimates that there are more than 100 potential risk indicators for physical abuse.[31] According to much of the earlier literature, rates of physical abuse were considered similar among boys and girls. Information from recent work by Wolfner and Gelles,[32] as well as from the OHSUP,[5] suggest that males are more at risk for physical victimization. Although children of all ages are at risk for physical abuse, pre-school children are most at risk for experiencing abusive violence.[32] Children of pre-school age are also over-represented in reports of serious physical injury and fatalities resulting from abuse.

Variables in the family that are associated with an increased likelihood of physical abuse include: poverty; young maternal age; large family; single-parent family; parent(s) with a history of physical abuse during childhood; spousal abuse; social isolation or lack of support; and unplanned pregnancy or negative parental attitude toward the pregnancy (for specific references to each of these variables, please refer to MacMillan et al, 1993).[33] With respect to the demographic variables such as poverty, one of the longstanding questions is whether physical abuse appears more prevalent in low socioeconomic families because of a reporting bias. Recent studies have indicated that while a reporting bias likely does exist for low income families, physical abuse probably does occur more often among families of low socioeconomic status.[34]

One of the most controversial issues in the literature is the question of intergenerational transmission of child physical abuse. Although there has been the widespread belief that victims of physical abuse during childhood inevitably go on to become abusive parents, the evidence suggests otherwise. It is estimated that approximately 30% of physically abused or neglected children abuse their offspring.[35]

Several variables commonly listed by other authors as risk indicators have been omitted purposely. These factors are categorized as characteristics of the child, and include prematurity, low birth weight, physical disability and temperament. For each of these variables the evidence is conflicting, and there are significant methodologic issues in evaluating the relationship with child physical abuse. In a critical review examining the risk status of prematurity and low birth weight for child physical abuse, Leventhal[36] emphasized that only three studies included a specific control group and adjusted for susceptibility factors. His group concluded that there was no association between these child characteristics and child maltreatment as an outcome. Other variables such as temperament and physical disability have been evaluated after physical abuse has occurred. Several authors point out that early infant problems or disabilities may be the result of abuse or poor parenting. There is insufficient evidence that any of these child variables precedes physical abuse.

Both drug and alcohol use are often included in a list of risk indicators for physical abuse, yet the evidence is not clear. In the 1985 US community survey on family violence, respondents were asked to report on their substance use.[32] When rates of violence were examined with respect to alcohol use, there were no significant differences in rates of abusive violence between those who used and did not use alcohol. In contrast, drug users reported 20% more minor violence and 46% more severe violence compared to those who did not use drugs. It has been common in the past to assume that any type of substance abuse plays a causal role in physical abuse, however this issue has not yet been investigated adequately. Although it makes sense to suppose that children should be raised in an environment free from caretakers who have problems with substance abuse, the nature of the relationship between parental substance abuse and child physical abuse needs further study in community samples.

In summary, the use of screening devices for identifying caretakers at risk for committing child physical abuse is not justified. However, it is useful for paediatricians to know the risk indicators for physical abuse so that interventions can be targeted at groups or communities at risk while avoiding the stigma of labelling an individual.

## PREVENTION OF CHILD PHYSICAL ABUSE

Many strategies and programmes have been proposed for the prevention of child physical abuse. MacMillan and colleagues carried out a systematic review

**Table 4.2** Effectiveness of interventions for prevention of physical abuse

| Intervention | Evidence of effectiveness | Reference |
|---|---|---|
| Home visitation During/after/during and after pregnancy | Beginning during or just after pregnancy **and** extending until two years was shown effective in preventing physical abuse during programme | Olds et al, 1986[39] Hardy & Streett, 1989[40] Olds & Kitzman, 1990[48] Olds et al, 1994[41] |
| Intensive pediatric contact with home visits | Insufficient evidence | Gray et al, 1979[38] |
| Extended parent-child postpartum contact With visits/without visits | Insufficient evidence but may be beneficial for other reasons | Siegel et al, 1980[42] O'Connor et al, 1980[43] |
| Drop-in centre | Insufficient evidence | Lealman et al, 1983[44] |
| Parent training program | Insufficient evidence but may be beneficial for other reasons | Resnick, 1985[46] Wolfe et al, 1988[45] |
| Free access to health care | No evidence | Olds et al, 1986[39] |
| Comprehensive health care program | No evidence | Brayden et al, 1993[47] |

of prospective controlled trials published between 1979 and 1993 evaluating interventions aimed at prevention of child physical abuse.[37] The interventions can be described broadly as perinatal and early childhood programmes. The seven main categories of interventions are listed in Table 4.2. The following section gives an overview of controlled trials which evaluated the effectiveness of preventive interventions for child physical abuse.

Because of the problem with defining and measuring child physical abuse, numerous and varied outcomes were reported across studies. In assessing effectiveness of the interventions, those outcomes considered most representative for the assessment of physical abuse were as follows: (1) official reports of suspected or verified child physical abuse; (2) hospitalizations; (3) injury rates; and (4) rates of visitation to emergency rooms. The latter three outcomes were considered 'proxy measures' of physical abuse. The trials each received a score for methodologic rigor. The quality of each study was considered when summarizing the results.

## Interventions evaluated by controlled trials

A randomized controlled trial (RCT) evaluated intensive paediatric contact plus home visitation by public health nurses and lay health visitors for mothers identified as being at risk for abnormal parenting practices.[38] The number of verified reports of child physical abuse did not differ significantly between the intervention and control groups, however the children of women in the control group were significantly more likely than those of women in the intervention group to require inpatient treatment for serious injuries. The study suffered from inadequate follow up; outcome was evaluated in only 50% of the families. Since the study examined a combined intervention of intensive paediatric contact plus home visitation, the lower number of seriously injured children in the intervention group cannot be attributed to intensive paediatric contact alone.

Several RCTs have evaluated home visitation as the primary preventive intervention. The two most rigorous studies with respect to sample size, outcome assessment and length of follow-up demonstrated a reduction in the incidence of child physical abuse and outcomes related to maltreatment in the intervention groups.[39,40] Olds and colleagues[39] evaluated home visits made by nurses to white, primiparous women who were primarily young or single or of low socioeconomic status. Women in the control group received no services during pregnancy or free transportation for prenatal and well-child care. There were two treatment groups; women in one group were visited by a nurse during pregnancy (pregnancy-visited group) and the second group received visits during pregnancy and after birth until the child's second birthday (infancy-visited group). Infants in the latter group had fewer emergency room visits in the first ($P = 0.04$) and second ($P = 0.01$) year of life, and were seen less frequently for injuries and poisonings in the second year of life ($P = 0.03$), than infants in the control group. In a subgroup of mothers considered at highest risk for physical abuse or neglect (poor, unmarried teens) 19% of those in the control group and 4% of those in the infancy-visited group had instances of verified physical abuse and neglect ($P = 0.07$). The incidence of outcomes in the pregnancy-visited group generally fell between the rates in the infancy-visited group and the control group.

Olds and colleagues examined whether the reduced rates of child abuse among high-risk families who received home visitation continued during the third and fourth years of life, after the programme ended.[41] There were no enduring treatment differences in rates of child abuse and neglect, however nurse-visited children lived in homes with fewer hazards and had 40% fewer injuries and ingestions. Although the programme effects on reduced rates of child maltreatment did not persist into the third and fourth years of life, it does not discount the fact that children in high-risk families were abused less frequently while the programme was in operation. In addition, ongoing reduction in injuries and ingestions points to improvement in abuse-related outcomes. Olds and colleagues concluded that it may be necessary to extend the length of the programme to produce lasting reductions in child maltreatment.

In an RCT carried out in Baltimore, black mothers of low socioeconomic status were assigned to receive either home visits beginning in the newborn period until the infant was 24 months old or no such intervention.[40] Most of the women were single and one-quarter were primiparous. The home visitor was a community woman with support provided through a health care programme for children and youth. Children in the intervention group had significantly fewer admissions to hospital ($P < 0.01$) and episodes of suspected physical abuse or neglect than those in the control group ($P < 0.01$). The incidence of closed head trauma was lower in the intervention group than in the control group although the difference was not significant.

Siegel and colleagues[42] evaluated the effects of three types of intervention; (1) early and extended hospital contact after delivery between women and their newborns; (2) home visits by paraprofessionals during the first three months after birth; and (3) both. At one year follow-up, the three intervention groups did not differ from the control group in the number of reports of abuse and neglect. The visits only continued during the first three months of the infant's life.

O'Connor and associates[43] compared the effects of extended postpartum hospital contact (rooming-in) with routine care. Although the experimental group showed a reduction in parenting inadequacy, no significant differences were found in the number of hospital admissions, injuries, emergency room visits or reports of physical abuse to child protective services. The outcome of parenting inadequacy was too broad to draw conclusions about prevention of child physical abuse.

A controlled trial without randomization and involving high-risk families evaluated contact by the project social worker after the mother's discharge from hospital and access to a drop-in centre.[44] Although the number of children seen in the emergency department was lower in the intervention group compared to the control group, there were no other differences in outcome. Since no statement was made about randomization or baseline comparison of groups prior to the intervention, no conclusions about the effectiveness of the intervention can be drawn from the trial.

Two trials evaluated the effectiveness of parent training programmes for mothers at risk of committing physical abuse.[45,46] Both studies focused on parent-child interactions; neither study evaluated reports of physical abuse or related events (such as hospital admissions). For these reasons, it was not possible to determine the effectiveness of these programmes in preventing physical abuse.

Olds and colleagues[39] also evaluated the intervention of free access to health care. This included free transportation to appointments for regular prenatal and well-child care. There was no difference between this group and the control group for any outcome. This intervention did not prevent any of the outcomes associated with child physical abuse.

A comprehensive health services programme was one type of intervention that was not included in the original review by MacMillan and colleagues because the results of this trial were published after the review was carried out.[47] Women seen for prenatal care were recruited for participation in the study and assessed for risk regarding physical abuse and neglect. Individuals considered high risk for committing physical abuse or neglect were assigned randomly to the high-risk intervention group or a control group which received standard care. Women in the high-risk intervention group received prenatal, postnatal and paediatric care at a clinic by a multidisciplinary team until their children were 2 years of age. Public agency documents were reviewed for reports of maltreatment 36 months after the birth of infants in the trial. The comprehensive care programme did not demonstrate any preventive effect for physical abuse. The investigators concluded that the intervention was not sufficiently intensive to offset adverse environmental circumstances. It is of note that the services were offered primarily in a health care facility, rather than in the home.

## Summary of programme effectiveness

In summary, the trials by Olds and associates and Hardy and Streett provide evidence that home visitation can prevent child physical abuse, or outcomes associated with maltreatment (e.g. injuries and emergency room visits) among disadvantaged families.[39,40] Both studies focused on mothers who were predominantly of low socioeconomic status and single. The evidence for intensive paediatric contact, home visitation over the short term (three months or less), early or extended postpartum hospital contact or both, use of a drop-in centre and parent training programmes remains inconclusive. Several of the studies lacked sufficient statistical power to detect a difference between the groups in the outcomes evaluated. Free access to health care did not result in any reduction in child physical abuse. One model of comprehensive health services did not prevent child physical abuse among high-risk parents.

## Home visitation programmes

The spectrum of preventive interventions for child physical abuse is extremely broad, but only home visitation has been demonstrated effective. Home visitation programmes vary in the duration of the intervention, the frequency of visitation, the curriculum and the qualifications of the intervenors. There are important similarities in the nature of the home visitation programmes evaluated by Olds et al and Hardy and Streett, which were both effective in preventing child physical abuse. In the trial by Olds and colleagues, nurses focused on three activities: (1) parental support; (2) parent education; and (3) establishment of links between family members and community services. The visits, which were 75 minutes long, occurred approximately ever two weeks during pregnancy, weekly during the six weeks after delivery and were followed by a schedule of tapering visits over the next two years.

In the second trial, visits were provided by a college-educated community woman. Visits, which lasted approximately one hour, began shortly after delivery and were scheduled every two months tapering to three months up until the infant's second birthday. The main areas of focus included: (1) parental support; (2) parental education; (3) teaching of preventive health care; and (4) reinforcement of regular clinic attendance.

In both studies, the authors stressed the need for the home visitor to establish a supportive relationship with the family before addressing the educational aspects of the programme. The visitors needed to be flexible in responding to family problems as they arose. Both programmes were aimed at families who were psychosocially disadvantaged. Olds has recommended targeting communities with high rates of poverty, and single and adolescent parenthood for such interventions.[48] One can emphasize to potential participants the benefits of such services when referring for home visitation to minimize the problems associated with mislabelling. An intervention offered to communities or groups of individuals on the basis of several needs avoids the hazards of labelling 'potential child abusers' as determined by a screening instrument.

What about the interventions that demonstrate improvement in parent-child interactions or parental knowledge of child development? Although some authors[45] view child physical abuse as one end of the continuum of parenting behaviour, one must be cautious in concluding that improved competence in parenting directly results in a reduction in child abuse. In addition, improvements observed in parent-child interactions under experimental conditions may not accurately reflect events in daily life. As Fink and McCloskey have emphasized,[49] programmes using such outcome variables as child-rearing measures must demonstrate two things to prove prevention of physical abuse: improvement in the outcome variable (e.g. dysfunctional parenting) due to the intervention and a reduction in the incidence of child physical abuse due to the improvement. Indeed, Gelles has challenged the assumption that physical violence is on a continuum from the mildest form (e.g. a slap) to the most severe forms (e.g. use of a knife). He suggests that there may be two distinct categories of violence: physical punishment and abusive violence.[32]

## FUTURE DIRECTIONS

Home visitation is the only intervention shown effective in preventing physical abuse. Other types of programmes may be effective; many simply have not undergone adequate evaluation. One approach to child abuse prevention that is currently undergoing evaluation is the community-based initiative. The central aim of a community intervention for child abuse is to build a supportive community which in turn empowers families to avoid abusive patterns of behaviour. Such programmes generally include an integrated system of services ranging from home visitors to a food bank. While such an approach to address child abuse is appealing, it is important that these initiatives undergo rigorous evaluation. Despite numerous programmes being developed throughout North America, very few have actually undergone any formal evaluation. Earls and colleagues recently reported the results of a pilot study designed to evaluate the impact of a community-based approach to preventing child maltreatment.[50] The authors advocate a system of assessing change at the neighbourhood level by collecting periodic survey data through cross-sectional sampling of neighbourhood residents.

The majority of the interventions evaluated to date have been directed toward women. Men are frequently abusive toward children, yet there is little information about strategies to prevent physically abusive behaviour by males.[51] Fathers are under-represented in the literature on prevention of child physical abuse, and this represents an important area of future investigation.

## WHAT CAN THE CLINICIAN DO?

With home visitation being the only intervention shown effective in preventing physical abuse, the clinician may be confused about his or her role with an individual patient or family. The evidence for home visitation to date is with high-risk families, yet earlier it was pointed out that screening individuals through instruments may do more harm than good. However, with a knowledge of risk indicators, the paediatrician is in a unique position to recommend home visitation for families who have these risk indicators. While there is no net benefit in screening individuals for such services, the positive aspects of the programme can be emphasized and the intervention recommended for disadvantaged parents. The clinician can encourage families to accept help through a home visitor, while reducing the potential for stigmatization.

The programmes of home visitation that were shown effective involved an intensive service extending for two years in both trials. What if a specific organized programme is not available in a community? It is risky to assume that a less intensive intervention would offer the same or even partial benefits. Nevertheless, the paediatrician is often faced with the question of how to intervene when a comprehensive service is not available. Olds and Kitzman[48] summarized the key elements in a home visitation intervention: (1) the programme should take into account multiple rather than single factors; (2) the visitor should visit often enough to establish an alliance with the families; and (3) the programme should be directed at families with psychosocial disadvantage. While more research is necessary to determine the elements of home visits which are essential to its effectiveness, the concept of providing intensive support to families in their homes by nurses or trained community workers appears effective. Several authors recommend that paediatricians and other physicians become involved in primary prevention of child abuse by increasing parents' knowledge of child development and addressing child management issues.[1] The American Medical Association Diagnostic and Treatment Guidelines on child physical abuse and neglect recommend that physicians employ strategies to improve parenting skills. Although this makes eminent sense, there is no evidence that such activities translate into reduction of child physical abuse. A paediatrician likely provides better services to a family by advocating for a home visitor that can work with a family intensively, than by direct service delivery.

## CONCLUSION

Historically, child physical abuse has been recognized as a public health problem only in recent years. While the physician's role in child physical abuse has generally been one of medical diagnosis, knowledge of prevention strategies has become an important issue in paediatric practice.

The use of screening devices for identifying caretakers at risk for committing child physical abuse is not recommended because of the high false-positive rate and the harm associated with labelling individuals as potential child abusers. Interventions can be targeted to groups of individuals or communities, while avoiding the stigma of labelling.

The spectrum of preventive interventions for child physical abuse is extremely broad, but there are few programmes that have been demonstrated effective. It appears that home visitation during the perinatal period through infancy can prevent child physical abuse for disadvantaged families. The evidence for other interventions such as intensive contact with a paediatrician, early or extended postpartum hospital contact or both, use of a drop-in centre, or parent training programmes remains inconclusive. Free access to health care was not effective in preventing physical abuse. A trial evaluating a comprehensive health care programme showed no reduction in child abuse during operation of the programme.

Future areas of research include: (1) developing interventions aimed at preventing child physical abuse by both men and women; and (2) determining those elements of a home visitation programme which are crucial for effectiveness.

## KEY POINTS FOR CLINICAL PRACTICE

- Children of all ages are at risk for physical abuse, although it is most common among those of pre-school age.
- Physicians need to be aware of risk indicators for physical abuse. These are factors associated with an increased likelihood of physical abuse, but are not necessarily causal.
- Indicators for physical abuse include: low socioeconomic status, social isolation, young maternal age, large family size, single parent family, spousal violence, parent's childhood experience of maltreatment and unplanned pregnancy or negative parental attitude toward pregnancy.
- There is no evidence that screening approaches for identifying individuals at risk for committing physical abuse do more good than harm.
- Interventions should be targeted toward groups of individuals or communities rather than labelling an individual through use of a screening interview or questionnaire.

- Home visitation is effective in preventing child physical abuse and outcomes associated with abuse while the programme is in operation.
- The characteristics of home visitation shown effective in preventing child physical abuse are as follows: (1) takes into account multiple rather than single factors; (2) the visitor visits often enough to develop an alliance with the family; and (3) the programme is directed toward families at greatest psychosocial disadvantage.
- Further research is necessary to determine which elements in a home visitation programme are essential in preventing child physical abuse.

## REFERENCES


1 American Medical Association. Diagnostic and treatment guidelines on child physical abuse and neglect. Arch Fam Med 1992; 1: 187–197

2 Reece RM, ed. Child abuse: medical diagnosis and management. Malvern: Lea and Febiger, 1994

3 Zigler E, Hall NW. Physical child abuse in America: past, present and future. In: Cicchetti D, Carlson V, eds. Child maltreatment: theory and research on the causes and consequences of child abuse and neglect. New York: Cambridge University Press, 1989: 38–75

4 Straus MA, Gelles RJ. Societal change and change in family violence from 1975 to 1985 as revealed by two national surveys. J Marriage Fam 1986; 48: 465–479

5 MacMillan HL, Fleming JE, Trocme N et al. Prevalence of child physical and sexual abuse in the community: results from the Ontario Health Supplement. Submitted

6 Malinosky–Rummell R, Hansen DJ. Long–term consequences of childhood physical abuse. Psychol Bull 1993; 114: 68–79

7 Dodge KA, Bates JE, Pettit GS. Mechanisms in the cycle of violence. Science 1990; 250: 1678–1683

8 Widom CS. The cycle of violence. Science 1989; 244: 160–166

9 Finkelhor D, Dziuba–Leatherman J. Children as victims of violence: a national survey. Pediatrics 1994; 94: 413–420

10 Boney–McCoy S, Finkelhor D. Psychosocial impact of violent victimization on a national sample of youth. Paper presented at the San Diego Conference on Responding to Child Maltreatment; January, 1994

11 Committee on Child Abuse and Neglect and Committee on Community Health Services. Investigation and review of unexpected infant and child deaths. Pediatrics 1993; 92: 734–735

12 Caplan G. Principles of preventive psychiatry. New York: Basic Books, 1964

13 Dubowitz H. Prevention of child maltreatment: what is known. Pediatrics 1989; 83: 570–577

14 Wolfe DA, Wekerle C. Treatment strategies for child physical abuse and neglect: a critical progress report. Clin Psychol Rev 1993; 13: 473–500

15 Helfer RE, Bristor M, Cullen B, Wilson A. The perinatal period, a window of opportunity for enhancing parent–infant communication: an approach to prevention. Child Abuse Negl 1987; 11: 565–579

16 Orkow B. Implementation of a family stress checklist. Child Abuse Negl 1985; 9: 405–410

17 Milner JS. Applications and limitations of the Child Abuse Potential Inventory. Early Child Dev Care 1989; 42: 85–97

18 Milner JS, Gold RG, Ayoub C, Jacewitz MM. Predictive validity of the Child Abuse Potential Inventory. J Consult Clin Psychol 1984; 52: 879–884

19 Schneider CJ. The Michigan Screening Profile of Parenting. In: Starr RH, ed. Child abuse prediction: policy implications. Cambridge: Ballinger, 1982: 157–174

20 Altemeier WA, O'Connor S, Vietze P, Sandler H, Sherrod K. Prediction of child abuse: a prospective study of feasibility. Child Abuse Negl 1984; 8: 393–400
21 Leventhal JM, Garber RB, Brady CA. Identification during the postpartum period of infants who are at high risk of child maltreatment. J Pediatr 1989; 114: 481–487
22 Daniel JH, Newberger EH, Reed RB, Kotelchuck M. Child abuse screening: implications of the limited predictive power of abuse discriminants from a controlled family study of pediatric social illness. Child Abuse Negl 1978; 2: 247–259
23 Solnit AJ. Too much reporting, too little service: roots and prevention of child abuse. In: Gerbner G, Ross CJ, Zigler E, eds. Child abuse: an agenda for action. New York: Oxford University Press, 1980: 135–146
24 Caldwell RA, Bogat GA, Davidson II WS. The assessment of child abuse potential and the prevention of child abuse and neglect: a policy analysis. Am J Community Psychol 1988; 16: 609–624
25 Kaufman J, Zigler E. The intergenerational transmission of child abuse. In: Cicchetti D, Carlson V, eds. Child maltreatment: theory and research on the causes and consequences of child abuse and neglect. New York: Cambridge University Press, 1989: 129–150
26 Steele BF, Pollock D. A psychiatric study of parents who abuse infants and small children. In: Helfer RE, Kempe CH, eds. The battered child. Chicago: University of Chicago Press, 1968: 103–148
27 Dubowitz H, Newberger E. Pediatrics and child abuse. In: Cicchetti D, Carlson V, eds. Child maltreatment: theory and research on the causes and consequences of child abuse and neglect. New York: Cambridge University Press, 1989: 76–94
28 Belsky J. Child maltreatment: an ecological integration. Am Psychologist 1980; 35: 320–335
29 Belsky J. Etiology of child maltreatment: a developmental–ecological analysis. Psychol Bull 1993; 114: 413–434
30 Department of clinical epidemiology and biostatistics, McMaster University. How to read clinical journals: IV. To determine etiology and causation. Can Med Assoc J 1981; 124: 985–990
31 Muir RC, Monaghan SM, Gilmore RJ, Clarkson JE, Crooks TJ, Egan TG. Predicting child abuse and neglect in New Zealand. Aust N Z J Psychiatry 1989; 23: 255–260
32 Wolfner GD, Gelles RJ. A profile of violence toward children: a national study. Child Abuse Negl 1993; 17: 197–212
33 MacMillan HL, MacMillan JH, Offord DR. Periodic health examination, 1993 update: 1. primary prevention of child maltreatment. Can Med Assoc J 1993; 148: 151–163
34 Trickett PK, Aber JL, Carlson V, Cicchetti D. Relationship of socioeconomic status to the etiology and developmental sequelae of physical child abuse. Dev Psychol 1991; 27: 148-158
35 Kaufman J, Zigler E. Do abused children become abusive parents? Am J Orthopsychiatr 1987; 57: 186–192
36 Leventhal JM. Risk factors for child abuse: methodologic standards in case-control studies. Pediatrics 1981; 68: 684–690
37 MacMillan HL, MacMillan JH, Offord DR, Griffith L, MacMillan A. Primary prevention of child physical abuse and neglect: a critical review. part I. J Child Psychol Psychiatr 1994; 35: 835–856
38 Gray JD, Cutler CA, Dean JG, Kempe CH. Prediction and prevention of child abuse and neglect. J Soc Issues 1979; 35: 127–139
39 Olds DL, Henderson Jr CR, Chamberlin R, Tatelbaum R. Preventing child abuse and neglect: a randomized trial of nurse home visitation. Pediatrics 1986; 78: 65–78
40 Hardy JB, Streett R. Family support and parenting education in the home: an effective extension of clinic–based preventive health care services for poor children. J Pediatr 1989; 115: 927–931
41 Olds DL, Henderson Jr CR, Kitzman H. Does prenatal and infancy nurse home visitation have enduring effects on qualities of parental caregiving and child health at 25 to 50 months of life? Pediatrics 1994; 93: 89–98
42 Siegel E, Bauman KE, Schaefer ES, Saunders MM, Ingram DD. Hospital and home support during infancy: impact on maternal attachment, child abuse and neglect, and health care utilization. Pediatrics 1980; 66: 183–190
43 O'Connor S, Vietze PM, Sherrod KB, Sandler HM, Altemeier III WA. Reduced incidence of parenting inadequacy following rooming-in. Pediatrics 1980; 66: 176–182

44 Lealman GT, Haigh D, Phillips JM, Stone J, Ord–Smith C. Prediction and prevention of child abuse – an empty hope? Lancet 1983; 1: 1423–1424
45 Wolfe DA, Edwards B, Manion I, Koverola C. Early intervention for parents at risk of child abuse and neglect: a preliminary investigation. J Consult Clin Psychol 1988; 56: 40–47
46 Resnick G. Enhancing parental competencies for high risk mothers: an evaluation of prevention effects. Child Abuse Negl 1985; 9: 479–489
47 Brayden RM, Altemeier WA, Dietrich MS et al. A prospective study of secondary prevention of child maltreatment. J Pediatr 1993; 122: 511–516
48 Olds DL, Kitzman H. Can home visitation improve the health of women and children at environmental risk? Pediatrics 1990; 86: 108–116
49 Fink A, McCloskey L. Moving child abuse and neglect prevention programs forward: improving program evaluations. Child Abuse Negl 1990; 14: 187–206
50 Earls F, McGuire J, Shay S. Evaluating a community intervention to reduce the risk of child abuse: methodological strategies in conducting neighbourhood surveys. Child Abuse Negl 1994; 18: 473–485
51 Wekerle C, Wolfe DA. Prevention of child physical abuse and neglect: promising new directions. Clin Psychol 1993; 13: 501–540

5

# Unintentional injury prevention

*E. M. L. Towner   S. N. Jarvis*

Unintentional injury in childhood is a major public health problem in all developed and an increasing number of developing countries.[1] However, despite its importance in terms of both health and socioeconomic impact, unintentional injury has, until recently, received relatively little attention at a national or international level.

In 1992 the *Health of the Nation, a strategy for health in England*, identified the reduction of 'the death rate of accidents amongst children aged under 15 by at least 33% by 2005' (baseline 1990) as one of its key targets.[2] Earlier, the Department of Transport had set targets for reductions in road traffic accident casualties in Great Britain by one third by the year 2000 (baseline average 1981-85).[3] Children were identified as a key target group and in 1990 the Department of Transport published *Children and roads: a safer way* which set out a plan of action for achieving the target reduction.

The annual NHS cost of unintentional injury to children in England and Wales has been estimated at £200 million per annum.[4] There is considerable potential for improvement. In the United States, Rivara has calculated that the introduction of twelve preventive strategies could reduce childhood injury deaths by 29%.[5] The purpose of this chapter is to examine how unintentional injury can be prevented. We consider why children are particularly vulnerable to injury, the scale of the problem, factors associated with unintentional injury and then examine different strategies in injury prevention. Finally, we look at the importance of data to stimulate action and to target interventions and consider the ways in which a paediatrician can be involved in injury prevention.

## CHILDREN'S VULNERABILITY TO UNINTENTIONAL INJURY

The type of accidents children have and where they occur reflect the child's age and stage of development and also their exposure to risk (of different hazards in different environments) at different ages.

Children are particularly vulnerable to unintentional injury because of their physical, psychological and behavioural characteristics. In terms of physical characteristics, the small stature of children can make them vulnerable to road accidents. The height of toddlers makes them hard to see as they play behind vehicles and drivers can reverse over them. A pedestrian's height can influence both the type and severity of injury. Pedestrians are mostly struck by the front of a vehicle rather than being run over: an impact that could result in an adult having a broken leg might result in a serious head or neck injury in a small child.[6] Another problem arising from a child's small stature is that the road becomes functionally wider than it is for adults. Five to six year olds take paces about half the size of adult steps and thus when they cross the road they take longer and are thus more exposed to traffic than adults.[7]

Apart from height and size, other physical characteristics of children can make them vulnerable to accidents. Children under the age of four are more likely to suffer from head injuries in falls downstairs than older children.[8] The skin of babies and toddlers burns more deeply and quickly and at lower temperatures than the thicker skin of adults.[9]

Children live in an environment designed principally for adults. Sandels, in her studies of children in traffic in Sweden, believes that it is 'impossible to adapt fully small children to the traffic environment. They are biologically incapable of managing its many demands'.[10] The complexity of the road crossing task needs to be stressed: in 1991, Rivara et al estimated that road crossing can involve up to 26 different tasks to negotiate traffic successfully.[11] Skills to perceive distance and velocity and the capacity to integrate this information are well developed in adults, but not in children. Children's judgements about the safety of gaps in traffic do not begin to approach those of adults until the age of about 11 years.[7] Skills do not develop uniformly in all children, and some children of the same age groups show greater overall performance than others.

The way in which children behave also differs markedly from that of adults and makes them more vulnerable to accidents. Wilson et al describe the play of pre-school children: 'they do not make time and space calculations before they run behind a swing or think about velocity when they get off a moving merry-go-round. They dismount from the see-saw without notice and let their companion fall'. They comment 'no amount of lecturing will produce safe play behaviour'.[6]

Play and exploration of young children within the home environment also brings them into contact with a range of different hazards. Sinnott describes children's use of the home: '(they) crawl about the floor, climb onto the window ledge, squeeze through stair balustrades, slide down the stair handrail, swing on the gate, run from room to room and ride bikes inside as well as out ... making use of their homes in ways that seem to them to be reasonable, but have not apparently been foreseen by the designer'.[12]

Older children and young adolescents range more widely than younger children and take more risks during play; for example, jumping the furthest from a swing, climbing the highest tree, etc.

## SCALE OF THE PROBLEM

In 1992, 563 children under the age of 15 in England and Wales died as a result of unintentional injury: 40% of these were children under five years,

**Table 5.1** Deaths in childhood from unintentional injury (ICD E800-E949)* in England and Wales in 1992

| | 28 days – 4 years | | 5 – 9 years | | 10 – 14 years | | 28 days – 14 years | | |
|---|---|---|---|---|---|---|---|---|---|
| | M | F | M | F | M | F | M | F | Total |
| Total (E800–E949) | 143 | 85 | 106 | 43 | 126 | 60 | 375 | 188 | 563 |
| Motor vehicle traffic accidents (E810–E819) | 34 | 22 | 63 | 22 | 81 | 45 | 178 | 89 | 267 |
| Involving collision with pedestrian (E814)† | 17 | 12 | 44 | 15 | 42 | 33 | 103 | 60 | 163 |
| Pedal cyclist involved in collision with MV (E813.6)† | 3 | 0 | 7 | 1 | 24 | 0 | 34 | 1 | 35 |
| Other transport accidents (E800–E807: E820–E848) | 0 | 0 | 3 | 2 | 2 | 5 | 7 | 7 | 14 |
| Fire and flames (E890–E899) | 33 | 21 | 13 | 10 | 1 | 4 | 47 | 35 | 82 |
| Drownings and submersion (E910) | 23 | 10 | 8 | 3 | 3 | 0 | 34 | 13 | 47 |
| Accidental falls (E880–E888) | 10 | 5 | 6 | 3 | 13 | 0 | 29 | 8 | 37 |
| Accidental mechanical suffocation (E913) | 14 | 6 | 4 | 0 | 17 | 0 | 35 | 6 | 41 |
| Inhalation and ingestion (E911 & E912) | 7 | 6 | 2 | 0 | 0 | 2 | 9 | 8 | 17 |
| Poisoning (E850–E869) | 5 | 1 | 0 | 0 | 1 | 3 | 6 | 4 | 10 |

Source OPCS (1994); 1992 Mortality Statistics, Childhood, England and Wales. London: HMSO.
*ICD Codes E800-E949 are used in this table. Injuries caused by violence and self-harm are excluded. This definition is used in the Health of the Nation Key area Handbook on accidents, Department of Health, 1993.
†Both included in motor vehicle traffic accidents.

26% were aged 5–9 years and 33% were aged 10–14 years. Boys were twice as likely to die as girls. Motor vehicle traffic accidents accounted for nearly half of the deaths, with pedestrian accidents accounting for 61% of these. The second major cause of death was fire and flames, with 15% of all unintentional injury deaths, followed by drowning, with 8% of deaths (Table 5.1).

For the period 1975–84 death rates in England and Wales showed considerable geographical and social variations: death rates were generally higher in the North and West and lower in the South and East and rates were higher in urban than in rural areas. There was more than a 5-fold difference between highest and lowest rates by districts. There was also a strong correlation with social deprivation.[13]

Over the years, injuries have been responsible for a growing proportion of all deaths in childhood and young adulthood. In the 40-year period from 1950 to 1990 in England and Wales, mortality from injuries at age 1–19 years fell by a quarter in contrast to mortality from other causes, which fell by nearly three-quarters.[14]

We now examine in more detail the patterns of mortality and morbidity from motor vehicle traffic accidents (particularly pedestrians) fire and flames and drowning.

## Motor vehicle traffic accidents

Motor vehicle traffic accidents cause half of all unintentional injury deaths in childhood. In 1992, 6249 children under the age of 15 in England and Wales

**Table 5.2** Child casualties in road accidents in England and Wales in 1992

| | 0–4 | | | 5–9 | | | 10–14 | | | Total | | |
|---|---|---|---|---|---|---|---|---|---|---|---|---|
| | M | F | Total | M | F | Total | M | F | Total | M | F | Total |
| **Pedestrian** | | | | | | | | | | | | |
| Fatal | 22 | 10 | 32 | 32 | 12 | 44 | 37 | 35 | 72 | 91 | 57 | 148 |
| Seriously injured | 425 | 216 | 641 | 1027 | 498 | 1525 | 1007 | 730 | 1737 | 2459 | 1444 | 3903 |
| Slightly injured | 1321 | 760 | 2081 | 3273 | 1709 | 4982 | 3206 | 2559 | 5765 | 7800 | 5028 | 12828 |
| Total | 1768 | 986 | 2754 | 4332 | 2219 | 6551 | 4250 | 3324 | 7574 | 10350 | 6529 | 16879 |
| **Pedal cyclist** | | | | | | | | | | | | |
| Fatal | 2 | 0 | 2 | 8 | 0 | 8 | 21 | 0 | 21 | 31 | 0 | 31 |
| Seriously injured | 21 | 0 | 21 | 240 | 32 | 272 | 532 | 109 | 641 | 793 | 141 | 934 |
| Slightly injured | 94 | 19 | 113 | 1235 | 260 | 1495 | 2972 | 696 | 3668 | 4301 | 975 | 5276 |
| Total | 117 | 19 | 136 | 1483 | 292 | 1775 | 3525 | 805 | 4330 | 5125 | 1116 | 6241 |
| **Car occupant** | | | | | | | | | | | | |
| Fatal | 10 | 7 | 17 | 9 | 4 | 13 | 5 | 10 | 15 | 24 | 21 | 45 |
| Seriously injured | 131 | 132 | 263 | 171 | 163 | 334 | 208 | 211 | 419 | 510 | 506 | 1016 |
| Slightly injured | 1523 | 1471 | 2994 | 1794 | 2014 | 3808 | 1688 | 2259 | 3947 | 5005 | 5744 | 10749 |
| Total | 1664 | 1610 | 3274 | 1974 | 2181 | 4155 | 1901 | 2480 | 4381 | 5539 | 6271 | 11810 |
| **Other vehicle* occupant** | | | | | | | | | | | | |
| Fatal | 2 | 1 | 3 | 1 | 0 | 1 | 0 | 4 | 4 | 3 | 5 | 8 |
| Seriously injured | 12 | 10 | 22 | 33 | 8 | 41 | 68 | 33 | 101 | 113 | 51 | 164 |
| Slightly injured | 196 | 182 | 378 | 200 | 201 | 401 | 415 | 378 | 793 | 811 | 761 | 1572 |
| Total | 210 | 193 | 403 | 234 | 209 | 443 | 483 | 415 | 898 | 927 | 817 | 1744 |

*Includes motorcycle, bus or coach, LGV, HGV and vehicle type unknown. Source: Mr P Wilding, Directorate of Statistics, Department of Transport.

were killed or seriously injured on the roads (Table 5.2). About one child in 15 is injured in a road accident before their sixteenth birthday.

There are great gender differences: nearly twice as many boys are killed or seriously injured in road accidents than girls. This difference is greatest for cycling, whereas for vehicle occupants the numbers are similar (Table 5.2) for both. Boys' and girls' pedestrian casualty rates rise from birth to peak at the age of 12.[15] Boys are much more at risk than girls because they tend to play more often in the street, especially between the ages of 6–10 years. After the age of 12, girl pedestrians are not much safer than boys.[15]

Child pedestrian accidents follow a different pattern from those of adults. The majority of accidents occur in built up areas (over 90%) and those involving children tend to be scattered across the road network, in contrast to those involving adults which are more clustered.[15] More road accidents occur at times coinciding with journeys to and home from school. There are also seasonal variations, with more children being injured in winter morning and evening peaks than in equivalent summer peak hours, reflecting more difficult weather and lighting conditions in the winter. Overall, however, there are 25% more child pedestrian accidents on school days in summer than in winter.[15]

There are steep social class gradients for pedestrian deaths: children in social class V are more than 4 times as likely to die than children in social class I.[16] Children from some ethnic groups may be more at risk: Lawson and Edwards found that young Asian pedestrians in Birmingham were over-represented in accidents by a factor of two, but this may be a reflection of social disadvantage: the Asian children in this example mainly lived in deprived inner city areas.[17]

When fatal casualty rates for road accidents are compared for different Organisation for Economic Cooperation and Development (OECD) countries, Great Britain's traffic safety record is one of the best, but the child pedestrian fatality rate is one of the worst and child fatality rates have been slower to decline than in comparable European countries. The reasons are not very clear, but major factors are likely to include level of urbanisation in different countries and exposure to traffic.

### Fire and flames

Fire and flames rank as the second highest cause of unintentional injury death in children under 15. In 1992, 82 children died. Children of any age may be caught in house fires, but younger children are more likely to have difficulty escaping:[18] two thirds of the deaths occur in children under 5 years. Fewer gender differences occur than for other causes of death, but there are very steep social gradients in deaths from house fires.[16] 40% of fatal house fires are due to ignition with cigarettes, but only a small fraction are associated with children's play with matches, etc. Deaths associated with ignition of clothing have fallen steeply since regulation of children's nightwear materials was introduced.[19]

### Drowning

Drowning is the third commonest cause of unintentional injury death in children. Not only is there high mortality after submersion incidents, but some children sustain severe neurological deficit.[20] Kemp and Sibert determined the pattern of drowning and near drowning of children in the UK in 1988 and 1989. In these two years, there were 306 confirmed submersion incidents; 149 died and 157 survived after a near drowning.[20] The annual incidence in England and Wales was 1.5/100 000 and mortality 0.7/100 000. This contrasts with a drowning rate of 3.1 in Honolulu, 3.2 in Georgia and 5.2 in Brisbane, where water exposure is much higher.[20]

The under 5 age group is the most vulnerable to drownings and drownings are most likely to occur in or very near the home. The young child is most at risk in the bath, garden ponds and domestic pools. As the child gets older, the area of risk moves away from the home to rivers, lakes, canals and the sea.[20] Gender differences in drowning increase with age (Table 5.1).

Most children who were drowned or nearly drowned were unsupervised at the time of the accident. High levels of supervision in public swimming pools are probably responsible for low mortality in these pools. In contrast, private pools had more deaths than public pools.

## FACTORS ASSOCIATED WITH CHILDHOOD INJURIES

Most injuries are caused by a mechanical, thermal or chemical energy impinging on the body. Energy is thus the agent which causes the disease (injury) in a susceptible host (the person).[21] Pearn stresses that accidents happen 'as a result of a chain of linked events set upon an underlying, predisposing baseline and initiated by a trigger'.[22] In childhood drownings, for example, sixteen different factors can be identified, and for every individual drowned, an average of four concurrent contributory factors are known to be present.[22]

There are a number of host factors which are related to different rates of injury, including gender, age, individual characteristics of the child, parent and family, risk taking and affluence/poverty. Boys have a higher rate of injury at all ages than girls, but the increased risk of injury in boys does not appear to be due to differences in motor skills.[23] Girls mature earlier and faster than boys, but boys at all ages are more coordinated than girls in gross motor skills, are stronger, and have faster reaction times.[23] Boys and girls behave in different ways, in where they play, in their range of behaviour, in risk taking activities. In Newcastle, the rate of A&E attendance for boys for cycling injuries is twice that of girls, but many of the differences appear to stem from different exposure rates.[24] Factors leading to increased risks for males are complex and difficult to untangle. They may include innate differences in behaviour as well as differences in exposure related to traditional male and female roles in society. The child's age is important in the type, severity and frequency of injury: this was discussed in more detail in the previous section.

A number of epidemiological studies have examined factors associated with high injury rates in childhood.[25] Behavioural factors relating to the characteristics of the child, the parent and the family have been identified. Characteristics of the child strongly associated with high injury rates include aggression, impulsivity and hyperactivity. Parental characteristics associated with a greater number of child accidents include poor maternal physical and mental health and young parental age, and family characteristics include family size, birth order, single parent families, step families and parental unemployment.

The concept of accident proneness in some individuals has some lay support, but little scientific foundation. Statistical correlation between past and future injuries are low, and the great range of potential confounding factors may account for the high injury rates in some groups.[23,26] There are some children who are repeatedly injured, but injuries are common events. Injury repetition may be due to chance alone or to the coincidence of other environmental and social factors.

Risk taking behaviour appears to play a major role in the increased rate of injuries amongst adolescence.[23] Risk taking behaviour may allow the adolescent to express a sense of control of his or her life, opposition to authority and allow adolescents to gain acceptance in a peer group.[23] Thuen et al, in Norway, found that risk seeking and a low level of safety seeking amongst adolescents were part of health compromising lifestyle, consisting of unhealthy food habits, smoking and alcohol consumption.[27]

Unintentional injury in childhood is strongly related to social and physical deprivation. The reasons for this are not clearcut and explanations can vary from a behavioural explanation at one end of the spectrum to a mainly structural or environmental explanation at the other. The behavioural argument stresses that children from deprived backgrounds take more risks, exhibit more unsafe behaviour and are less supervised than affluent children, while the environmental explanation considers the excess number of hazards in the environment that deprived children encounter. They have less access to safe play areas in gardens, are more likely to play in the streets and are exposed to more hazards within their homes because safety equipment is expensive to buy and cheaper furniture for example is more flammable.

## PREVENTIVE STRATEGIES

In 1986, a World Health Organization report commented that despite the importance of unintentional injury prevention there was a lack of evaluated studies on the effectiveness of injury prevention measures.[28] Seven years after the WHO report, a literature review published by the Health Education Authority found very little concrete evidence of effectiveness: 'unintentional childhood injury has been little researched and is the subject of only a limited number of preventive programmes'.[29] Unintentional injury cannot be regarded as one 'disease': for each injury type a number of interventions are possible. For instance, Table 5.3 shows possible countermeasures to prevent bicycle injuries. There are three main approaches to injury prevention – education,

**Table 5.3** Possible countermeasures to prevent bicycle injuries

**Changing the physical environment**
- Broad planning policies, e.g. location of schools, shopping centres
- Broad transport policies, e.g. change from private to public transport
- Engineering or traffic calming schemes (speed humps, banned right turns, etc)
- Traffic speed reduction (speed limits, speed cameras, etc)
- Separate bicycle from motor vehicles through bicycle ways, physical barriers
- Improve the riding surface

**Product design**
- Improvements in bicycle design
- Improvements in car design (to reduce impact with bicyclists, pedestrians)

**Increasing bicycle helmet use**
- Bicycle helmet legislation
- Promotion of helmet use
- Improve helmet design to enhance comfort and appeal
- Reduce price and increase availability of helmets

**Increase visibility**
- Promote wearing of reflective clothing
- Requirements for bicycle lights after dark

**Changing child and adult behaviours**
- Provision of bicycle proficiency training
- Education – discouraging stunt riding, etc
- Make drivers more aware of bicyclists
- Regular parental inspection of bicycles

Adapted from Wilson et al[6]

environmental modification and legislation. Examples of effective interventions include local traffic calming schemes, child safety restraints in cars, the prevention of falls from windows by window bars and child resistant packaging of drugs.

## Educational approaches

An example of a well designed and evaluated study employing an educational approach to injury prevention is a home safety campaign conducted in a disadvantaged community in the Riverside area of Newcastle upon Tyne.[30] This study compared the effects of a mass media campaign on its own (the BBC *Play it Safe* programme) with the mass media campaign in combination with targeted advice by health visitors during planned home visits. Only 9% of the first group of families took any action to make their home safer, compared to 60% of the second group, who received a home visit and specific advice. This group fitted fireguards and safety gates and other safety devices to make their homes safer. The authors felt that the failure of health education often reflected the inappropriateness of the educational method. Here, advice was heeded by families because it was 'specific, detailed and concrete at a pre-arranged home visit'. Local information about the availability of safety devices was an essential ingredient as well.

In the US, a small scale behavioural programme in two schools encouraging seat belt use in cars was expanded to a larger scale programme in 25 schools.[31] The project used behavioural procedures and involved rewards, modelling, prompting and feedback. Rewards, such as stickers, car bumper strips and prizes of pizza dinners were used to reinforce the messages of the programmes. Seat belt use in children rose from 18% before the programme to 60% after the programme and even when the incentives were withdrawn the compliance declined to only 49%. The authors felt that basic information and publicity was helpful, but insufficient to achieve a great impact on behaviour 'the clear and dramatic effect of rewards lent credence to the use of incentives to motivate safety behaviour'.[31]

A bicycle helmet campaign conducted in Seattle in the US included the main ingredients that characterise the most successful interventions. The campaign targeted elementary schoolchildren and their parents. It sought to overcome three obstacles to helmet use, parental awareness, the cost barrier to helmet use and peer influence not to wear helmets.[32] The campaign used a Healthy Alliance approach to employ a range of methods. Parents and children thus heard about helmets on television, radio, in newspapers, in their doctor's surgeries, at school and at youth clubs. Discount coupons reduced the price of helmets to half. The campaign resulted in an increase in helmet use from less than 5% in 1987 to 33% in 1990. Children modelled their behaviour on their parents. 95% of children riding with helmeted parents wore bicycle helmets in contrast with one third of children riding with unhelmeted parents.[23] This programme was successful because it had a single aim (increasing helmet wearing rates), a narrow target group and the educational measures used reinforced one another and it also increased the availability and reduced the cost of the safety equipment involved.

## Environmental measures

Children's accidents on urban roads differ from those of adults. Instead of occurring in clusters they are more widely spaced across the whole road network. With this pattern of accidents, single site or 'black spot' treatments are not possible and instead area wide measures have been experimentally introduced in the 1970s and 1980s in a number of countries. Packages of measures tailored to suit individual areas, to slow traffic, to redistribute traffic and to improve the safety of individual sites were introduced. These included more roundabouts, banned right turns, closure of roads, sheltered parking bays, right turn bays and central refuges in roads to reduce speeds, discourage overtaking and provide a central reservation for pedestrians. In Britain, the Urban Safety Project was evaluated by the Transport and Road Research Laboratory in five locations, Reading, Sheffield, Nelson, Bradford and Bristol.[33] Using road traffic accident (STATS 19 data) collected over a 7 year period, 5 years before and 2 years after the implementation of measures, an overall accident reduction of 13% occurred in the experimental areas compared with the control areas for all ages and all types of injury. Vulnerable road users, such as child pedestrians and cyclists, benefited from the schemes. The lessons learnt in these experimental sites have now been incorporated in a strategy for urban safety management in the UK and traffic calming and environmental measures are now widely used throughout the country.

Another example of modifying the environment relates to the fitting of window bars in the *Children can't fly* campaign to reduce deaths and injuries from window falls in New York.[34] A total of 16 000 window guards were provided to 4200 families living in high rise apartments in the City. A free protection device was provided, and in many cases fitted, where children were at risk. The authors reported a 50% decline in falls from windows in the Bronx area, 31% decrease City wide and a 35% decrease in mortality due to falls. In addition to the environmental modification in the shape of a window bar, the campaign was supported by a variety of approaches, (a mass media campaign, individual education and home inspection) and by the range of agencies involved (community organisations, schools and clinics) which reinforced the clear message of the importance of window bars to prevent falls.

## Regulation and legislation

Sinnott (1977)[12] and Gloag (1988)[35] describe a number of features of domestic architecture which have been regulated since the 1960s to enhance home safety. Measures include the prohibition of open tread stairs and the control of the opening distances of windows in high rise buildings. In 1966, handrails on stairs became compulsory and steepness of stairs limited. Architectural glass can cause lacerations in children and interior glazing in new buildings is now regulated. Direct correlation between these measures and reduction in injury rates have not been produced, but there is direct evidence of legislation relating to child resistant containers leading to a fall in poisonings in children. In 1976 in the UK, all children's aspirin and paracetamol preparations were required to have child resistant closures or dark tinted packaging. In the year following the Act, there was a highly significant fall in childhood admissions for poisoning for these preparations from 7, 000 admissions per annum to less than 2000.[36]

In Victoria, Australia, bicycle helmet legislation was passed in 1990. Before legislation, education was very important in influencing public opinion and the opinion of policy makers. A concerted 10 year campaign to increase bicycle helmet wearing preceded the legislation, which included a wide range of community and professional organisations. Over this time, there was a steady increase in wearing rates from 5–70% in primary school children and 2–20% in secondary school pupils. After legislation, these rates increased 70–90%.[37]

Education, environmental measures and legislation all have a part to play and their effect in combination is important. Health education has a wider role than one solely directed at individualised behaviour change. It can also be directed at local and national policy makers and thus underpins both environmental change and legislation.[25]

## THE IMPORTANCE OF DATA

In countries such as Sweden, Australia and the US, which have taken the lead in research and practice in injury prevention, the systematic use of population based surveillance systems appears to be the key to effective interventions. Surveillance systems can be used to target local interventions, to stimulate interest in the subject of injury prevention and to evaluate the impact of those interventions.

The Child Accident Prevention Trust has recently reviewed the data collection systems relating to childhood injury at both local and national levels in Britain and found that there is very little compatibility between existing systems.[38] For most District Health Authorities, the only accurate source of local data available are mortality data, but an average of five deaths a year cannot be used to set priorities. Instead, data on non-fatal injuries are required, but it is also important to define the severity of injury. In addition to information on injury events, some measure of exposure to injury risk is also useful.

Risk data have been collected for pre-school and 11–14 year old schoolchildren in a series of surveys in north east England.[24] These data can provide the basis for local planning. An example from the preschool survey in Newcastle can help to illustrate this. Parents of 3-year-old children were asked about whether they used different items of safety equipment. Table 5.4 shows

**Table 5.4** Study of injury risk in 3-year-old children in Newcastle upon Tyne in 1990

| | City Challenge area n = 173 | Rest of Newcastle n = 1084 |
|---|---|---|
| All 3 items used | 6% | 13% |
| 1 or 2 items used | 42% | 57% |
| None used | 51% | 30% |
| Unemployed | 56% | 23% |
| Home owners | 20% | 56% |
| First floor flat and above | 18% | 6% |

Preliminary results relating to use of home safety equipment, fireguards, safety gates and smoke detectors.

the responses of parents for the most deprived Riverside area of Newcastle, which forms part of the *City Challenge* area, compared to responses from parents of children living in the rest of the City and their use of three important items of safety equipment, fireguards, safety gates and smoke detectors. Within the *City Challenge* area, 51% of families used none of these items compared with 30% for the rest of Newcastle. Results of this survey were used in a proposal coordinated by Newcastle *Healthy City* project to seek funding for a safety equipment loan scheme and safety project workers from the *City Challenge* funding. Funding was obtained for this scheme, demonstrating the use of data in identifying locations where safety equipment was required.

## THE WAYS IN WHICH A PAEDIATRICIAN CAN BE INVOLVED IN INJURY PREVENTION

There are a number of ways in which a paediatrician can play a significant role in the prevention of childhood injuries: individualised advice and counselling, through research activities and supporting local data collection systems, through advocacy and public policy.

Paediatricians have the opportunity to discuss injury prevention with parents and help them to modify individual behaviour, for example in encouraging the use of infant car safety restraints, smoke detectors and bicycle helmets. Bass et al conducted a literature review to see whether health education through primary care based counselling was effective in preventing childhood unintentional injury and found sufficient evidence to support the American Academy of Pediatrics (AAP) to include injury prevention counselling as part of routine health surveillance.[39]

A second way in which paediatricians can enhance injury prevention activities is in research and in actively supporting the collection of local data to inform and stimulate local action. The previous section stressed the importance of data collection. Paediatricians also have a critical public policy role: 'paediatricians have been at the helm behind most legislative initiatives to reduce injury among all people'.[23] Notable examples are the introduction of child resistant containers in Britain and bicycle helmet legislation in Victoria, Australia.

Successful injury prevention involves a range of different approaches and the coming together of different individuals and agencies in a Healthy Alliance has the potential to promote the adoption of complementary approaches. An injury prevention campaign in Falköping, Sweden helps to illustrate the advantages of inter-agency working.[40] A surveillance system was used to identify the main problems in a local community and the campaign relied on a Healthy Alliance to plan and coordinate local injury prevention activities. This 'reference group' came from health, local authority, voluntary, commercial and media agencies and journalists, who helped to publicise the campaign locally. Great emphasis was placed on the education of local policy makers and health workers. In association with this campaign, home accidents in young children decreased by 27% in the intervention area compared to the control area. The paediatrician played the key role in stimulating this successful alliance.

## KEY POINTS FOR CLINICAL PRACTICE

- Unintentional injury causes nearly half of all deaths for children aged 1–14 years. It is also an important cause of morbidity and long-term disability.

- The child pedestrian death rate in the UK is one of the highest in Europe.

- Boys are more likely to die as a result of an unintentional injury than girls, at all ages and for all injury types.

- Deaths from unintentional injury have a steeper social gradient than for any other disease.

- The types of unintentional injuries that children have and where they occur reflect the child's age and stage of development and exposure to risk at different ages.

- Children's physical, psychological and behavioural characteristics make them particularly vulnerable to injury.

- Unintentional injuries can be prevented by a wide range of educational, environmental and legislative measures and combinations of these.

- Countermeasures for which there is strong evidence of effect include child resistant containers to prevent poisoning, bicycle helmets, child car safety restraints, seat belts, smoke detectors, traffic calming measures, speed reduction, window bars to prevent window falls and barriers for private swimming pools.

- There is a need for good local data to stimulate interest in the problem of injuries, to target effectively and to evaluate the impact of preventive measures.

- Paediatricians can play a significant role in the prevention of childhood injuries: through individualised advice and counselling, through research activities and supporting local data collection systems, through advocacy and public policy.

## REFERENCES

1 Manciaux M, Romer C. Accidents in childhood and adolescence. The role of research. Geneva: WHO, 1991
2 DoH (Department of Health). The health of the nation. A strategy for health in England. London: HMSO, 1992
3 DoT (Department of Transport). Road safety: the next steps. London: HMSO, 1987
4 CAPT (Child Accident Prevention Trust). The NHS and social costs of children's accidents. A pilot study. London: CAPT, 1992: 49
5 Rivara F. Traumatic deaths of children in the United States: currently available prevention strategies. Pediatrics 1985; 75: 456
6 Wilson MH, Baker SP, Tenet SP, Shock S, Gabarino. Saving children. A guide to injury prevention. Oxford: Oxford University Press, 1991
7 Thomson J. The facts about child pedestrian accidents. London: Cassell Educational, 1991
8 Joffe M, Ludwig S. Stairway injuries in children. Pediatrics 1988; 82: 457
9 Feldman K. Help needed on hot water burns. Pediatrics 1983; 71: 145
10 Sandels S. Children in traffic. (Revised edn) Surrey: Elek Books Ltd, 1975
11 Rivara F, Booth C, Bergman A, Rogers L, Weiss J. Prevention of pedestrian injuries to children: effectiveness of a school training program. Pediatrics 1991; 88: 770
12 Sinnott W. Safety aspects of domestic architecture. In: Jackson RH, ed. Children, the environment and accidents. London: Pittman Medical, 1977: 76
13 Avery J, Vaudin J, Fletcher J, Watson J. Geographical and social variations in mortality due to childhood accidents in England and Wales 1975–84. Public Health 1990; 104: 171
14 Woodroffe C, Glickman M, Barker M, Power C. Children, teenagers and health. The key data. Bucks: Open University Press, 1993
15 O'Reilly D. Child pedestrian safety in Great Britain. In: Road Safety Division Department of Transport, ed. Road accidents Great Britain 1993. The Casualty Report. London: HMSO, 1994: 33
16 OPCS (Office of Population Censuses and Surveys). Occupational Mortality: childhood supplement. London: HMSO, 1988 DS; vol 8
17 Lawson S, Edwards P. The involvement of ethnic minorities in road accidents: data from three studies of young pedestrian casualties. Traffic Engineering + Control 1991; January: 12
18 Avery J, Jackson R. Children and their accidents. London: Edward Arnold, 1993
19 McLoughlin E, Crawford J. Burns. Pediatr Clin North Am 1985; 32: 61
20 Kemp A, Sibert J. Drowning and near drowning in children in the United Kingdom: lessons for prevention. BMJ 1992; 304: 1143
21 Haddon WJ. Advances in the epidemiology of injuries as a basis for public policy (Landmarks in American Epidemiology). Public Health Reports 1980; 95: 411.

22 Pearn J. Current controversies in child accident prevention. An analysis of some areas of dispute in the prevention of child trauma. Aust N Z J Med 1985; 15: 782
23 Grossman D, Rivara F. Injury control in childhood. Pediatr Clin North Am 1992; 39: 471
24 Towner E, Jarvis S, Walsh S, Aynsley-Green A. Measuring exposure to injury risk in 11–14 year old school children. BMJ 1994; 308: 449
25 Towner E. The role of health education in childhood injury prevention. Injury Prevention 1995; 1:53
26 Langley J. The international classification of diseases codes for describing injuries and the circumstances surrounding injuries: a critical comment and suggestions for improvement. Accid Anal Prev 1982; 14: 195
27 Thuen F, Klepp K, Wold B. Risk-seeking and safety-seeking behaviors. A study of health-related behaviors among Norwegian school children. Health Education Res 1992; 7: 269
28 World Health Organization. Accidents in children and young people. Geneva: WHO, 1986 World Health Statistics Quarterly; vol 39
29 Towner E, Dowswell T, Jarvis S. Reducing childhood accidents. The effectiveness of health promotion interventions: a literature review. London: HEA, 1993
30 Colver A, Hutchinson P, Judson E. Promoting children's home safety. BMJ 1982; 285: 1177
31 Roberts M, Fanurik D, Wilson D. A community program to reward children's use of seat belts. Am J Community Psychol 1988; 16: 395
32 Bergman A, Rivara F, Richards D, Rogers L. The Seattle children's bicycle helmet campaign. Am J Dis Child 1990; 144: 727
33 Mackie A, Ward H, Walker R. Urban safety project. 3. Overall evaluation of area wide schemes. Crowthorne: Transport and Road Research Laboratory, 1990 TRRL DoT, ed. Research Report RR 263
34 Spiegel C, Lindaman F. Children can't fly: a program to prevent childhood morbidity and mortality from window falls. Am J Public Health 1977; 67: 1143
35 Gloag D. Strategies for accident prevention: a review of the present position. In: Dept Health & Social Security, ed. Strategies for accident prevention: A colloquium. London: HMSO, 1988: 65
36 Sibert J, Craft A, Jackson R. Child-resistant packaging and accidental child poisoning. Lancet 1977; August 6: 289
37 Vulcan A, Cameron M, Watson W. Mandatory bicycle helmet use: experience in Victoria, Australia. World J Surg 1992; 16: 389
38 Benson A. The collection and dissemination of accident data. In: CAPT and Faculty of Public Health Medicine, 1993
39 Bass J, Christoffel K, Widome M et al. Childhood injury prevention counseling in primary care settings: a critical review of the literature. Pediatrics 1993; 92: 544
40 Schelp L. The role of organizations in community participation – prevention of accidental injuries in a rural Swedish municipality. Soc Sci Med 1988; 26: 1087

6

# Television violence and its effects on children's behaviour

*M. M. Davies*

Television's effects on children's behaviour may result in them being brought to a doctor with a variety of presenting problems – although, according to a 1994 report produced by Young Minds (The National Association for Child and Family Mental Health), much mental ill-health in children goes undiagnosed.[1] The report cites a 1993 Mental Health Foundation finding that GPs identify mental health problems in only one child in 50, when it is known to be present in up to one child in four attending GPs' surgeries. Examples of children's mental ill-health cited in the report include emotional and conduct disorders, eating disorders, suicide, crime (offenders under 21 commit 45% of all known crimes), drug use and depression. Much of this is associated with family discord and economic hardship and with other sorts of ill health, including chronic illness.

Nevertheless, exposure to mass media in a variety of forms may also be an implicating factor in disturbed behaviour in children. The most frequently canvassed area of concern has been the effect of film and television violence. In the words of a recent *Lancet* editorial: 'After forty years of research and an international bibliography of over 3000 studies, reviews, commentaries and meta-analyses, it is clear that television violence can lead to harmful aggressive behaviour'.[2] In Britain, this concern was recently focused by a particularly horrific case: the murder of 2-year-old James Bulger in 1993, by two 10-year-old boys. The judge at their trial suggested that they had been influenced by a video of the horror film, *Childsplay 3* (although no evidence was presented in court that they had been). This suggestion was sufficient to initiate a long-running public debate about the harmful effects of the media, with provisions limiting the availability of violent videos being incorporated into the 1994 Criminal Justice and Public Order Act.

The proposed link between media and delinquency is not a new one. As the *Lancet* points out, it has been discussed and researched extensively since television became a universally available medium in the USA in the 1950s. Reviews of this vast research literature can be found in Friedrich-Cofer & Huston (1986)[3] and Wood et al (1991).[4] Although television, in particular, has been seen as almost uniquely problematic in generating disturbance in children, partly because of its universal accessibility, and partly because of its apparent realism, there is historical evidence that all media which represent human behaviour, from epic poetry, through theatre, the novel and cinema to, currently, computer games, have aroused passionate public concern about the potentially harmful effects of displaying 'bad examples' to the young.[5] Television is not the only medium to have an effect on legislation; in the mid-1950s US psychiatrist, Frederic Wertham, published a book based on case studies of children who had been psychologically damaged and influenced to commit criminal acts by reading horror comics, which led to these comics being banned in the UK.[6]

This generalised cultural concern, often involving intense academic and political arguments among broadcasters, scholars, legislators, and public campaigners, has not generally involved clinicians, although Young Minds, formed in 1994, has the backing of professional associations for psychiatrists and clinical psychologists. Thus, clinicians confronted with disturbed or violently aggressive children, may not always be aware of possible media influences. In the case of such disturbed children, there is evidence from a number of studies to suggest that media consumption, as well as other factors, should be investigated.

## MEDIA CONSUMPTION

Children in the UK watch around 21 hours of television a week, and audience ratings produced by the British Audience Research Board (BARB) show that, as a group, their favourite viewing consists of soap operas such as *East Enders* and *Neighbours*, and situation comedies. They have their own programmes in the afternoon on both BBC1 and ITV, which are also popular; these are carefully vetted and regulated for suitability of content.[7] British broadcasting has for many years operated a 'watershed' policy of not showing adult material, such as explicit sex, and graphic violence, until after 9 pm when young children are assumed to be in bed. Thus, there is evidence that children in Britain have not been routinely exposed to a great deal of media violence – unlike the situation in the US, referred to in the *Lancet.*

However, a number of recent developments are causing this situation to change. The deregulation of British broadcasting in 1990, and the increase in the number of channels available to viewers, with the consequent pressure to find audiences by whatever means are commercially profitable, has led to greater availability of what could be unsuitable material for children on the airwaves all round the clock. Similarly, the increased popularity of the videorecorder in the last decade, with around 70% of all households owning one,[8] means that films given adult ratings can be viewed by children in the home. Research has suggested that as many as 40% of children under 12 claim to have seen adult films classified as 'video nasties'.[9] Even though research based on self-report by children is not always reliable, [10] it seems likely that many young children are exposed to televised or video material which is not intended for them, and which may contain scenes of adult behaviour, particularly violence, including sexual violence, which could influence their behaviour and/or cause them distress.

There are a number of areas of clinical concern in evaluating the potential impact of this material on young children. This paper will review three of them: first, the impact of violent and horrific representations on aggressive behaviour; second, the impact of such representations on fear behaviour; third, factors which can mitigate harmful impacts. It goes without saying that the first questions arising from any exposure of a young child to disturbing TV or film material, should be to the parents or guardians: how was it possible that the child had access to upsetting, adult-rated material? And what sort of supervision arrangements are being made to protect him or her from repeating the damaging experience (and maybe other damaging experiences, if the child is regularly left alone)? A further relevant question is about the parents' own viewing habits. Social modelling is one of the main mechanisms proposed by researchers in television's influence on children (e.g. Bandura[11]). If modelling (or imitation) is accepted as a cause of children's behaviour, then imitation of parents is likely to be just as powerful an influence as the influence of the media. If parents regularly watch and enjoy violent and horrific entertainment, it is likely that their children will want to watch it too. Peer group pressure is another source of such influence.

## DEFINITIONS OF VIOLENCE

Before outlining examples of effects of television on children's behaviour, it is helpful to define what is generally meant by screen violence in the research literature. The most widely used definition is that of George Gerbner and his colleagues at the Annenberg School for Communication, University of Pennsylvania, who have been monitoring the content of American prime-time television, and children's programming since 1967; their Cultural Indicators programme involves regular sampling of TV channels, in which content analysis procedures are used to determine the number of violent incidents that occur every hour.

The Cultural Indicators definition of a violent incident is 'the overt expression of physical force, (with or without a weapon), against self or other... being hurt or killed or actually hurting or killing'. Such events include violent accidents, or natural catastrophes, used intentionally for dramatic purposes.[12] Gerbner's definition makes no distinction between different kinds of dramatic genre, or artistic quality, and it does not include news. The definition of extreme horror films – or 'video nasties' – adopted in a UK study by Barlow and Hill[13] is any films that 'contain scenes of such violence and sadism involving either human beings or animals that they would not be granted a certificate by the British Board of Film Censors for general release for public exhibition in Britain'. A list of such films is kept by the Director of Public Prosecutions. Incidents in such films quoted by Barlow & Hill include dismemberment, cannibalism, violent rape, castration, stabbings, and humans and animals being drilled with an electric drill. These are unlikely to be seen on broadcast TV, but may be seen in videos.

There are problems in defining screen violence in such a precise way as to produce agreement between teams of content analysts, looking for high inter-coder reliability correlations; such scientific precision can leave out wider cultural considerations. American culture generally exalts violence in its national myths about war and the conquest of the frontier, and in actual military activity and expenditure. Television violence is a reflection of this, and as such, reinforces values already present in the culture. However, there is evidence from a Canadian study carried out by Tannis Macbeth Williams[14] that television viewing, when introduced into a community that did not have it before, was associated with increased levels of aggression in children's playground behaviour. Thus, even if the culture already provides influences towards aggression, Williams' study has provided evidence that the impact of television can exacerbate them.

## RESEARCH EVIDENCE

Most of the evidence about the impact of aggression comes, not in the form of clinical studies, but from studies on samples drawn from the general population: these include experimental laboratory studies; observational studies in naturalistic settings such as schools and playgrounds; and longitudinal surveys and interviews, measuring children's media tastes and aggressive behaviour over time, and looking at the correlations between them. These studies do not concern themselves with children who have actually come before the courts, or into pyschiatric care, because of their aggression – although in some cases, e.g. Belson,[15] boys who demonstrated delinquent behaviour happened to be included in the sample.

Nevertheless, there is anecdotal evidence of individual cases in which aggressive behaviour appears to be linked with TV or film viewing. Wilson[16] cites incidents in Cardiff in which three youths were convicted of kicking a man to death after seeing the video *Juice*. American examples include the reported impact of *Natural Born Killers* in 1994, which was supposed to have influenced copycat murders in both the US and France, and a widely reported case in the USA in 1993 involved a 5-year-old who burned down the family home, killing his younger sister, supposedly as a result of seeing two cartoon characters, Beavis and Butthead, playing with fire. (In this case, the children had been left unsupervised, and later evidence suggested that the home – a caravan trailer – did not have cable television, so the child was unlikely to have seen the programme. As with the Bulger case, and others, there are problems with identifying all the background information in such cases; exposure to violent videos is a comparatively easy influence to spotlight.)

A further caveat about academic studies on the impact of media violence, is that many of them, such as Belson's study, were carried out on boys only – and demonstrations of effects also tend to be confined to boys. Girls in general neither share boys' tastes for violent television programmes, nor do they display the same levels of aggression in their behaviour. Hence, it is important to recognise that the debate about the effects of television violence on children, is primarily a debate about the effects of television violence on boys.

## Laboratory studies of imitation/modelling

The most widely cited experimental evidence on the effects of screen violence are still the studies of Albert Bandura and colleagues in America in the 1960s.[17] Bandura showed young children a film of adults hitting a 'bobo' doll (a doll that bounces back after being hit) and then gave them the opportunity to play with toys which included such a doll. Compared to control groups who saw the same adult behaving non-violently, or who saw no film at all, the children who saw the aggressive film were significantly more likely to hit the doll, just as the adult had done. In subsequent experiments, this behaviour became even more likely when children saw the aggressor being rewarded for his aggression. Similar studies were carried out by Leonard Berkowitz with American college students – again, primarily male. In this case students were given the opportunity to 'get even' with somebody who had annoyed them (an experimental 'stooge') by giving the stooges bogus electric shocks. Students who had seen an aggressive film about boxing were more likely to display increased aggression towards their 'victims' than were controls.[18]

Laboratory studies have been criticised for their artificiality, and these kinds of experiments are now rarely carried out by media researchers. Nevertheless, the social learning model of TV effects underpinning experimental studies – that children automatically imitate what they have seen – continues to be a powerful one in public debate about the effects of screen violence. Imitation – as evidenced by the anecdotal evidence outlined above – is still seen as the primary mechanism of influence, and a major cause of concern, whereas, as described below, there is evidence to suggest that effects on children's fears and anxieties might be a greater cause of concern.

## Observational studies

Observation of children's normal play behaviour can be a more reliable measure of their tendencies towards aggression, or otherwise, than experimentally-engineered tasks. Jerome and Dorothy Singer[19] carried out a two-year study of pre-school children during which their behaviour in their nursery school was measured at four points in time. Measures of television viewing, including viewing of aggressive action-adventure drama, were correlated with measures of aggression towards other children and towards toys, as the children played in the nursery. The Singers were interested in the 'direction of effect' – that is the question of whether children who are already aggressive are drawn to violent television, or whether television leads to aggressive behaviour. They found that children with higher measures of aggression at the beginning of the study did not significantly increase their aggression at the end of it, despite watching action-adventure programmes. However, children with lower measures of aggression who also watched action-adventure programmes, did increase their level of aggressive play over the two years. The differences found were small – and aggression was not life-threatening, but within the bounds of rough play, for instance, knocking over other children's bricks. Again, although there was an effect in both boys and girls, the effect was smaller in girls, except at one out of the four measurement points.[19]

One of the most interesting aspects of the Singers' study was their observations of family backgrounds. From interviews with parents in the home, they were able to identify four different groups of children, associated with different styles of child-rearing. High levels of aggression were observed in both high-TV viewing and low-TV viewing families. Aggression was most likely to be associated with parental disorganisation and indiscipline, and lack of direction towards other activities for their children. The Singers' analysis of family child-rearing styles emphasised the interaction of factors such as discipline and domestic organisation with television-viewing, in producing different outcomes in children. Television-viewing could not be seen as an influence in isolation.

## Longitudinal studies

Longitudinal studies avoid the criticism directed against experiments – that they only produce a short-term effect, in an artificial setting, and thus cannot 'prove' anything about how children would normally behave at home, over extended periods of time. The most thorough and widely cited of Longitudinal studies in this field was carried out by Leonard Eron and his associates in the 1970s and 1980s on elementary schoolchildren in upstate New York.[20–22] Because of the difficulties and expense of carrying out studies on large populations of children over extended periods of time, the literature on television violence still relies on these earlier studies in a way that would perhaps not be acceptable in other scientific fields. There is also the problem of cultural differences with these studies. Nearly all the research on screen violence has been carried out in the US, which has been prepared to devote the necessary massive financial resources to the field – more research funding than on all other areas of communication research combined according to Cumberbatch.[10] Hence, British researchers have to rely on data produced in the very different cultural environment of the USA, where, for instance, the right to bear arms is vocally defended and handguns are freely available. One exception to this rule is the study carried out in London by William Belson – which was, however, partially funded by American money. Belson's study demonstrated an association between preferences for violent television and aggressive and delinquent behaviour in adolescent boys over a period of time. Again, Belson did not study girls[15].

In the Eron et al study, boys rated as aggressive by parents, peers and themselves, at the age of eight were more likely to be aggressive in their behaviour at the age of 18 if they had persistently displayed a taste for violent television programming. (This relationship was not found for girls.) The later follow up, reported in 1984, indicated a significant correlation between the seriousness of crimes for which the male subjects were convicted by the age of 30, and their aggression ratings, and taste for violent programmes at the age of eight. These researchers have also proposed that the extent to which children *identify* with the characters committing aggressive acts on television, can increase the likelihood of imitation – although not all researchers accept this (e.g. Cook et al, 1983[23]).

Many of the objections to the research findings in this field, as in this case, come from re-analysis of the statistical correlations, which, even where they are significant, tend to be weak.[24] This is one reason why it has proved so difficult for the debate about the effects of television violence to be brought to any convincing conclusions. It continues to the present day – a recent example being the Young Minds campaign (1994), organised by a group of mental health professionals, which included a season of films and a panel at the National Film Theatre, exploring the topic once again, and calling for greater awareness among clinicians and policy makers about the possible effects of screen violence on the young.

## Fear, distress and disturbance

The definition of screen violence produced by Gerbner and his associates is the one most widely used in studies about the impact of violence on the young. However, the sorts of dramatised violence seen in, for instance, television police series, are rather different from the kinds of supernatural fantasy violence found in the horror film genre – this kind of violence is often blatantly impossible, and there is evidence that the less realistic violent representations are, the less their effect.[25] Discussion of the effects of screen violence and horror has not always made a distinction between different kinds of material or genres. Concern about television violence focuses, as has been said, on modelling – the danger of children imitating aggressive behaviour. The impact of horror and fantasy violence is more likely to be related to fear.

A report in the *British Medical Journal*[26] describes two cases of 10-year-old boys who were referred (separately) by their respective GPs to the child psychiatry unit at Gulson Hospital, Coventry, UK. Simons and Silveira propose that the children were suffering from recognisable symptoms of post-traumatic stress disorder: amnesia, psychic numbing, intrusive flashbacks, panic attacks, sleeplessness and school refusal. The symptoms appear to have arisen from seeing the horror film *Ghostwatch* on television on Hallowe'en, 1992. In both cases, the fear symptoms began directly after viewing this film. They persisted for the four months between the viewing of the film, and the boys first being seen in the psychiatric unit.

The first child was described as 'a sensitive child and a worrier'. His parents had separated when he was 4 years old. The treatment in his case was a behavioural programme – keeping a diary of flashbacks; help for the mother in 'regaining control in their relationship' and encouragement not to discuss ghosts and their terrors. The boy was discharged after eight weeks, 'happier and confident and free of symptoms'.

The second child – also described as 'a worrier' – began to feel sick immediately after watching *Ghostwatch*, and became excessively clingy, refusing to sleep without his parents' reassurance. A behavioural programme reassuring him and encouraging him to sleep in his own room resulted in improvement after only three weeks. Again, discussion of the film was vetoed as part of the treatment. Simons and Silveira argue for behavioural and cognitive strategies specifically addressing the children's preoccupations and anxieties in cases such as these. They point out that post-traumatic stress disorder due to watching TV has not been reported previously.

## DEVELOPMENTAL FACTORS

Nevertheless, there is a growing research literature which examines children's fears at watching violent and horrific television and film representations, in contrast to earlier preoccupations with imitations of aggression, as cited above. This literature helps to shed light on some of the mechanisms whereby children can be affected by media representations. Cantor, [27] has carried out a number of studies at the University of Wisconsin, Madison, addressing the questions: 'what types of mass media stimuli and events frighten children the most, and what are the best methods of preventing or reducing children's media-induced fears?' (p 140). She argues that developmental considerations are central: 'we have found that a child's age is a major determinant of the things that will be frightening and the techniques that will be most effective in counteracting emotional disturbances' (p 140).

Cantor proposes that, as a function of cognitive development, younger children respond to 'perceptible' aspects of stimuli and older children respond more to 'conceptual' aspects. For example, Sparks and Cantor (1986) carried out a study examining children's fear responses to the TV show, *The Incredible Hulk*, in which a mild-looking young man is regularly transformed into a monstrous-looking, green-coloured giant; the research found that pre-school children experienced most fear at the actual transformation. Older children in elementary school reported the *least* fear at this time, because they knew that the Hulk's transformation meant he was going to rescue some innocent victim, and to restore moral order.

In another study of children's responses to a realistic drama, *The Day After*, which showed the aftermath of a nuclear attack, in a recognisable setting (Kansas), Cantor et al predicted that, contrary to public concern, the youngest children would be least affected by the drama, whereas older children would be very disturbed by it.[28] This prediction was borne out. Cantor argues that the impact of the film on teenagers came from their ability to comprehend 'the potential annihilation of the earth, a concept that is beyond the grasp of the young child' (p 143). Cantor's general point is that most children over the age of 9 or 10 will not be lastingly frightened by blatantly fantastic material, as often appears in horror movies, whereas younger children are, because of the concrete 'perceptible' salience of the physical representation. Nevertheless, case studies such as those of Simon and Silveira indicate that, where there are other predisposing factors, such as an anxious personality, or family disruption, frightening events on screen may trouble older children too.

In the studies cited by Cantor, realistic material – which may seem innocuous to an adult and meaningless to a pre-schooler – can disturb older elementary (junior) school children. Cantor cites *The Little House on the Prairie* as an example; this series, which idealises the rugged life of the American prairie homesteaders in the 19th century, routinely deals with upsetting themes such as child molestation, kidnapping and accidental death, and as such generated distress in child viewers. None of the subjects in these studies reported by Cantor were clinical cases; some children were disturbed, but not pathologically so. Nevertheless, developmental considerations are clearly generally important in evaluating the impact of media material on children, and in deciding what is, or what is not, appropriate viewing for different age groups. Advice on this can be given to parents at clinics and in the course of developmental check-ups, and in parentcraft classes.

## HORROR AS THERAPY

Derdeyn and Turley describe a case study of a 13-year-old boy who was admitted to a psychiatric unit after a drunken outburst in which he destroyed the home of the guardians with whom he was living (his childless uncle and aunt) with an axe.[29] The boy, Carl, had been abandoned by his mother – who had a psychiatric history of her own – at the age of nine. At first he seemed to thrive in the stricter discipline of his uncle's home. Then – as the authors suggest, with the onset of puberty, (another example of a developmental factor) – Carl's behaviour became more disturbed. Previously a good and well-behaved student, he became involved in theft, truancy, alcohol abuse and the company of 'unsuitable' friends. During therapy, it emerged that a particular source of resentment in Carl was his uncle and aunt's refusal to let him indulge his passion – almost an 'addiction' – for watching horror movies.

The therapist used one of Carl's favourite horror films, *A Nightmare on Elm Street*, as a way of exploring Carl's own anger at being abandoned by his mother (the monster/hero of the Nightmare series, Freddy Kreuger, had also been abandoned by his mother). According to Derdeyn and Turley, the films enabled Carl to discover his general feelings of anger at adults who do not protect their children properly, such as the parents whose children are attacked by Freddy in the films. Carl admired 'the guys who make these stories up' and the therapist suggested that he make up his own film in which his uncle was Freddy and Carl the heroic teenager who destroys him. The therapeutic programme used the themes of the films to help Carl and his guardians recognise the sources of the conflict between them. After several family sessions, the patient was discharged to the care of his guardians and was 'free of symptoms and functioning well' at six month follow-up. He no longer felt compelled to watch horror movies, although he still enjoyed them. Derdeyn and Turley invoke Bettleheim's[30] psychoanalytic account of the 'uses of enchantment' in fairy tales as means to help children to 'manage the fears and anxieties they experience' in their 'developmental tasks'. Theirs is a psychodynamic approach, although it has some similarities to the behavioural programme reported by Simons and Silveira, and appears to have had a similar outcome.

## Mitigating factors

In evaluating the impact of televised anti-social behaviour on children, it is important to recognise the complexity of the interacting factors which can be operating. Personality needs to be taken into account, as in the case studies of fear reactions described above; there is some evidence that children with generous, altruistic personalities can use anti-social examples to strengthen these attitudes.[31] Noble found that 'unselfish' children liked villains such as J.R. Ewing because they enjoyed disapproving of them. As already mentioned, gender is a powerful predictor of the likelihood of aggressive behaviour, with femaleness being the greatest protector against anti-social activity. Boys are much more at risk of turning into violent delinquents than are girls, and this holds true of television influences, as for other areas of activity. The Singers' study demonstrates the importance of family child-rearing styles in the study of children's behaviour and television viewing.

A number of experimental studies have also been carried out which demonstrate that children can learn examples of good behaviour from television modelling, e.g. Stein and Bryen,[32] Wolfe and Cheyne.[33] In these studies, children (again mostly boys) who had seen televised examples of good behaviour, such as keeping to the rules of a game, or obeying adult injunctions not to touch toys, were more likely than control groups to behave with similar self-control. Other studies, e.g. Durkin,[34] have demonstrated that pre-school children can be taught to have more liberal and open-minded attitudes from watching counter-stereotypical programmes which show women working at 'men's' jobs and men looking after home and family. These experimental studies suffer from the same objections to their short-term impact as do the studies on violence. Nevertheless, where there is a sustained portrayal of positive attitudes towards other races, or to disabled people, given to children over time, as in the case of the pre-school programme, *Sesame Street*, improvements in children's tolerance towards others can be demonstrated.[35] Pro-social, educational television, allied with 'media literacy' programmes in school, teaching children about the differences between reality and fantasy and how they are portrayed on television (the ability to 'read' television and film appropriately is another protective factor[36]) are seen by many researchers and educators as a more constructive way of helping children come to terms with media violence than futile campaigning for stricter censorship laws. Limiting freedom of speech, and the free market in media products, particularly in the US, is unlikely to meet with much success. A review of research on positive and educational effects of television viewing is found in Davis (1989).[37]

## KEY POINTS

- Media violence may be implicated in some behavioural problems seen by doctors.
- Regular exposure to violent and aggressive television programming is associated with aggressive behaviour over time, and into adulthood, especially in boys.
- Exposure to horrific film and video material may result in excessive fear reactions, which can be classified as the Post Traumatic Stress Syndrome.
- The impact of particular graphic horrific scenes can vary with personality factors, for instance, horror films may be used therapeutically in appropriate cases.
- Aggressive behaviour, television viewing, and the relationship between them are mitigated by parental child-rearing styles. Large amounts of TV viewing, including aggressive material, are less likely to have harmful effects on children with orderly, secure, affectionate family backgrounds, which provide other sorts of leisure activity as well as TV.
- Television can be used pro-socially to help children learn good behaviour and positive attitudes.
- There are very large gender differences, with most of the studies and demonstrated harmful effects coming from boys, not girls.
- Most of the studies have been done in the US and allowances need to be made for different cultural values, and for the wider values of the culture as a whole, in evaluating the contribution of televised violence. For instance, as I write today, the newspapers are full of accounts of the racist violence of English football fans, which led to a soccer match between England and the Republic of Ireland being stopped. Such behaviour seems to be peculiar to England, and unknown in US sports grounds. It does not appear to have its antecedents in television or film.
- Exposure to harmful and frightening scenes on film and television is a function of parental supervision, which is an important protective factor in all areas of child health and behaviour.

REFERENCES


1 Violence and young minds: screen violence and child mental health. Report by Young Minds, the National Association for Child and Family Mental Health. London: 1994
2 Editorial. Reel violence. Lancet 1994; 343: 8890
3 Friedrich-Cofer L, Huston AC. Television violence and aggression: the debate continues. Psychol Bull; 100: 364-371
4 Wood W, Wong F, Chachere J. Effects of media violence on viewers' aggression in unconstrained social interactions. Psychol Bull; 109: 371-383
5 Starker S. Evil influences. New Jersey: Transaction, 1991
6 Wertham F. The Seduction of the Innocents. 1954
7 Home A. Into the box of delights: a history of children's television. London: BBC, 1993
8 Barwise P, Ehrenberg A. Television and its audience. London: Sage, 1992
9 Nelson GK. The findings of the national viewers' survey [on exposure to video nasties]. In: Barlow G, Hill A. eds. Video violence and children. London: Hodder and Stoughton, 1985
10 Cumberbatch G, Howitt D. A measure of uncertainty: the effects of the mass media. London: John Libbey, 1989
11 Bandura A. Aggression: a social learning analysis. Englewood Cliffs, NJ: Prentice Hall, 1973
12 Gerbner G, Gross L, Morgan M, Signorielli N. Living with television: the dynamics of the cultivation process. In: Bryant J, Zillman D. eds. Perspectives on media effects. Hillsdale NJ: Lawrence Erlbaum, 1986
13 Barlow G, Hill A. eds. Video violence and children. London: Hodder & Stoughton, 1985
14 Williams TM. ed. The impact of television: a national experiment in three communities. New York: Academic Press, 1986
15 Belson W. Television violence and the adolescent boy. Farnborough: Saxon House, 1976
16 Wilson P. Violence and young minds: screen violence and child mental health. Report by Young Minds. London, December 1994
17 Bandura A, Ross D, Ross SA. Imitation of film-mediated aggressive models. J Abnormal Social Psychol 1963; 66: 3-11
18 Berkowitz L. Some aspects of observed aggression. J Personal Social Psychol 1965; 2: 359-369
19 Singer J, Singer DG. Television, imagination and aggression: a study of pre-schoolers. Hillsdale, NJ: Lawrence Erlbaum, 1981
20 Eron LD, Walder LO, Lefkowitz MM. Learning of aggression in children. Boston MA: Little Brown, 1971
21 Lefkowitz MM, Eron LD, Walder LO, Huesmann LR. Growing up to be violent. New York: Pergamon, 1977
22 Huesmann LR, Eron LD, Lefkowitz MM, Walder LO. Stability of aggression over time and generations. Dev Psychol 1984; 20: 1120-1134
23 Cook TD, Kendzierski DA, Thomas SV. The implicit assumptions of television research: an analysis of the 1982 NIMH Report on Television and Behavior. Public Opin Q 1983; 47: 161-201
24 Wober M, Gunter B. Television and social control. Aldershot: Gower, 1988
25 Gunter B, Wakshlag J. TV viewing and perceptions of crime among London residents. Paper to International Television Studies Conference, London: 1986
26 Simons D, Silveira WR. Post-traumatic stress disorder in children after television programmes. BMJ 1994; 308: 389-390
27 Cantor J. Confronting children's fright responses to mass media. In: Zillman D, Bryant J, Huston AC. eds. Media, children and the family: social scientific, psychodynamic and clinical perspectives. Hillsdale, NJ: Lawrence Erlbaum, 1994
28 Cantor J, Wilson BJ, Hoffner C. Emotional responses to a televised nuclear holocaust film. Commun Res 1986; 13: 257-277
29 Derdeyn AP, Turley JM. Television, films and the emotional life of children. In: Zillman D, Bryant J, Huston AC. eds. Media, children and the family: social scientific, psychodynamic and clinical perspectives. Hillsdale, NJ: Lawrence Erlbaum, 1994
30 Bettelheim B, The uses of enchantment: the meaning and importance of fairy tales. New York: Random House, 1975
31 Noble G. Social learning from everyday television. In: Howe MJA. ed. Learning from television: psychological and educational research. London: Academic Press, 1981

32 Stein G, Bryen JH. The effect of a television model upon role adaptation behaviour of children. Child Dev 1972; 43: 2061-2065
33 Wolfe TM, Cheyne JA. Persistence of effects of live behavioural, televised behavioural and live verbal models on resistance to deviation. Child Dev 1972; 43: 1429-1436
34 Durkin K. Television, sex roles and children. Milton Keynes: Open University Press, 1985
35 Lovelace V, Scheiner S, Dollberg S, Segui I, Black T. Making a neighborhood the *Sesame Street* way: developing a methodology to evaluate children's understanding of race. J Ed Television 1994; 20: 69-77
36 Brown J. Television 'critical viewing skills' education. Hillsdale, NJ. Lawrence Erlbaum, 1991
37 Davies MM. Television is good for your kids. London: Hilary Shipman, 1989

# 7

# Advanced practice nurses in neonatal intensive care

*J. Pinelli B. Paes*

The demand for highly specialized care givers in neonatal intensive care units (NICU) has created opportunities for expanding the traditional role of registered nurses. Reductions in the numbers of physicians-in-training and paediatric specialists/consultants are creating a need for alternative care providers in a clinical area with increasing acuity and technological complexity.

## PHILOSOPHY OF THE NEONATAL NURSE PRACTITIONER ROLE

The role of the neonatal nurse practitioner (NNP) developed in the US in the early 1970s because of a number of demands and changes in the delivery of neonatal intensive care.[1] This development has also been influenced by changes in medical education and practice.[2] Infant survival and parent satisfaction with the quality of care their infants' receive is in part dependent on consistent evidence-based practice standards delivered by health professionals. These goals are becoming more difficult to achieve with recent medical trends. There is an increasing emphasis on paediatric residency programmes to broaden their educational objectives, to encompass greater ambulatory care experiences, while ensuring training opportunities for research and scholarship. The ability of physicians-in-training to develop advanced technical skills is limited due to brief experiences in neonatal critical care. The level of commitment and interest in neonatology by physicians-in-training is variable unless residents plan to pursue this area as a subspecialty.[1] Moreover, the rotation of physicians on a monthly or bi-monthly basis may interrupt the continuity of care, especially for infants with chronic diseases. Reliance on physicians-in-training to provide all of the day-to-day care in a NICU on a 24 hour basis is no longer a viable option in many programmes.

Registered nurses who wish to advance their knowledge and skills in clinical care are seeking new challenges and opportunities to expand their level of practice. Over the years, many nurses became frustrated with their traditional roles in neonatal intensive care units, assuming additional responsibilities for which they were not theoretically or technically prepared. These 'unofficial' roles were not recognized outside of the institution in which the nurses practised so that there was little organized support for such roles.[2] Concomitantly with the development of expanded nursing roles in neonatal critical care came the development of educational programmes to prepare nurses to function in these roles. Post-basic specialty education was believed to be necessary in order to positively influence the role of a NNP. The form that this education should take, however, remains controversial.

A number of authors have described the role of NNPs, and the formal education and training that these nurses received in the past.[1–5] The education of NNPs was initially offered within the hospital setting.[5] This educational preparation was in keeping with the preparation of nurse practitioners in other specialties, including primary care.[6] The reason for this type of training resulted from three factors: the urgent need for practitioners; lack of funding for educational programmes; and lack of support for the role within the university setting. Faculties of nursing were not convinced that the nurse practitioner (NP) role was an appropriate one for nurses to assume.[6] Over time, hospital-based continuing education or certificate programmes have been replaced with university-based or master's degree programmes.[5] Professional organizations in the US support the movement of increased educational preparation for the NP and graduate preparation in nursing as the entry-level requirement.[7–9] However, lack of funding, lack of qualified NNP graduate-level faculty and lack of geographically available programmes in the face of an increasing demand for NNPs has hampered the movement toward establishing a standard of graduate education.[10]

In addition to the controversy related to educational preparation, the definition and titling of the neonatal practitioner remains an issue. The two predominant titles in the US are neonatal nurse practitioner (NNP) and neonatal nurse clinician (NNC).[5] In Canada, the title clinical nurse specialist/neonatal practitioner (CNS/NP) has been adopted.[11] Other titles used are neonatal critical-care nurse practitioner (NCCNP) and neonatal clinical specialist (NCS).[5] Despite the variability in title, many of the skills, tasks and general role function are similar. Some of the titling difficulties arise from the variation in educational preparation. The title of clinical nurse specialist (CNS) has traditionally been associated with graduate level preparation while the titles of nurse practitioner and nurse clinician have been associated with certificate preparation. Generally, the CNS has been associated with secondary and tertiary level care and the NP with primary care. A number of studies have demonstrated the increasing similarity in the function and attributes among CNSs and NPs, as well as in the curricula which prepare them.[11–22] The National Association of Neonatal Nurses has recommended that the term neonatal nurse clinician be eliminated and that, presently, both CNS and NP be used to delineate advanced practice nurses in neonatology.[8]

## ROLE OF THE CLINICAL NURSE SPECIALIST/NEONATAL PRACTITIONER

With respect to the specific role functions of the advanced practice or expanded role nurse in neonatology, the NNP and CNS/NP provide tertiary care for neonates in ICUs and stabilize sick neonates being transferred to referral centres.[5,11] NNPs are also used in community hospitals to attend deliveries or examine newborns in normal nurseries. They provide follow-up care for high-risk infants and consult with multidisciplinary health care professionals offering services to this population.[5]

To limit the view of the NNP or CNS/NP to a 'physician replacement' will result in a number of negative consequences. Firstly, the preparation of a graduate-prepared neonatal practitioner includes more than the knowledge and skills needed to provide physical or emergency care to the ill neonate. Graduate level NNPs bring to their role a wealth of knowledge and experience related to infants' responses to illness and treatment, parental responses and needs, and the growth and development of premature and term neonates. They also receive preparation in critical appraisal and basic research methodology which allows them to incorporate appropriate research findings in clinical decision-making and participate on project teams. Graduate level NNPs can be active participants in clinical teaching for all disciplines and an invaluable resource to the hospital staff. Their participation on research teams, presentations at conferences, and publications in refereed journals make them much more than replacements for physicians-in-training. The competence of NNPs in the medical management of ill neonates make them an excellent alternative care-provider but their nursing experience, knowledge and skills make them invaluable members of health care teams whose foci are on provision of high quality care, as well as on education and research.

## INTRODUCTION AND ESTABLISHMENT OF THE ROLE

In 1985, a multidisciplinary research team at McMaster University in Hamilton, Ontario, Canada adapted Spitzer's[23] strategy of evaluation to introduce advanced practice nurses into neonatal intensive care units. The first phase involved a determination of the needs of medical staff in NICU settings. In the next phase, the role of the practitioner was defined, the educational level of preparation determined and the educational programme was developed. The third phase of this research involved an evaluation of the educational programme in terms of knowledge, problem-solving, communication and clinical skills. A controlled trial was recently conducted to evaluate the role in terms of safety, efficacy, quality of care, parent satisfaction and costs. Lastly, the job satisfaction of CNS/NPs; and their impact on the job satisfaction, autonomy and quality of work-life of other health care team members was investigated. The results of this research programme is presented in subsequent sections.

## ASSESSMENT OF NICU STAFF

The determination of the adequacy of medical staffing in neonatal ICUs was the first step in the introduction of advanced practice nurses in neonatology in Ontario, Canada.[24] A survey of medical directors, head nurses and staff physicians in nine tertiary level NICUs and the directors of five postgraduate paediatric residency programs was conducted in July, 1985. The ideal neonatologist:patient staffing ratio of 1:6 was based on current recommended guidelines assuming the availability of adequate support from allied health care professionals.[25] Factors affecting the supply of medical personnel in these NICUs were: time spent by neonatologists, neonatology trainees and paediatric residents in direct patient care, education, research and administration; staffing ratios per work shift; and the number of neonatology trainees graduating in practice in Canada. Factors affecting the demand on medical personnel in NICUs were: admission to the NICU by birth weight; length of stay in NICU by birth weight (patient-days); ventilator patient-days; rates of transfer out of the NICU; and occupancy rates. These data provided a measure of changes in acuity, patient population and workload. Results of this survey indicated that most of the NICUs were understaffed. This problem would be exacerbated by continuing reductions of paediatric residency positions and restrictions on immigration of foreign medical trainees.

The heavy workload reported in the results of this survey was believed to compromise the structured educational objectives of paediatric residents, as mandated by the Royal College of Physicians and Surgeons of Canada, and to affect the desirability of this subspecialty for medical graduates because of negative lifestyle implications. The increase in proportion of critically ill to convalescent infants in the NICU has also contributed to the increased workload and stress level of presently employed physicians. The authors of the survey concluded that the main requirement to improve the under-staffing was for bedside care-givers. They recommended replacement of 'resident-dependent activity with resident-independent service'.[24] Exploration of acceptable alternative personnel was the basis of the next phase of the research programme. It was recognized that caregivers selected for this role should have specific assets. These assets would include a dedicated commitment to neonatology, advanced critical thinking, problem-solving and communication skills, technical expertise necessary in the management of critically ill newborns and familiarity with the psychosocial dimensions of intensive care. The research team felt that there should be a pool of caregivers to choose from and once functional, these personnel would not constitute an economic burden to the health care system. The role of both 'complement' and 'substitute' personnel was entertained and critically reviewed with regard to availability, acceptability, feasibility and cost effectiveness. The CNS/NP was felt to best meet the requirements for the new role.

## DEFINITION OF THE ROLE AND EDUCATIONAL PROGRAMME

The focus of the second survey was to determine the perception of need for an expanded role nurse in the NICU, the role definition, and level of knowledge and skill required for competent function in the role.[11] Self-administered questionnaires were mailed to medical directors, head nurses, directors of nursing, staff registered nurses and staff physicians in all tertiary level Ontario NICUs. Data were also obtained from certified NNP/NNCs in the US ($n$ = 189) and in one Canadian province ($n$ = 22), from medical directors ($n$ = 50) and head nurses ($n$ = 50) in the US who employ NNP/NNCs.

The survey results indicated that the role of the advanced practice neonatal nurse should include clinical, educational, research and administrative responsibilities; with the majority of time devoted to clinical practice (70-75%). The role was consistent with a graduate level preparation of advanced practice nurses. The authors describe the details of the activities within each of the four subroles.[11]

The clinical practice of the CNS/NP is viewed as collaborative and 'is based on a strong team philosophy with the belief that an emphasis on demarcation of what is nursing and what is medicine in a critical care area only serves to fragment care and accentuate territoriality'.[11] The unique contributions from team members are based on their respective backgrounds, but there is considerable overlap of knowledge and skills among these professionals. This overlap is depicted in Figure 7.1, which has been adapted from the authors' previous work.[11] The clinical role of the CNS/NP involves assessment, diagnosis, planning, intervention and evaluation of care. The preparation for and focus of the role of the CNS/NP produces a 'hybrid' nursing professional which blends the medical and nursing aspects of care into a distinctive whole.

The educational activities include sharing responsibility for teaching rounds and conferences, and participating in the clinical education of students from

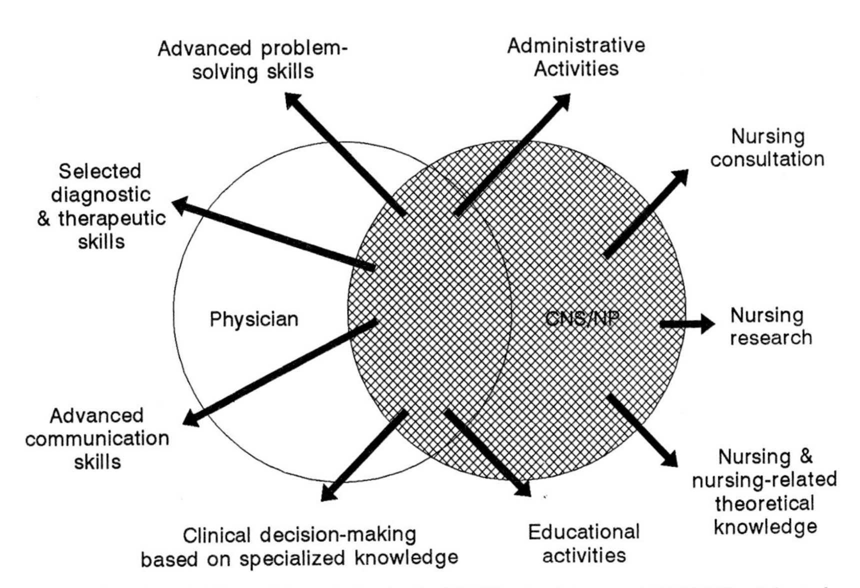


**Fig. 7.1** Overlap of skills and knowledge in the NICU: physicians and CNS/NPs. Adapted with permission from Hunsberger et al.[11]

various disciplines. Research activities include evidence-based practice, identification of relevant research questions, and participation on projects as principal and co-investigators. Administrative responsibilities include participation on selected NICU, hospital and community committees; developing and revising policies, procedures and protocols in collaboration with physicians and other health care professionals; and participating in quality care reviews.[11]

An educational programme to prepare nurses to function in this role did not exist in Canada at the time of the survey. A programme was developed by three members of the research team: a CNS, a neonatologist and a nurse educator, all of whom held faculty appointments. The programme was designed using a problem-based learning format and self-directed learning style which are consistent with the approaches used at McMaster University Faculty of Health Sciences. The details of the educational programme are described elsewhere,[26] but include general graduate level courses as well as specialty specific content. The specialty specific content includes pathophysiology, pharmacology, and neonatology courses. In addition, procedural skills are taught and practised using simulated infant and animal models. The programme, which is 16 months in length, encompasses over 700 hours of supervised clinical practice. Supervision is provided jointly by neonatologists and advanced practice nurses. This educational stream is part of the graduate health sciences programme at McMaster University and produces approximately four advanced practice neonatal nurses each year. Applicants must have a baccalaureate degree in nursing and two years of tertiary level neonatal experience in order to be considered for admission to the programme.

## EVALUATION OF THE ROLE

In order to evaluate the graduates of the new programme, a prospective cohort study was conducted which compared all of the NNP graduates from the first three years of the programme ($n$ = 10) and 13 (87%) second-year paediatric residents.[27] One hundred multiple-choice questions and 20 radiographic slides were used to test knowledge; a semi-structured oral examination tested problem-solving skills; three simulated interactions with parents appraised communication skills and seven simulated procedures evaluated clinical skills. Graduating NNPs scored similarly to the paediatric residents on all assessed outcomes. The authors concluded that this equivalency would likely enable the NNPs to deliver comparable care in the clinical setting.[27] Graduating NNPs were also compared on all outcomes, except clinical skills, to first year NNP students.[26] The results demonstrated a statistically significant difference, favouring the graduating NNPs, on all outcomes except communication skills. It was concluded that the educational programme was successful in preparing experienced neonatal nurses to become advanced practice nurses.[26]

Because of the paucity of rigorous studies which evaluate the efficacy of NNPs, a controlled trial was conducted as part of the research programme at McMaster.[28] All infants admitted to the NICU at McMaster over a 1-year period were randomized to care by a Clinical Nurse Specialist/Neonatal Practitioner team or a paediatric resident team. Outcome measures included: mortality, morbidity, quality of care, parent satisfaction with care, long-term outcomes and patient care costs. Results indicated that the two teams were comparable with respect to all measures of performance. The quality of care, as measured by indicator conditions, were comparable in all instances except for the evaluation of jaundice and clinical documentation, both of which favoured the CNS/NPs. Another outcome of interest was the amount of time spent with each team by the attending neonatologist. The time was significantly lower with the CNS/NP group. The authors concluded that CNS/NPs provide care which is comparable to current practice standards and, therefore, can be used on a more widespread basis.[28]

The research involving the CNS/NP would not be complete without a measure of satisfaction with the role by health professionals who work directly with CNS/NPs and by the CNS/NPs themselves. CNS/NPs have been surveyed each year since the programme began with respect to their satisfaction with the role. They have consistently reported a high level of satisfaction and a number of positive aspects of the role.[29] Positive aspects of the role include: increased autonomy, diversity of job function, access to knowledge, caring for infants from admission to discharge, challenging clinical experiences, being able to support and educate staff nurses, working with CNS/NP colleagues, acceptance as valued members of a multidisciplinary health care team, having flexibility in work-patterns through self-scheduling and involvement in non-clinical activities. Negative aspects of the role included insufficient financial compensation, being overworked, the political struggle between nursing and medicine, a heavy clinical component which leaves little time for research and educational activities and working independently in centres without CNS/NP colleagues.

The impact of the NP role on staff nurse quality of work-life in a neonatal intensive care unit was demonstrated in the recent study by Mitchell et al.[29] 85% of the staff nurses who were surveyed reported that the CNS/NP increased their level of job satisfaction. Staff nurses reported that they felt comfortable working with the CNS/NPs; were confident in their abilities; that the CNS/NPs consulted and shared information with them and were readily available. CNS/NPs give nursing a higher level of respect than other health professionals, challenge nurses, communicate effectively and give positive feedback. The survey indicated that the CNS/NPs included the staff nurses in patient care decision-making to a greater degree than with medical staff and treated them as equal partners.[29]

There is no doubt that the role of the CNS/NP is a powerful influence on staff nurses in terms of education, professionalism and clinical leadership. As the numbers of CNS/NPs increase on a particular unit, the potential extent of this influence becomes even more impressive. The positive influence on staff nurses' job satisfaction, autonomy and quality of life will likely, in turn, influence retention. As clinical role models, the CNS/NPs may also influence the career paths of staff nurses who wish to remain involved in direct patient care.

In addition to nursing staff, the impact study by Mitchell and colleagues included medical staff residents, and allied health professionals.[29] The medical staff and residents reported a number of positive influences with respect to the CNS/NP role. They indicated that the care provided by CNS/NPs was competent, efficient, reliable and consistent. Their own role as medical staff was enhanced because the presence of CNS/NPs allowed them to ideally focus on education, research and more global issues in patient care rather than providing direct care, without compromising the quality of care. The CNS/NPs are valued by medical staff because they provide a service which the physicians perceive as equivalent to senior residents, who are in short supply and in the long-term, may be more cost effective to the health care system. The medical staff also recognize the differences between the CNS/NPs and residents which is reflected in their desire to maintain a mixture of the two groups within the NICU. The residents and the CNS/NPs provide the medical staff with opportunities to meet their professional and educational needs which the medical staff report as important to their job satisfaction.

The CNS/NPs are perceived by residents as facilitating their education directly and decreasing their workload, allowing more time for educational activities. A negative impact on the resident education is the decreased opportunities for practical experiences, such as technical procedures. 80% of the residents who were surveyed, however, reported that the CNS/NPs make a positive difference to the satisfaction with their role.[29]

The survey did reveal an overall negative impact with one group of health professionals in the NICU, that is the respiratory therapists (RTs). Respiratory therapists are graduates of accredited programs with a licence to practise in accordance with designated standards. They are available on a 24-hour basis to neonatal intensive care units in Canada and the US and are responsible for the provision of oxygen and ventilator therapy, cardiorespiratory monitoring and the assessment and treatment of cardio-respiratory and associate disorders. They trouble-shoot acute ventilator problems as they arise and liaise with health care professionals offering advice on ventilation strategies for complicated respiratory disorders. Respiratory therapists in some centres are now qualified to assume total ventilator care for all neonates admitted to NICU's including intubation, ordering of blood gases and adjustments of ventilation based on results obtained. More senior staff hold geographic full time appointments with academic, administrative and research responsibilities. They, therefore, are not ideal candidates for global patient care but rather offer a very select service in the management of the newborn. RTs view the CNS/NPs as encroaching on their area of expertise. They indicated through the survey that a physician should be in charge of the patient, and that the CNS/NPs and RTs could do certain aspects of care, mainly procedural. The respiratory therapy approach to care is based on the traditional model which fragments total care into components, whereas, the CNS/NP role is founded on continuous holistic care. It is not surprising, therefore, that the CNS/NPs are perceived as negatively influencing the job satisfaction of RTs. The RTs expertise is limited to respiratory disease and therapy, whereas the CNS/NPs expertise includes a wide variety of body system pathology and therapeutic strategies/interventions, as well as knowledge of growth and development. An important implication of these findings is to ensure that the role of the CNS/NP is communicated to all health professionals with whom they work. Any misunderstanding of the CNS educational preparation and role definition, as well as the overall philosophy of the approach to patient care in an area, may lead to dissatisfaction, and could negatively influence the overall impact of the CNS/NP role.[29]

The positive impact of CNS/NPs has been demonstrated with respect to direct patient/family care, through the increased profile of the nursing profession in the provision of health care and by the influence on the role satisfaction of the majority of health professionals with whom CNS/NPs work. As more of these advanced practice nurses are utilized in the provision of care in a variety of health care settings, the power of this role will be more fully realized.

## KEY POINTS FOR CLINICAL PRACTICE

- The demand for highly specialized care givers in neonatal intensive care units has created opportunities for expanding the traditional role of registered nurses.

- Reductions in the numbers of physicians and recent medical educational trends make reliance on physicians to provide all of the day-to-day care in a neonatal intensive care unit on a 24-hour basis a less viable option.

- Viewing the role of the neonatal nurse practitioner or clinical nurse specialist/neonatal practitioner solely as a 'physician replacement' results in under-utilization of the knowledge and skills that these practitioners possess.

- In 1985, a multidisciplinary research team at McMaster University in Hamilton, Ontario, Canada adapted Spitzer's strategy of evaluation to introduce advanced practice nurses into neonatal intensive care units in Ontario.

- A needs survey determined that there was a lack of bedside medical care-givers in neonatal intensive care units in Ontario and that clinical nurse specialists/neonatal practitioners would best meet the requirements of an alternative care-provider.

- A second survey determined that the role of the clinical nurse specialist/neonatal practitioner should include clinical, educational, research and administrative responsibilities; with the majority of time devoted to clinical practice (70-75%). The preparation for and focus of this role produces a 'hybrid' nursing professional which blends the medical and nursing aspects of care into a distinctive whole.

- Although controversy exists over the appropriate level of education for neonatal nurse practitioners, the trend is toward graduate preparation. An educational programme to prepare clinical nurse specialists/neonatal practitioners did not exist in Canada at the time of the survey so one was developed at McMaster University in 1986. The programme includes general graduate level courses as well as specialty specific content; that is, pathophysiology, pharmacology and neonatal courses.

- A prospective cohort study was conducted which compared all of the neonatal nurse practitioner graduates from the first 3 years of this programme and second-year paediatric residents. Graduating neonatal nurse practitioners scored similarly to the residents on knowledge, problem-solving, communication and clinical skills.

- A controlled trial comparing care given by a clinical nurse specialist/neonatal practitioner team and a paediatric resident team resulted in no significant differences on a number of outcomes; including mortality, morbidity, quality of care, parent satisfaction with care, long-term outcomes and patient care costs.

- A positive impact of clinical nurse specialists/neonatal practitioners has been demonstrated with respect to direct patient/family care, through the increased profile of the nursing profession in the provision of health care and by the influence on the role satisfaction of the majority of health professionals with whom clinical nurse specialists/neonatal practitioners work.

REFERENCES

1 Barnett SI, Sellers P. Neonatal critical care nurse practitioner: a new role in neonatology. MCN Am J Matern Child Nurs 1979; 4: 279-286
2 Bellig L. The expanded nursing role in the neonatal intensive care unit. Clin Perinatol 1980; 7: 159-171
3 Harper RG, Little GA, Sia CG. The scope of nursing practice in level III neonatal intensive care units. Pediatrics 1982; 70: 875-878
4 Barton L. Neonatal nurse clinician: a qualitative evaluation of an expanded nursing role. Neonatal Netw 1983; 2: 23-35
5 Zukowski K, Coburn CE. Neonatal nurse practitioners: who are they? J Obstet Gynecol Neonatal Nurs 20: 128-132

6 Bullough B. Alternative models for specialty nursing practice. Nurs Health Care 1992; 13: 254-259
7 American Nurses' Association. A social policy statement. (Publ. No. NP-68A). Kansas City, MO: American Nurses' Association, 1980: 23
8 National Association of Neonatal Nurses. Press release. Advanced Practice Role Definition. Petaluma, CA: National Association of Neonatal Nurses, 1989: 1-2
9 Price M, Martin A, Newberry Y, Zimmer P, Brykczynski K, Warren B. Developing national guidelines for nurse practitioner education: An overview of the product and the process. J Nurs Educ 1992; 31: 10-15
10 Erdmann T, Lynam L, DeArmond D, Robertson D, Trotter C. More on NNPs. Neonatal Intensive Care 1992; 5: 8-9
11 Hunsberger M, Mitchell A, Blatz S et al. Definition of an advanced nursing practice role in the NICU: the clinical nurse specialist/neonatal practitioner. Clin Nurs Spec 1992; 6: 91-96
12 Lynaugh J, Gerrity P, Hagopian G. Patterns of practice: master's prepared nurse practitioners. J Nurs Educ 1985; 24: 291-295
13 Riegel B, Murrell T. Clinical nurse specialist in collaborative practice. Clin Nurs Spec 1987; 1: 63-69
14 Kitzman H. The CNS and the nurse practitioner. In: Hamric A, Spross J, eds. The clinical nurse specialist in theory and practice. Toronto, ON: WB Saunders. 1989
15 Elder R, Bullough B. Nurse practitioners and clinical nurse specialists: are the roles merging? Clin Nurs Spec 1990; 4: 78-84
16 Forbes K, Rafson J, Spross J, Kozlowski D. The clinical nurse specialist and nurse practitioner: core curriculum survey results. Clin Nurs Spec 1990; 4: 63-66
17 Gleeson R, McIlvain-Simpson G, Boos M et al. A model of collaborative care. MCN Am J Matern Child Nurs 1990; 15: 9-12
18 Hanson C, Martin L. The nurse practitioner and clinical nurse specialist: should the roles be merged? J Am Acad Nurse Pract 1990; 2: 2-9
19 Schroer K. Case management: clinical nurse specialist and nurse practitioner, converging roles. Clin Nurs Spec 1991; 5: 189-194
20 Patterson C, Haddad B. The advanced nurse practitioner: common attributes. Can J Nurs Adm 1992; 5: 18-22
21 Fenton M, Brykczysnki K. Qualitative distinctions and similarities in the practice of clinical nurse specialists and nurse practitioners. J Prof Nurs 1993; 9: 313-326
22 Keane A, Richmond T. Tertiary nurse practitioners. Image 1993; 25: 281-284
23 Spitzer WO. Evidence that justifies the introduction of new health professionals. In: Slayton P, Trebilcock MJ, eds. The professions and public policy. Toronto, ON: University of Toronto Press, 1978
24 Paes B, Mitchell A, Hunsberger M et al. Medical staffing in Ontario neonatal intensive care units. Can Med Assoc J 1989; 140: 1321-1326
25 American Academy of Pediatrics, Committee on Fetus and Newborn, Committee of the Section on Perinatal Pediatrics. Estimates of need and recommendations for personnel in neonatal pediatrics. Pediatrics 1980; 65: 850-853
26 Mitchell A, Watts J, Whyte R et al. Evaluation of an educational program to prepare neonatal nurse practitioners. J Nurs Educ 1993; In press
27 Mitchell A, Watts J, Whyte R et al. Evaluation of graduating neonatal nurse practitioners. Pediatrics 1991; 88: 789-794
28 Mitchell A, Guyatt G, Marrin M et al. A controlled trial of nurse practitioners in neonatal intensive care. Pediatrics 1994; in press
29 Mitchell A, Pinelli J, Southwell D. Introduction and evaluation of an advanced nursing practice role in neonatal intensive care. Series on Nurs Adm 1995; 4-8: In press

# 8

# Pathophysiology of respiratory distress syndrome

*H. M. Berger  R. M. W. Moison  D. van Zoeren-Grobben*

Respiratory distress syndrome is a major cause of morbidity and mortality in newborn babies. The pathogenesis, clinical picture and treatment have recently been reviewed in detail.[1–3] Although it predominantly occurs in preterm babies, the disease can manifest in term babies and we will use the phrase neonatal respiratory distress syndrome (NRDS). The pathophysiology of adult respiratory distress syndrome (ARDS)[4] was recently compared with NRDS[5] and will only be alluded to.

The phrase NRDS triggers thoughts of surfactant deficiency but other factors are also involved because of the 'global immaturity'.[1] Pulmonary oedema is a major second factor[3] and problems such as pulmonary hypertension[3, 6] and ventilatory pump failure[7] also contribute. Reactive oxygen species (ROS, including free radicals, such as superoxide [$^{\cdot}O_2^-$], nitric oxide [$^{\cdot}NO$] and hydroxyl radical [$^{\cdot}OH$] which have an unpaired electron in their outer orbit, as well as metabolites, such as hydrogen peroxide [$H_2O_2$], hypochlorous acid [HOCl] and peroxynitrite [ONOO-] can influence these problems and is an interlinking factor.[5, 8] NRDS has physiological (decreased pulmonary compliance), clinical (grunting), radiological (reticulogranular appearance), and biochemical (decreased $PaO_2$ and increased $PaCO_2$) hallmarks.[1] This review will be based on the hypoxaemia and hypercapnia: simple input/output and flow models[5, 9] will be used to analyse the underlying pathophysiological mechanisms (Fig. 8.1).

Normal $PaO_2$ and $PaCO_2$ levels are maintained by balancing their inputs and outputs to and from the plasma, and thus abnormal values can be analysed as disturbances along these pathways. A low $PaO_2$ may be caused by decreased input (ventilation/diffusion/perfusion problems) or excess output (consumption due to an increased metabolic rate), and a raised $PaCO_2$ by an increased input (increased production) or decreased output (perfusion/-diffusion/ventilation problems). The dominant mechanism in respiratory distress is, of course, the disturbed pulmonary gas exchange (decreased $O_2$

Abbreviations: NRDS, neonatal respiratory distress syndrome; ARDS, adult respiratory distress syndrome; ROS, reactive oxygen species; SP, surfactant proteins; TNF, tumour necrosis factor; ANF, atrial natriuretic factor; PDA, patent ductus arteriosus; PPHN, persistent pulmonary hypertension of the newborn; GSH, glutathione; TRAP, total peroxyl radical trapping capacity; PUFA, polyunsaturated fatty acids; FRC, functional residual capacity.

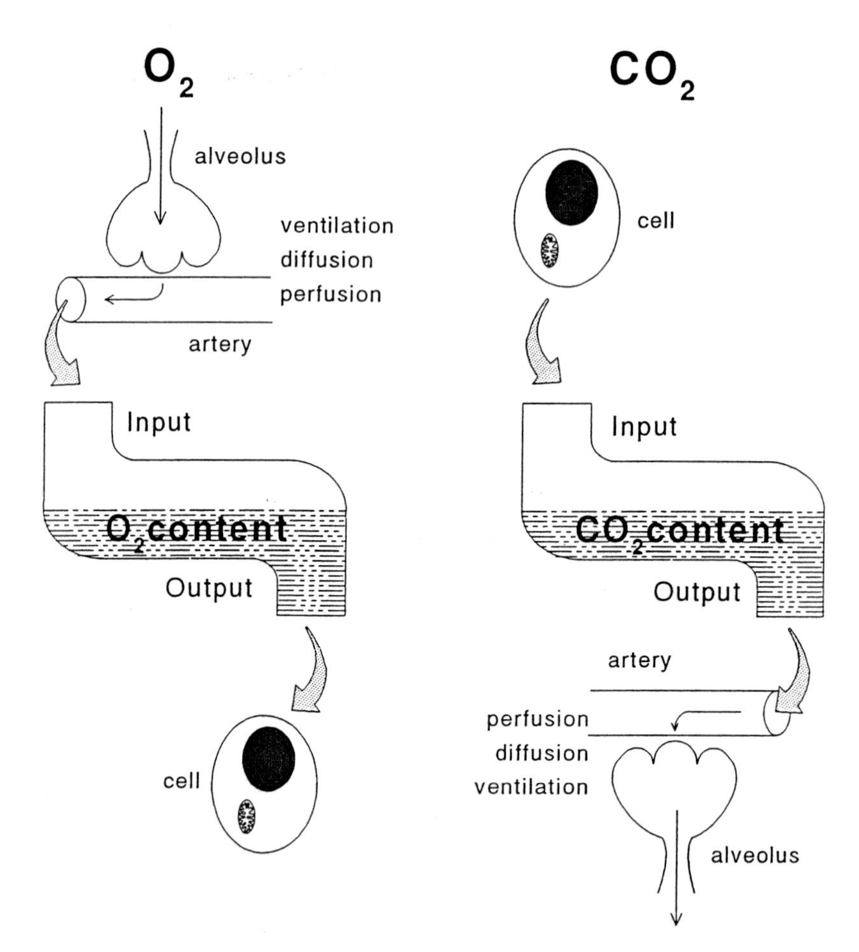


**Fig 8.1** Schematic presentation of how the $O_2$ and $CO_2$ levels in arterial blood are influenced by their respective inputs and outputs.

input and decreased $CO_2$ output). Normal pulmonary gas exchange depends on adequate and matched flows of ambient air (pulmonary ventilation) and blood (pulmonary perfusion) to the alveoli and adequate diffusion across the alveolar capillary membrane.[10,11] Air and blood flow depend on the pressure gradient and resistance (Poiseuille's law: flow is proportional to [pressure x radius$^4$]/[viscosity x length]). Viscosity (in blood), length, and especially the radius of vessels and airways determine resistance to flow. The factors influencing gas diffusion are surface area and thickness of the alveolar capillary membrane, and the diffusion constant and partial pressure gradient of the gas (Fick's law: diffusion rate is proportional to [area x gas diffusion constant x partial pressure]/[thickness]). The diffusion constant of $CO_2$, related to its solubility, is much greater (23x) than $O_2$ and its diffusion is rarely impeded.

In the following section, the factors influencing ventilation, diffusion, and perfusion will be discussed.

## DISTURBANCE OF VENTILATION

In NRDS, inadequate ventilatory pressure and/or increased resistance to air flow could affect gas transport into and out of the lung.

### Ventilatory pressure

Adequate ventilation requires coordinated stimulation of the diaphragm and intercostal muscles by the respiratory centre. Preterm babies with NRDS may be unable to sustain these tasks.[7] Although immaturity of neurological control by the respiratory centre plays a role, muscle dysfunction due to immaturity, fatigue, e.g. due to acidosis, [1,7] or ROS damage[12] are more important factors. Increased oxygen consumption by stressed muscles increases ROS levels and impairs muscle function.[12] Deficient antioxidant defences may magnify this problem in immature babies.[5]

### Airway resistance

Reduced air flow due to bronchiolar obstruction[13] has not been considered a problem in NRDS. However, it may sometimes play a role. Surfactant deficiency makes airway mucus more rigid and this impairs ciliary transport and may produce obstruction.[14] Furthermore, interstitial emphysema, usually due to use of excessive ventilatory pressure, may compress terminal bronchioles.[13] A nasogastric tube for feeding or air removal will increase upper airway resistance.[15]

## DISTURBANCE OF DIFFUSION

Normally the large alveolar capillary surface area allows $CO_2$ and $O_2$ (mixed venous levels) in the blood perfusing the alveolar capillaries to rapidly equilibrate with the gases in the alveoli. Therefore, the alveolar-systemic arterial difference in $PO_2$ and $PCO_2$ is small. Alveolar development, e.g. number and septation, is a prolonged antenatal and postnatal process and structural immaturity can limit diffusion.[1] However, atelectasis, which decreases surface area, and pulmonary oedema, which increases membrane thickness, are the main factors limiting diffusion in NRDS.[3]

### Atelectasis of alveoli

This occurs when the expanding force in the alveolar space (air pressure) is less than the retractile (i.e. surface tension and elastic fibres) and compressing (e.g. intrabdominal gas) forces in the lung. Mucus obstruction[14] may decrease air input and thus air pressure but increased surface tension is the main cause of the atelectasis, i.e. surfactant deficiency decreases lung compliance.

*Intra-alveolar surfactant pool in normal subjects* (Fig. 8.2)

According to Laplace's law (pressure is proportional to tension/radius: unlike the tension in elastic material, e.g. a balloon, which increases when stretched, the tension in air fluid surface remains constant – thus the formula shows that the pressure required to keep an alveolus open increases as its radius decreases), the smaller the radius of an alveolus the greater the pressure needed to keep it expanded. However surfactant, in the alveolar space, reduces the pressure required as the radius decreases because the molecules resist compression, i.e. they lower surface tension. Type II pneumocytes synthesize surfactant,[16] a lipid-protein complex of phospholipids such as phosphatidylcholine, phosphatidylinositol, phosphatidylglycerol and specific surfactant proteins (SP-A, -B, -C and -D). Synthesis, which requires nutrients such as fatty acids and inositol, is stimulated by cortisol and thyroxine and inhibited by insulin and testosterone. Phosphatidylcholine is the major component and contains mainly palmitic acid and smaller amounts of unsaturated fatty acids. Phosphatidylglycerol gradually replaces phosphatidylinositol as the foetus matures.

Intracellular surfactant, condensed into lamellar bodies, is released[16] into the alveolar space where it unravels into tubular myelin structures which, aided by SP-B and SP-C, spread and adsorb into the phospholipid monolayer of the air-liquid interface. The baby's adrenaline surge, induced by birth stress, triggers the release of surfactant by pneumocytes II, whose β-adrenergic receptor development is induced by cortisol. The surfactant constantly recycles, with SP-A aiding uptake, and losses via circulation are insignificant.

*Intra-alveolar surfactant pool in NRDS* (Fig. 8.2)

The decrease may be relative due to dilution by oedema[17] or absolute due to a fall in input and/or rise in output.[5] If surfactant is deficient, the surface tension is increased and high inspiratory pressure is required to initiate lung expansion (poor compliance) while expiration continues until atelectasis and a low functional residual capacity (inset Fig. 8.2).[1] [Even though the tension physics of alveolar fluid surface and rubber balloons differ, the analogy of blowing up a balloon is helpful as a memory aid for pressure-volume relationships in surfactant deficiency. Initially much effort is needed to start inflating the balloon and then it becomes a lot easier.]

(a) ***Dilution***: excess fluid in the alveolar space dilutes surfactant.[17] This may explain the increased incidence of NRDS after caesarian sections. However, decreased synthesis and/or increased inactivation are the main causes of decreased surfactant activity in NRDS.

(b) ***Decreased input***: this can be due to decreased synthesis or decreased release into the alveolar space.

*Decreased synthesis:*

(i) Genetic regulation: inborn errors of surfactant synthesis and acquired inhibition of gene expression have been detected.[18,19] SP-B deficiency has been reported in three term siblings with NRDS[19]. Inhibition of mRNA will also interfere with surfactant metabolism and this mechanism plays a role in ARDS. Tumour necrosis factor (TNF), which is produced by macrophages and can inhibit expression of SP-A and SP-B,[20] has also recently been detected in NRDS.[21]

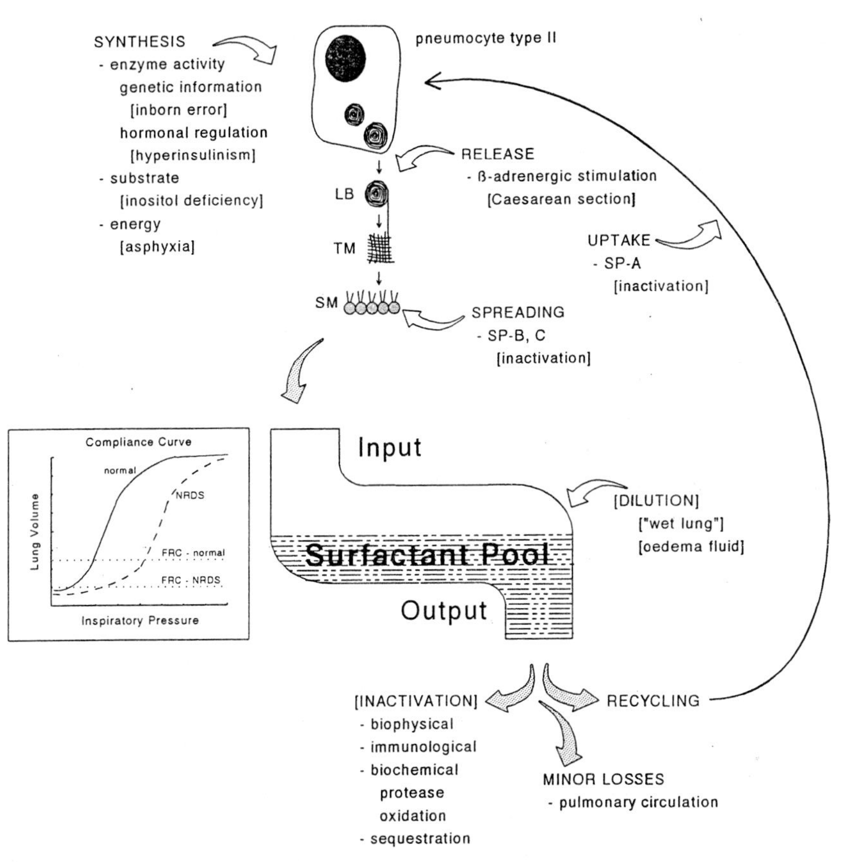


**Fig. 8.2** Input/output model showing physiological and pathophysiological factors (in square brackets) influencing the alveolar surfactant pool. Input of surfactant by a pneumocyte type II is shown, i.e. factors influencing surfactant synthesis and release. The conversion of the lamellar bodies (LB) via the tubular myelin network (TM) to the surfactant monolayer (SM) is shown. Output of active surfactant occurs via recycling, inactivation and minor losses. The concentration of surfactant can also be decreased by dilution. The inset shows the typical compliance curves and functional residual capacity (FRC) in lungs of normal babies and babies with NRDS.

(ii) Hormonal control: various hormones influence surfactant production.[16] Cortisol and thyroxine are well-recognised inducers of surfactant phospholipid and protein synthesis. Cortisol levels rise in late gestation and lack of this stimulus is a major factor in the pathogenesis of NRDS in premature babies. Lower thyroxine levels are present in NRDS, which also occurs more frequently in babies with congenital hypothyroidism. Atrial natriuretic factor (ANF) also stimulates surfactant production.[22] On the other hand, testosterone and insulin inhibit surfactant production. NRDS is more frequently seen in males, and in babies with foetal hyperinsulinism due to maternal diabetes.[1]

(iii) Nutrient supply: in animals, a maternal diet deficient in calories, essential fatty acids or inositol, decreases surfactant production and lung compliance of the newborn.[23] In man, both antenatal and postnatal nutrition, e.g. inositol and fatty acid intake, may influence the course of NRDS.[24]

(iv) Energy supply: asphyxia neonatorum increases the risk of NRDS.[1] Decreased ATP and acidosis do inhibit surfactant synthesis; however, resuscitation initiates rapid recovery of surfactant synthesis experimentally[25] and diminishes the severity of NRDS clinically.[1] Thus the occurrence of postasphyxial NRDS may not be due to anoxia but subsequent ROS damage from both excessive oxygen therapy and ischemia reperfusion injury: the pathophysiology of NRDS and ARDS may overlap more than is currently appreciated.[5]

*Decreased release into alveolar space:* decreased adrenalin release because of decreased birth stress (elective caesarian section[1]) or decreased β-adrenergic receptors' sensitivity on pneumocytes II (prematurity[16]) increase the risk of NRDS. ROS damage can decrease adrenalin release and β-adrenergic receptor sensitivity.[4] However, antenatal (betamethasone, labour inhibition with β-adrenergic agents[26]) and postnatal therapy (elective ventilation[1]) increase surfactant release.

(c) ***Increased output***: this can be due to inactivation of surfactant or decreased uptake of surfactant.

*Inactivation of surfactant:*[5]

(i) Biophysical mechanism: leaked plasma proteins may inhibit phospholipid adsorption into the air-liquid interface by competing for the available space.

(ii) Immunogenic process: leakage of surfactant proteins into the circulation may induce production of SP-B autoantibodies, which interfere with tubular myelin. Antibodies have been detected in babies who had not received exogenous surfactant.

(iii) Biochemical inactivation: could be produced by surfactant protein digestion by neutrophil proteases[27] or by peroxidation of lipids and proteins[5, 28] (see ROS section). These factors are important in ARDS and the evidence suggests that neutrophil induced damage also plays multiple roles in NRDS (see pulmonary oedema).

(iv) Sequestration of surfactant: the characteristic alveolar hyaline membrane is produced by conversion of leaked fibrinogen to fibrin. Surfactant is

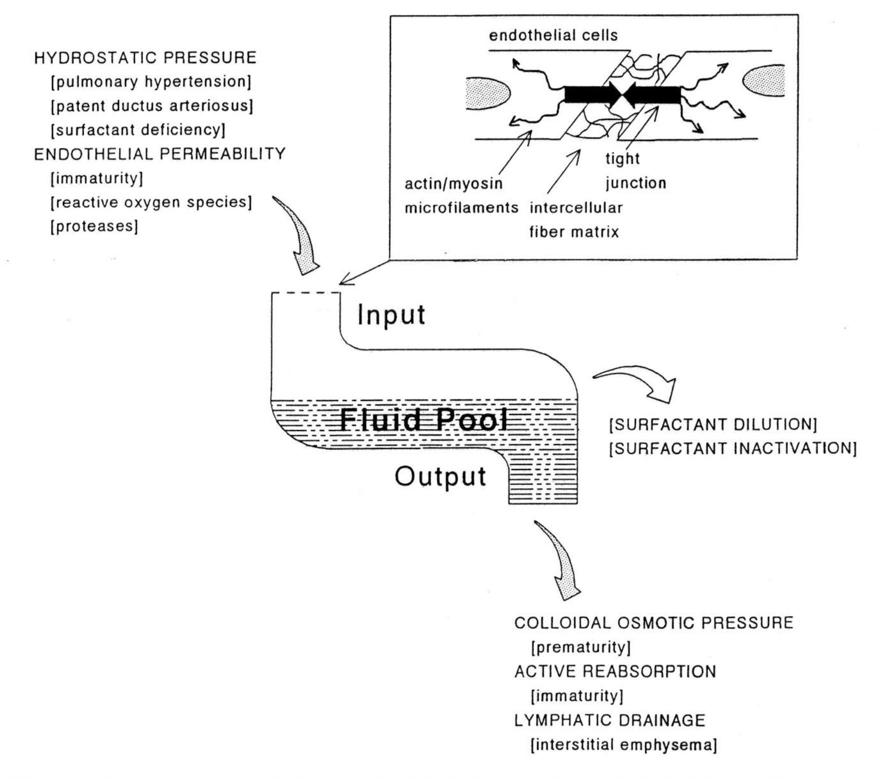


**Fig. 8.3** Input/output model showing physiological and pathophysiological factors (in square brackets) influencing the pool of pulmonary oedema. Input is influenced by hydrostatic pressure and endothelial permeability. The inset schematically illustrates the opposing forces that influence permeability, i.e. tight junctions, actin/myosin microfilaments and intercellular fibre matrix. Output is effected by colloidal osmotic pressure, active reabsorption and lymphatic drainage. Oedema can dilute and inactivate surfactant.

sequestered within fibrin strands. These persist because levels of plasminogen, precursor of the fibrinolytic enzyme plasmin, are low in NRDS.[29]

*Decreased uptake of surfactant*: inactivation of SP-A by antibodies, proteases, and peroxidation interferes with surfactant recycling, and alveolar capillary membrane damage may allow surfactant leakage into the circulation.

## Oedema of alveoli

This occurs if the balanced input and output of fluid is disturbed.

*Intra-alveolar fluid pool in normal subjects* (Fig. 8.3)

Back and forth flow of water between blood and tissue spaces depends on the balance between hydrostatic and osmotic forces and the resistance in the microchannels in the endothelial and epithelial intercellular spaces (Starling's law).[30,31] The permeability of intercellular 'pores' depends on the ability of intercellular protein adhesion molecules, linked as ridges of 'tight junctions', to prevent cells being pulled apart when actin/myosin microfilaments in the cytoskeleton contract (inset Fig. 8.3). Microfilaments contract if intracellular $Ca^{2+}$ increases but relax if $Ca^{2+}$ is lowered by increased cAMP or cGMP levels following β-adrenergic or ANF stimulation, respectively.

Lymphatics drain the interstitial space, and active reabsorption of water helps keep the alveolar space 'dry'. At birth, the adrenaline surge activates the $Na^+/K^+$ ATPase pump of alveolar cells which revert from chloride secretion to sodium absorption.[30,31] This reverses the osmotic gradient and foetal alveolar fluid, which aided pulmonary growth, is therefore reabsorbed.

*Intra-alveolar fluid pool in NRDS* (Fig. 8.3)

Pulmonary oedema, the major factor in ARDS, also plays an important role in NRDS. According to Starling's law oedema develops if hydrostatic pressure and alveolar capillary membrane permeability increase and colloid osmotic pressure decreases. However, diminished active reabsorption and lymph drainage may also contribute to pulmonary fluid accumulation.

(a) ***Increased input***: this can be due to increased hydrostatic pressure or increased membrane permeability.

*Increased hydrostatic pressure*: when pulmonary arteriolar vasoconstriction induces pulmonary hypertension (see perfusion section) not all arterioles constrict and interstitial oedema develops in high pressure capillary beds supplied by dilated arterioles.[32] Surfactant deficiency raises surface tension and this 'suction' synergistically increases transpulmonary hydrostatic pressure and thus oedema formation. Overfilling of the pulmonary circulation due to misjudged intravenous fluid volumes or left to right shunting across a patent ductus arteriosus (PDA) may aggravate the oedema. A PDA with bidirectional shunting frequently develops in NRDS; the pressure gradient between the pulmonary and systemic circulations determines the direction of the shunt.[6] (Letters by Evans and Skinner & Hey, which debate the shunt direction on the basis of their own findings, add perspective to this issue.[43]) Left to right flow can complicate the early clinical picture of NRDS ('silent PDA') but it is especially troublesome when pulmonary arterial pressure falls because of an increased $PaO_2$ due to spontaneous or surfactant therapy induced improvement.[33]

*Increased membrane permeability:* both high hydrostatic capillary pressures due to pulmonary hypertension and high alveolar distending pressures due to ventilation 'stretch' the tight junctions.[32] Tight junctions also leak if actin/myosin contracts or the adhesion proteins are damaged. ROS induced membrane damage, TNF and leukotrienes increase actin/myosin contractility by raising intracellular $Ca^{2+}$ levels[31] and neutrophil proteases can digest the adhesion proteins.[31] Extensive oedema is a well-recognised finding in NRDS and a generalised delay in tight cell junctions or β-adrenergic receptor maturation may be responsible,[13] however asphyxia does not increase the oedema.[13] ANF levels, raised in NRDS, peak at the same time that lung function improves; however, this may be related to its diuretic effect rather than its effect on endothelial permeability.[22]

(b) ***Decreased output***: plasma protein levels correlate with gestational age and colloidal osmotic pressure is low in preterm babies, particularly those with NRDS.[30] This decreases fluid reabsorption. Immaturity of β-adrenergic receptors will hamper active fluid reabsorption and decreased adrenaline release after an elective caesarian section may produce a 'wet lung'. Decreased lymph drainage can occur if interstitial emphysema blocks lymphatics (see[5]).

## DISTURBANCE OF PERFUSION

In NRDS, inadequate right ventricular pressure and or increased resistance to pulmonary blood flow may decrease blood transport of $CO_2$ to and $O_2$ from the alveoli. Normally, perfusion and ventilation rates are matched.[10,11] Pulmonary blood flow depends on adequate venous return and is positively related to the right ventricular pressure and inversely to pulmonary vascular resistance (Poisseuille's law). Pulmonary hypertension may produce right to left extrapulmonary shunting across the PDA and foramen ovale.

### Right ventricular pressure

In contrast to the clinically more accessible left ventricle, little is published on right ventricular function in NRDS.[43] Clinical signs of right ventricular failure are uncommon unless severe pulmonary hypertension is present. Perhaps the right ventricle, which pumps against high pulmonary resistance in low oxygen conditions for months in utero, is uniquely equipped to maintain blood flow when hypoxia and pulmonary hypertension persists postnatally. However Doppler flow studies indicate that tricuspid regurgitation often occurs.[33] This is an early sign of right ventricle decompensation but function could deteriorate further if there is an inadequate supply of oxygen and/or glucose. Systemic hypotension and anaemia will decrease the oxygen supplied via the right coronary artery. Systemic hypotension is frequently encountered in NRDS.[1,43] The aetiology is uncertain and disturbed autonomic nerve or cardiac muscle dysfunction (immaturity and anoxia), blood volume decrease (excess blood sampling, generalised oedema) or redistribution (decreased venous return due to inappropriate ventilation, PDA 'steal') may contribute. We suggest that ROS damage of muscle and adrenergic receptors[4] also plays a role in hypotension in NRDS.

### Pulmonary vessel resistance (Fig. 8.4)

NRDS is a secondary cause of persistent pulmonary hypertension of the newborn (PPHN).[3,6] The neurological, chemical, and hormonal factors

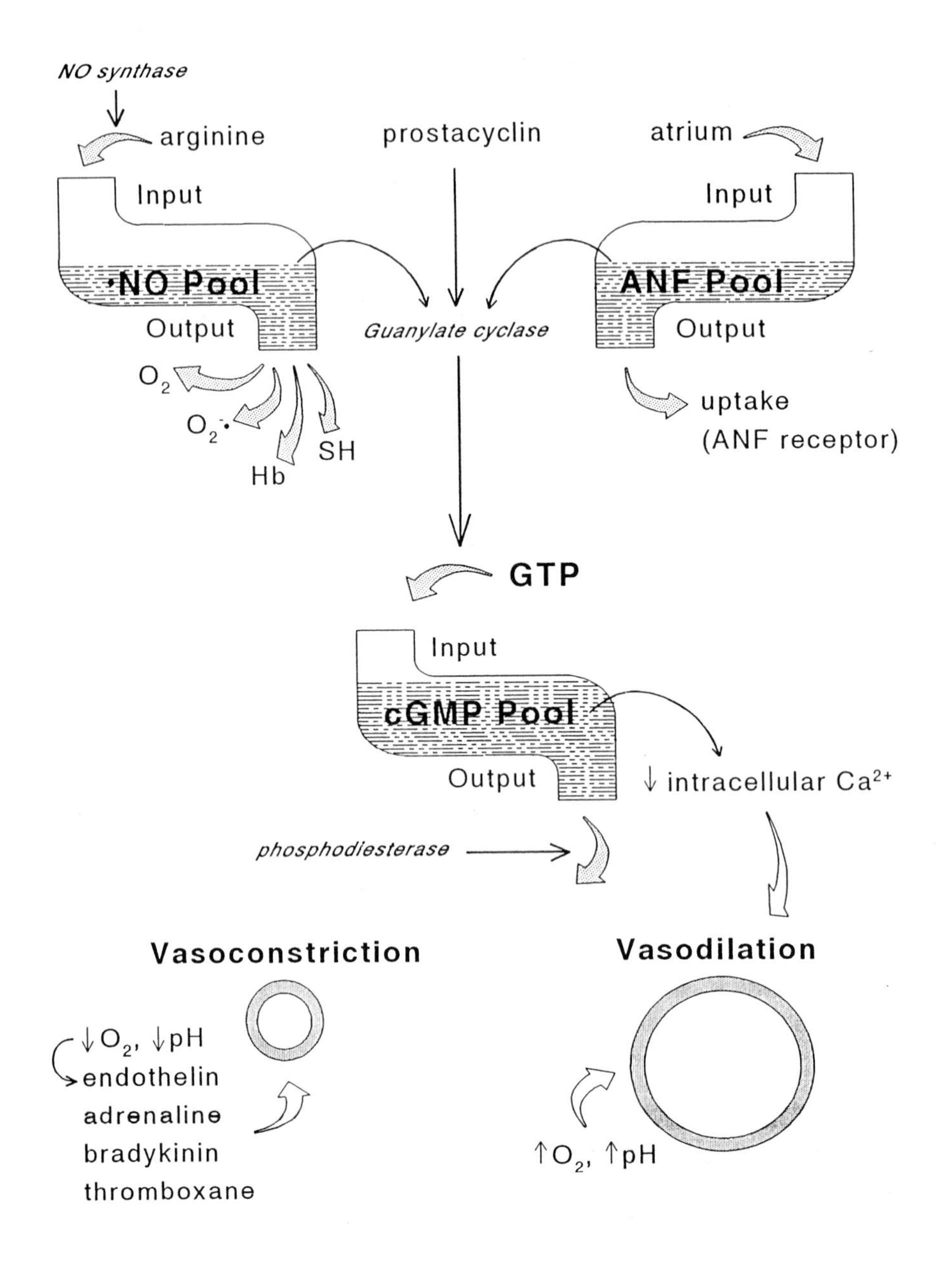


**Fig. 8.4** Vasoactivity of pulmonary arterioles depends on the balance between constricting and dilating stimuli. Increasing the pool of ˙NO, prostacyclin ($PGI_2$), and ANF activates guanylate cyclase, which converts guanosine triphosphate (GTP) to cyclic guanosine monophosphate (cGMP). Raising the cGMP pool induces vasodilation by lowering intracellular $Ca^{2+}$. The factors shown influencing the input and output of ˙NO, prostacyclin, and ANF are discussed in the text.

controlling pulmonary vasoactivity are being investigated. Pulmonary vessels are richly supplied with adrenergic and cholinergic nerves and receptors but their role in coordinating ventilation/perfusion matching is not understood. On the other hand, knowledge on the local control of vasoactivity by substances such as ˙NO and ANF is making rapid progress.[22, 34] The degree of contraction of the arteriolar wall muscle will depend on the balance of vasoconstricting and vasodilating factors. $O_2$ and pH levels are major factors and are used therapeutically to counter vasoconstriction. More recently acetylcholine and adrenaline, ROS (˙NO, $H_2O_2$, $˙O_2^-$ ), peptides (ANF, endothelin, angiotensin, and bradykinin), and eicosanoids (prostacyclin, thromboxane, leukotrienes) have been identified as important vasoactivators.[35] We will only discuss the regulation and action of ˙NO, ANF, and eicosanoids to illustrate how alterations in input and/or output change their pool size. ˙NO, ANF and prostacyclin induce dilation and thromboxane constriction by lowering or increasing intracellular $Ca^{2+}$, respectively. The three vasodilators activate guanylate cyclase[3] which converts GTP to cGMP, which induces vasodilation by lowering intracellular $Ca^{2+}$ (see analogous mechanisms in oedema). ˙NO is produced in endothelial cells from L-arginine by NO synthase after triggering by acetylcholine or shear forces and removed via reactions with haemoglobin, oxygen and superoxide and sulphydryl groups. Immaturity of NO synthase and low arginine levels may limit ˙NO production but the role of these deficiencies in PPHN in NRDS is undetermined.[3] ANF's vasodilatory action is endothelium independent and it binds to receptors on arteriolar muscle to activate guanylate cyclase. Its concentration depends on the rate of production in the atrium and lung tissue and rate of clearance via uptake (specific receptors) and degradation by the endothelium.[22] Trying to fit in the role of ROS[36] makes it even more difficult to understand: $H_2O_2$ activates guanylate cyclase and induces vasodilation but other peroxides and $˙O_2^-$ induce vasoconstriction: peroxides increase thromboxane production by activating phospholipase to release arachidonic acid from membranes and $˙O_2^-$ reacts with and lowers the level of ˙NO.

Manipulation of these systems will offer many therapeutic possibilities, but first the ins and outs of all these intricate systems must be understood. It must be stressed that simpler but no less important problems such as capillary compression due to inappropriate distending pressure and increased blood viscosity due to polycythaemia must not be forgotten. They are easier to diagnose and treat.

## MISMATCHING OF VENTILATION AND PERFUSION (Fig. 8.5)

Atelectasis and oedema do not significantly hinder the diffusion of $CO_2$ and raising the $O_2$ concentration of ambient air easily compensates for this gas's lower diffusion rate.[10,11] Therefore, the gas disturbances in NRDS are more related to ventilation/perfusion mismatching because of physiological dead space (no perfusion of ventilated alveoli) or intrapulmonary shunting (perfusion of non ventilated alveoli).

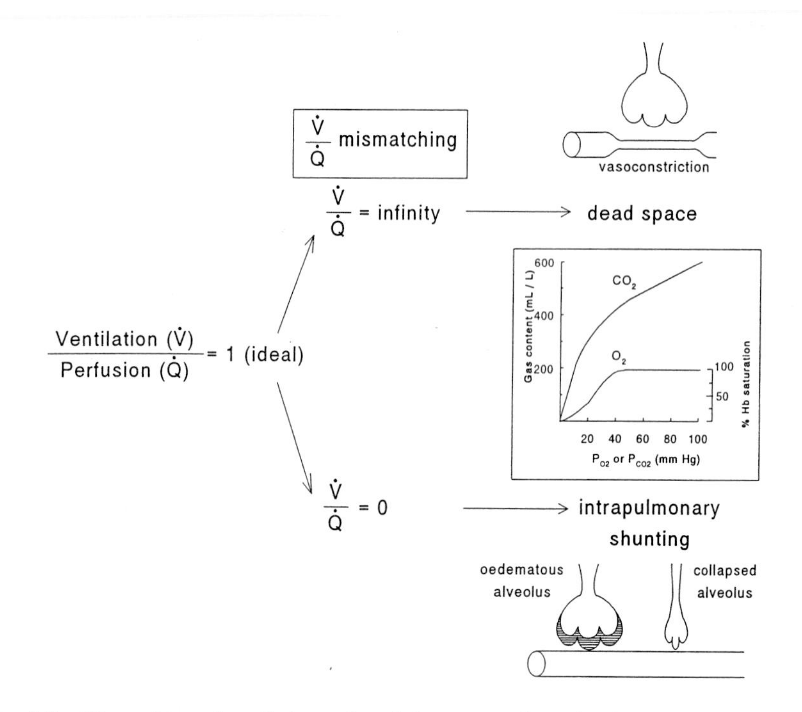


**Fig. 8.5** Mismatching of ventilation and perfusion can produce alveolar dead space or produce intrapulmonary shunting. The inset shows the effect of gas pressures on blood gas content. $O_2$ is mainly transported attached to haemoglobin, which is 100% saturated at a $PO_2$ of 6kP, whereas $CO_2$ is transported in plasma mainly as bicarbonate and never reaches saturation.

Increased physiological dead space, like increased dead space from an endotracheal tube, has a greater effect on $CO_2$ than $O_2$ in ventilated babies. Small increases in ambient $O_2$ will compensate for the dilution of the inspired $O_2$ by gas in the enlarged dead space. On the other hand, shunting affects $PaO_2$ much more than $PaCO_2$ levels in NRDS[10,11]. The inset of Figure 5 shows the $CO_2$ dissociation curve ($PaCO_2$ vs blood $CO_2$ content): it is very steep in the physiological range and never reaches saturation because $CO_2$ dissolves so easily in plasma to form bicarbonate. On the other hand, the oxyhaemoglobin dissociation curve ($PaO_2$ vs blood $O_2$ content) is sigmoid because $O_2$ is poorly soluble in plasma and is mainly transported as oxyhaemoglobin. Thus, increased ventilation of the remaining alveoli can compensate for poor $CO_2$ exchange in alveoli with shunts. However, it is not possible to increase the $O_2$ content in the normal alveoli with increased ventilation or increased ambient $O_2$: the foetal haemoglobin of the erythrocytes flowing to this area is already 100% saturated at a $PaO_2$ of around 6 kP. This greater effect on $O_2$ compared to $CO_2$ is analogous to the situation with extrapulmonary shunting due to PPHN or Tetralogy of Fallot. In PPHN, the mixed venous blood returning to the right heart is diverted via the foramen ovale and patent ductus arteriosus to the systemic circulation.[6]

## Role of reactive oxygen species in NRDS

ROS damage plays a major role in adult RDS[4,5] and Frank and Sosenko hypothesized that it may be the third factor in the pathogenesis of NRDS.[8] An extensive reference list for these aspects which are discussed below has been given previously.[5] ROS induced damage will be proportional to their concentration and susceptibility of the target molecules. ROS 'overflow' can oxidize lipids, proteins and DNA (Fig. 8.6). Lipid peroxidation disrupts cell membranes, inactivates surfactant, and produces toxic and chemotactic agents. The peroxides, by influencing eicosanoid metabolism ('peroxide tone') induce pulmonary hypertension and chemotaxis. Protein damage includes inactivation of β-adrenergic receptors,[4] enzymes, $\alpha_1$-antitrypsin (inhibitor of neutrophil proteases)[27] and muscle dysfunction.[12]

*Intra-alveolar ROS pool in normal subjects* (Fig. 8.6)

ROS are normally produced in respiratory tract and ventilatory muscles by mitochondrial metabolism and eicosanoid synthesis: molecular oxygen is reduced to $^{\cdot}O_2^-$ from which $H_2O_2$ is generated. The lung constantly exposed to oxygen, has intracellular antioxidant enzymes and substances which act with those in surfactant, alveolar lining fluid and blood to balance the input (production) and output (removal by scavenging or breakdown) of ROS. Superoxide dismutase reduces $^{\cdot}O_2^-$ to $H_2O_2$, which is reduced to water by catalase and glutathione peroxidase. The latter enzyme oxidises glutathione (GSH) to GSSG which is recycled (i.e. reduced) by glutathione reductase. Antioxidant substances, such as vitamins E and C, uric acid and bilirubin, act synergistically (analogous to buffers in pH regulation) in scavenging ROS and secondary peroxidation products to break oxidative chain reactions.

*Intra-alveolar ROS pool in NRDS* (Fig. 8.6)

(a) ***Increased input***: after birth, mitochondrial $^{\cdot}O_2^-$ production increases in the higher oxygen environment of terrestrial life and oxygen therapy intensifies this. In NRDS, the extra respiratory muscle activity consumes more oxygen and generates more ROS by the mitochondria.[12] Preceding hypoxia, e.g. birth asphyxia exacerbates $^{\cdot}O_2^-$ production in injured mitochondria, and activates xanthine oxidase[28] to oxidise hypoxanthine and produce $^{\cdot}O_2^-$. Other potentially important ROS are $H_2O_2$ and hypochlorous acid (HOCl) from activated neutrophils, and $^{\cdot}NO$ from endothelium, macrophages and neutrophils. $^{\cdot}NO$ can react with $^{\cdot}O_2^-$ to form another powerful oxidant, the peroxynitrite anion ($^-OONO$).[34] Neutrophils accumulate in large numbers in NRDS and they may contribute to the pathogenesis of NRDS.[27] In the presence of reduced non protein-bound iron (ferrous ion, $Fe^{2+}$) $H_2O_2$ can be converted to $^{\cdot}OH$, an extremely reactive oxygen radical. In the preterm baby, plasma transferrin is iron saturated and non-protein-bound iron occurs.[37] This potentially dangerous prooxidant status is aggravated by the babies' high vitamin C and

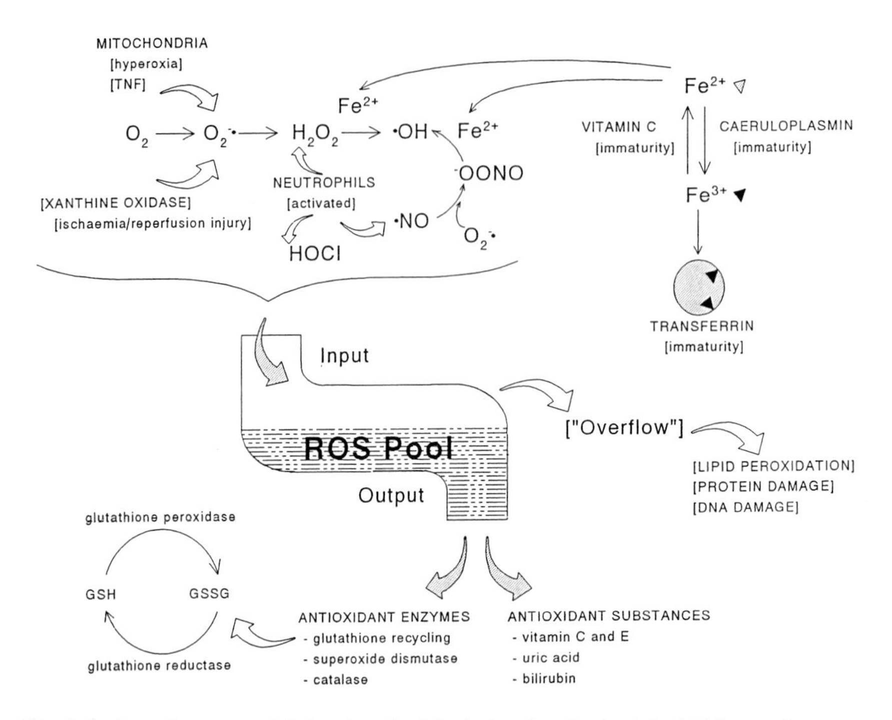


**Fig. 8.6** Input/output model showing physiological and pathophysiological factors (in square brackets) influencing the pulmonary pool of reactive oxygen species (ROS). Mitochondria, neutrophils, and xanthine oxidase produce ROS which are removed by antioxidant enzymes and substances. Excess production, e.g. hyperoxia and presence of nonprotein bound iron ($Fe^{2+}$), and decreased removal, e.g. catalase inactivity result in an 'overflow' of ROS damaging lipids, proteins and DNA. The high vitamin C and low caeruloplasmin and transferrin levels favour the presence of $Fe^{2+}$. This favours $^{\cdot}OH$ production from $H_2O_2$ or $^{-}OONO$ (formed from $^{\cdot}NO$ and $^{\cdot}O_2^{-}$.

low caeruloplasmin levels. Vitamin C, a powerful reducing agent, antagonises the ferroxidase activity of caeruloplasmin and keeps the non-protein-bound iron reduced (Fig. 8.6). In vitro, this plasma oxidizes surfactant and leakage of plasma into the alveolar space could damage surfactant.[37]

(b) ***Decreased output***: maturation of the pulmonary antioxidant enzymes parallels the surfactant system, and is diminished in preterm babies.[8] Glucocorticoids accelerate both processes but thyroxine, in contrast, activates the surfactant system but inhibits antioxidant enzyme maturation.[38] Natural surfactant has significant amounts of superoxide dismutase and catalase; however, preparation of animal surfactant for therapeutic use inactivates these enzymes. In vitro addition of vitamin E to commercial surfactant inhibits peroxidation damage.[37] Alveolar lining fluid contains all the major antioxidant enzymes and substances, for example catalase, GSH (140x higher level than plasma), and uric acid.

The antioxidant capacity of red blood cells and plasma contributes to the lung's defences. Plasma antioxidants diffuse into the alveolus and help protect endothelium and epithelium. The total peroxyl radical trapping capacity (TRAP) of plasma, which assesses the interaction of chain breaking anti-oxidants, is higher in newborns than in adults and may partly compensate for the lung's temporarily immature antioxidant enzyme defences. However, the TRAP and its contributors' uric acid and vitamin C levels fall postnatally due to a decreased input and/or an increased output (oxidative or urinary losses). Erythrocytes have high concentrations of catalase and glutathione peroxidase and they are believed to protect the lung against ROS. Erythrocyte catabolism of $H_2O_2$ by glutathione recycling is efficient in newborns and this may also compensate for their deficient pulmonary antioxidant capacity.

(c) ***Increased susceptibility to ROS damage***: babies with NRDS have increased unsaturated fatty acids (oleic, linoleic, and arachidonic) in their pulmonary surfactant. The susceptibility of phospholipids in surfactant (and cell membranes) to peroxidation should increase as the concentration of poly-unsaturated fatty acids (PUFA) rises. However, conflicting evidence is available. In animal studies, antenatal supplementation with PUFA protects cells against oxygen toxicity while postnatal parenteral nutrition with PUFA may increase the risk.[39]

## CURRENT AND FUTURE THERAPY OF DISTURBED VENTILATION AND PERFUSION IN NRDS

Methods to prevent premature delivery are being sought. Refinements in both antenatal therapy to induce lung maturity and postnatal therapy to optimize gas exchange while decreasing complications are also required. Analogous to our structured analysis of the pathophysiological disturbances the Table 8.1 summarises present and possible future therapies according to their effect on the input and output of blood gases. Permitting higher $PCO_2$ values may decrease iatrogenic lung damage;[40] nasal continuous positive airway pressure with or without use of surfactant appears to reduce the need for ventilation in even very small babies with NRDS.[3] However, dangers exist, for example intraventricular haemorrhage due to cerebral vasodilation, and further assessment is needed. If assisted ventilation is needed, spontaneous respiratory effort and assisted ventilation should be synchronised. This can best be achieved with rapid ventilation rates and low inspiratory:expiratory time ratios and/or triggering. This causes air trapping, which can precipitate oedema or pneumothorax.[1–3] High frequency ventilation and liquid ventilation are also undergoing trials.

Despite these supportive methods, the morbidity and mortality are still high and more specific therapies to counter the pathophysiological mechanisms are required. Theoretically, the possible steps are correction of the inappropriate inputs and outputs in surfactant and alveolar fluid and improvement of blood

**Table 8.1** Possible therapeutic steps in a baby with hypoxia and hypercapnia due to NRDS

| | | | |
|---|---|---|---|
| Permit poorer blood gas levels | permissive hypercapnia limits iatrogenic lung damage* | | |
| Improve blood gas levels | | | |
| Increase input $O_2$ and output $CO_2$ | | | |
| Ventilation | | | |
| (a) spontaneous | diaphragm function | <gastric distention, nurse prone*, +antioxidants* | |
| (b) assisted | relate PIP, PEEP, and I:E ratio to compliance | | |
| | synchronize ventilation | >rate | |
| | | <I:E ratio, triggering | |
| Diffusion | | | |
| (a) >gas diffusion gradients | high frequency ventilation | | |
| (b) >surface area | alveoli maturation | >growth (+ steroids) | |
| | surfactant | | |
| | | >endo- (+ steroids), + exogenous source | |
| | | <activation* (antioxidants, liquid ventil.) | |
| | oedema | <hydrostatic press | <fluid intake, <PDA |
| | | <permeability | <distention alveoli, + steroids, <myosin contract* <neutrophil, * <ROS * |
| Perfusion | | | |
| (a) >perfusion pressure | venous return | <PEEP (+ inadvertent) | |
| | cardiac output | +β-adrenergics | |
| (b) vascular resistance | vasoconstriction | >$PO_2$ and pH, <handling & pain, + α-adrenergic blockade, >·NO (+ exog. or endog.*) | |
| | capillary compression | <PEEP | |
| Decrease input $CO_2$ and output $O_2$ | | | |
| (a) <respiratory quotient | | <glucose and >lipid intake* | |
| (b) <$O_2$ consumption | | optimal environmental temperature | |

*is therapy that is undergoing clinical or preclinical trials; is >increase and <decrease; + is use as therapy. Abbreviations: PIP peak inspiratory pressure, PEEP positive end expiratory pressure, I:E inspiratory to expiratory time ratio, PDA patent ductus arteriosus.

flow. Surfactant deficiency may be alleviated by increasing endogenous production by antenatal hormone therapy, [3,26,41] or by exogenous replacement therapy.[1–3] Intra-uterine induction is now being finely tuned, e.g. combined use of betamethasone and thyrotropin releasing hormone.[41] These hormones may have side effects, e.g. thyroxine inhibits maturation of antioxidant enzymes.[38] Antenatal and postnatal supplementation of the diet, e.g. inositol, PUFA, vitamins E and C may influence NRDS by influencing production of surfactant,[24] and sensitivity of surfactant and tissues to ROS induced damage.[37] Addition of antioxidants[37] or removal of inhibitory proteins using liquid ventilation with fluorocarbons[42] may prevent inhibition of surfactant activity. Careful $PaO_2$ monitoring, inhibiting xanthine oxidase activity with allopurinol, and decreasing

$Fe^{2+}$ by exchange transfusions or chelating agents may decrease ROS damage.[28,37] Diminishing neutrophil recruitment with monoclonal antibodies to TNF may decrease ROS and protease induced damage.[27] Glucocorticoid therapy[13] and adrenergic drugs, e.g. the phosphodiesterase inhibitor pentoxifylline,[31] may prevent excess lung permeability.

If pulmonary perfusion cannot be improved by decreasing arteriolar vasoconstriction (increasing $PaO_2$ and pH) and decreasing capillary compression (lower end positive pressures) then pulmonary vasodilators are indicated. However, their systemic administration (e.g. tolazoline) can induce hypotension and increase intrapulmonary shunting by dilating arterioles supplying poorly ventilated alveoli. Inhaled ·NO, on the other hand, only dilates vessels supplying ventilated alveoli and does not cause systemic hypotension (extremely short half life),[3,34] however, oxidative damage may complicate its use.

## KEY POINTS FOR CLINICAL PRACTICE

- In all babies with apparent neonatal respiratory distress syndrome, remember that lung oedema due to infection or congenital heart disease (especially total anomalous pulmonary venous drainage) may mimic neonatal respiratory distress syndrome.

- In term babies, with possible neonatal respiratory distress syndrome, consider inherited and endocrine causes, e.g. diabetic mother, and the possibility of neonatal adult respiratory distress syndrome, e.g. following asphyxia or shock.

- History and examination are essential for correct interpretation of the continually changing biochemical and radiological picture in a baby with neonatal respiratory distress syndrome.

- Attempt to decrease interobserver differences in interpretation of clinical signs and chest x-rays.

- Minimal handling is essential but must not lead to minimal clinical assessment.

- Painful procedures may cause pulmonary vasoconstriction and excessive investigation must be eliminated. However, overzealous use of analgesics may prevent use of less aggressive respiratory therapy, e.g. nasal CPAP instead of ventilation.

- Surfactant therapy rapidly changes the status of the lung. Therefore, the optimal degree of therapy, e.g. the level of end positive pressure, must continuously be fine tuned.

- The complex stereogram of all the pathophysiological points created must not prevent medical and nursing staff from focusing on the simpler causes of hypoxia and hypercapnia. The contribution of pneumothoraces, abdominal distention, and the 'four toos' ('endotracheal tube too high or too deep, too narrow, or too dirty') must constantly be kept in the picture.

- Simple input output and flow models make it a lot easier to explain the basic pathophysiology and therapy of neonatal respiratory distress syndrome (and all related problems) to the baby's family.[9]

## REFERENCES

1 Greenough A, Morley CJ, Robertson NRC. Acute respiratory disease in the newborn. In: Roberton NRC. ed. 2nd edn. Edinburgh: Churchill Livingstone 1992: 385-504
2 Cooke RWI. Developments in the management of respiratory distress syndrome. Rec Adv Paediatr 1991; 9: 157-169
3 Hutchinson AA. Respiratory disorders of the neonate. Curr Opin Pediatr 1994; 6: 142-153
4 Doelman CJA, Bast A. Oxygen radicals in lung pathology. Free Rad Biol Med 1990; 9: 381-400
5 Berger HM, Moison RMW, Van Zoeren-Grobben D. The ins and outs of respiratory distress syndrome in babies and adults. J R Coll Physicians Lond 1994; 28: 24-35
6 Walther FJ, Benders MJ, Leighton JO. Persistent pulmonary hypertension in premature neonates with severe respiratory distress syndrome. Pediatrics 1992; 90: 899-904
7 Watchko JF, Balsan MJ. Ventilatory pump failure in premature newborns. Pediatr Pulmonol 1994; 17: 231-233
8 Frank L, Sosenko IRS. Development of lung antioxidant enzyme system in late gestation: possible implications for the prematurely born infant. J Pediatr 1987; 110: 9-14
9 Berger HM, Van Den Berg JM. An approach to integrating medical teaching and increasing medical competence: 'SOOPA MD'. In: Bender W, Hiemstra RJ, Scherpbier AJJA, Zwierstra RP. eds. Teaching and assessing clinical competence (Proceedings of the Third International Conference on Teaching and Assessing Clinical Competence). Groningen: Boekwerk Publications, 1990: 55-60
10 Cragg PA. Respiration. In: Bray JJ, Cragg PA, Macknight ADC, Mills RG, Taylor DW. eds. Lecture notes in human physiology. 3rd edn. London: Blackwell, 1994: 466-553
11 Boynton BR, Hammond MD. Pulmonary gas exchange: basic principles and effects of mechanical ventilation. In: Boynton BR, Carlo WA, Jobe AH. eds. New therapies for neonatal respiratory failure: a physiological approach. Cambridge: Cambridge University Press, 1994: 115-130
12 Anzueto A, Supinski GS, Levine SM, Jenkinson SG. Are oxygen-derived free radicals involved in diaphragmatic dysfunction? Am J Respir Crit Care Med 1994; 149: 1048-1052
13 Jobe AH. Pathogenesis of respiratory failure in the preterm infant. Ann Med 1991; 23: 687-691
14 Rubin BK, Ramirez O, King M. Mucus rheology and transport in neonatal respiratory distress syndrome and the effect of surfactant therapy. Chest 1992; 101: 1080-1085
15 Stocks J. Effect of nasogastric tubes on nasal resistance during infancy. Arch Dis Child 1980; 5: 17-21
16 Rooney SA. Regulation of surfactant-associated phospholipid synthesis and secretion. In: Polin RA, Fox WW, eds. Fetal and neonatal physiology. Philadelphia: WB Saunders, 1992: 971-985
17 O'Brodovich H, Hannam V. Exogenous surfactant rapidly increases $PaO_2$ in mature rabbits with lungs that contain large amounts of saline. Am Rev Respir Dis 1993; 147: 1087-1090
18 Rannels R, Rannels SL, Sneyd JG, Loten EG. Fetal lung development in rats with a glycogen storage disorder. Am J Physiol 1991; 260: L419-L427

19 Nogee LM, DeMello DE, Dehner LP, Colten HR. Deficiency of pulmonary surfactant protein B in congenital alveolar proteinosis. N Engl J Med 1993; 328: 406-410
20 Wispé JR, Clark JC, Warner BB et al. Tumour necrosis factor-alpha inhibits expression of pulmonary surfactant protein. J Clin Invest 1990; 86: 1954-1960
21 Murch SH, MacDonald TT, Wood CBS, Costeloe KL. Tumour necrosis factor in the bronchoalveolar secretions of infants with the respiratory distress syndrome and the effect of dexamethasone treatment. Thorax 1992; 47: 44-47
22 Perreault T, Gutkowska J. Role of atrial natriuretic factor in lung physiology and pathology. Am J Respir Crit Care Med 1995; 151: 226-242
23 Longmore WJ, Moxley MA. Metabolism of pulmonary surfactant: model systems. In: Robertson B, Van Golde LMG, Batenburg JJ. eds. Pulmonary surfactant: from molecular biology to clinical practice. Amsterdam: Elsevier, 1992: 229-253
24 Hallman M, Bry K, Hoppu K, Lappi M, Pohjavuori M. Inositol supplementation in premature infants with respiratory distress syndrome. N Engl J Med 1992; 326: 1233-1239
25 Berry D, Jobe A, Ikegami M, Seidner S, Pettenazzo A, ElKady T. Pulmonary effects of acute prenatal asphyxia in ventilated premature lambs. J Appl Physiol 1988; 65: 26-33
26 Kwong MS, Egan EA. Reduced incidence of hyaline membrane disease in extremely premature infants following delay of delivery in mother with preterm labour: use of ritodrine and betamethasone. Pediatrics 1986; 78: 767-774
27 Speer CP, Ruess D, Harms K, Herting E, Gefeller O. Neutrophil elastase and acute pulmonary damage in neonates with severe respiratory distress syndrome. Pediatrics 1993; 91: 794-799
28 Jenkinson SG, Roberts RJ, DeLemos RA et al. Allopurinol-induced effects in premature baboons with respiratory distress syndrome. J Appl Physiol 1991; 70: 1160-1167
29 Ambrus CM. Prevention of hyaline membrane with plasminogen. J Am Med Ass 1977; 237: 1837-1841
30 Bland RD. Formation of fetal lung liquid and its removal near birth. In: Polin RA, Fox WW. eds. Fetal and neonatal physiology. Philadelphia: WB Saunders Company, 1992: 782-789
31 Albelda SM. The alveolar-capillary barrier in the adult respiratory distress syndrome. In: Fishman AP, ed. Update: pulmonary diseases and disorders. New York: McGraw-Hill, 1992: 197-211
32 West JB, Mathieu-Costello O. Stress failure of pulmonary capillaries: role in lung and heart disease. Lancet 1992; 340: 762-767
33 Seppänen MP, Kääpä PO, Kero PO, Saraste M. Doppler-derived systolic pulmonary artery pressure in acute neonatal respiratory distress syndrome. Pediatrics 1994; 93: 769-773
34 Gaston B, Drazen JM, Loscalzo J, Stamler JS. The biology of nitrogen oxides in the airways. Am J Respir Crit Care Med 1994; 149: 538-551
35 Soifer SJ, Fineman JR, Heyman MA. The pulmonary circulation. In: Gluckman PD, Heymann MA. eds. Perinatal and pediatric pathophysiology. London: Edward Arnold, 1993: 519-525
36 Gurtner GH, Burke-Wolin T. Interactions of oxidant stress and vascular reactivity. Am J Physiol 1991; 260: L207-L211
37 Moison RMW, Palinckx JJS, Roest M, Houdkamp E, Berger HM. Induction of lipid peroxidation of pulmonary surfactant by plasma of preterm babies. Lancet 1993; 341: 79-82
38 Chen Y, Whitney PL, Frank L. Negative regulation of antioxidant enzyme gene expression in the developing fetal rat lung by prenatal hormonal treatments. Pediatr Res 1993; 33: 171-176
39 Pitkänen OM. Peroxidation of lipid emulsions: a hazard for the premature infant receiving parenteral nutrition? Free Rad Biol Med 1992; 13; 239-245
40 Feihl F, Perret C. Permissive hypercapnia. How permissive should we be? Am J Respir Crit Care Med 1994; 150: 1722-1737
41 Ballard RA, Ballard PL, Creasy RK et al. TRH Study Group. Respiratory disease in very-low-birthweight infants after prenatal thyrotropin-releasing hormone and glucocorticoid. Lancet 1992; 339: 510-515
42 Richman PS, Wolfson MR, Shaffer TH. Lung lavage with oxygenated perfluorochemical liquid in acute lung injury. Crit Care Med 1993; 21: 768-774
43 Evans N, and Skinner JR, Hey EN, Letters. Pediatrics 1993; 92: 737-738

# Advances in epilepsy: seizures and syndromes

*P. S. Baxter C. D. C. Rittey*

The term 'epilepsy' conceals an impressive and increasing variety of conditions – the epilepsies. This review centres on their diagnostic classification. Recent attempts to define the epilepsies aim to provide more clarity in diagnosis, better understanding of causes, more accurate prognoses and more rational treatment. New classifications have also been associated with the description of previously un- or under-recognised entities.

## NEW IDEAS ON SEIZURE TYPES

Seizures are a symptom, either of primary ('epileptic') or of secondary (e.g. infective, post traumatic, degenerative) cerebral disorders. The ideal clinical approach is to first diagnose the seizure type or types experienced by a patient and then the epilepsy syndrome. Accurate definition of seizure type or types is thus essential. The current classification, published by the International League against Epilepsy (ILAE) in 1981, uses clinical and EEG features (Table 9.1).[1–3] Terms such as grand mal and petit mal are obsolete because they are too vague. The classification has been generally accepted, but there are still some problems, such as the lack of localisation in partial seizures, the

**Table 9.1** Summary of the 1981 International League against Epilepsy seizure classification, which relies only on clinical features of the fit and on the ictal and interictal EEG

| | |
|---|---|
| *I* | *Partial (focal, local) seizures* |
| | Simple partial |
| | Complex partial |
| | Secondarily generalised |
| *II* | *Generalised seizures* |
| | Absence |
| | Atypical absences |
| | Myoclonic |
| | Clonic |
| | Tonic |
| | Tonic-clonic |
| | Atonic |
| *III* | *Unclassified epileptic seizures* |
| | Inadequate or incomplete data |
| | Some neonatal seizures |

percentage that fall into the unclassifiable category, or the differentiation of partial seizures into simple and complex, which has provoked controversy over the meaning of 'consciousness'.[4] Over the last 5 years, an international library of video–EEG recordings of seizures has been collected and a subcommittee of the ILAE is expected to recommend further refinements.[5]

### Partial seizures

Partial seizures arise from a localised focus in the cortex and can be 'simple', without impairment of consciousness, or 'complex', with impairment of consciousness which can vary from mild confusion to complete unconsciousness. Events during either type include motor changes, such as focal movements or posturing, version (turning of gaze, head and/or body), vocalisation or speech arrest; sensory experiences, both of peripheral sensation and of special senses such as smell, taste or vertigo, and autonomic symptoms such as gastric sensation or colour change. In complex partial seizures, psychic features, such as deja vu or fear, and automatisms (de novo complex movements or continuation of previous activity in a fugue state) can also occur. The ILAE may add other more recently recognised phenomena, such as partial seizures with motor arrest, perceptual change, unilateral neglect or speech disturbance. In simple partial seizures the EEG, taken between (interictal) or during (ictal) seizures, may show a focal discharge from the appropriate part of the cortex for the symptoms. In complex partial seizures the interictal EEG can show unilateral or bilaterally asynchronous discharges, often from the frontal or temporal regions, while the ictal EEG can show unilateral or bilateral discharges, either diffuse or focal.

### Primary and secondary generalisation

The term 'generalised' means that seizure activity is arising from both hemispheres simultaneously. EEG changes are therefore also generalised, i.e. synchronous and present in all the recording leads. Clinical accompaniments are loss of consciousness, since all the cortex is involved, with or without bilateral motor changes. 'Primary generalisation' means that the seizure activity begins everywhere simultaneously, although the mechanism for this is still unknown. 'Secondary generalisation' means that a generalised seizure, with the EEG features described above, follows another seizure. The initial seizure is usually a partial one, so that the EEG shows discharges in one part of the cortex leading into a generalised discharge, but recently it has been realised that secondary generalisation can follow other primary generalised seizures, so that for instance an absence can lead to a generalised tonic-clonic seizure. Tonic-clonic, tonic or clonic seizures have been considered the usual types of secondary generalised seizures, but myoclonic and absence seizures can also be seen. In a recent study, one third of seizures classified by paediatricians as primary generalised had focal clinical or EEG features, suggesting that they were in fact secondarily generalised and therefore would have quite different pathology.[6]

## Absences versus complex partial seizures

A brief impairment of consciousness, previously termed minor seizures or petit mal, can be due to a complex partial seizure or to an absence. Both can be provoked by hyperventilation. Complex partial seizures of temporal lobe origin are relatively slow to begin and end, are usually followed by confusion and either have focal or no discharges on the surface EEG. However, typical absences have a very abrupt beginning and ending without significant postictal confusion, are usually brief (62% <15 seconds, 83% <30 seconds), and are always accompanied by generalised regular 2–4 Hz spike-wave on the EEG. Rarely, some complex partial seizures of frontal lobe origin have an identical clinical and EEG appearance and can only be distinguished by the later appearance of other focal features.[7] Other differentials include daydreaming, which can resemble an absence or complex partial seizure, but does not interrupt speech; staring, which can accompany gratification phenomena such as masturbation, sometimes with only subtle associated movements, and tics, which can suggest partial seizures: all can usually be distinguished by a careful history of the circumstances in which they occur.

Both complex partial seizures and absences can be accompanied by autonomic changes or automatisms. The more prolonged the absence, the more likely are automatisms (95% if >16 seconds), in which case it is called a 'complex absence'. Penry and colleagues[8] found that less than 10% of typical absences were 'simple', i.e. unaccompanied by other phenomena, which also include eyelid flutter, head turning, head nods or even loss of body posture.

Atypical absences are distinguished by EEG features, such as asymmetry, irregularity, or slower rhythms and mainly occur in Lennox-Gastaut syndrome and other severe epilepsies. Clinically, onset and recovery are also less abrupt.

## Generalised tonic-clonic seizures

Most unprovoked non febrile generalised tonic-clonic seizures in children are due to secondary generalisation. Mistakes are common if the onset is missed. An aura is characteristic of this seizure type and is caused by the simple partial seizure, which is remembered because consciousness is not lost until the secondary seizure begins. The aura may have localising value: psychic, olfactory, auditory and visceral phenomena are often temporal, while diffuse warm feelings, lightheadedness and dizziness are often frontal.[9] Similarly, a postictal Todd's palsy indicates a focal origin. The EEG may also show focal features. Primary generalised tonic-clonic seizures appear rare in isolation[10] and should prompt a search for other generalised seizure types, such as absences or myoclonic seizures. Unless these features are sought the underlying syndrome will be misdiagnosed.

Generalised tonic-clonic seizures are sometimes confused with tonic seizures, which can have an identical onset of stiffening, loss of posture, etc., and can be accompanied by tongue biting, incontinence, a rapid generalised tremor and/or a few myoclonic jerks.[3] In a generalised tonic-clonic seizure the clonic movements are less rapid than myoclonic jerks, increase in amplitude, and slow down during the fit.[2] The distinction is important because tonic seizures in otherwise normal children are much more likely to be non-epileptic. The most common cause is syncope, particularly reflex anoxic seizures.[3] Raised intracranial pressure ('hydrocephalic attacks') is another non-epileptic cause.

## Myoclonic, tonic and atonic seizures; 'drop attacks'

Clonic seizures comprise repetitive rhythmic jerking of part or all of the body, which do not decrease in amplitude as the frequency decreases. The ictal EEG often shows fast activity and slow waves but can show spike and wave patterns. Pure clonic seizures are rare and most isolated single or recurrent jerks are myoclonic. Myoclonic seizures are sudden brief shock-like contractions which can involve part or all of the body, even sometimes part of a muscle group, with polyspike and wave discharges on the ictal EEG. Massive myoclonus can throw the patient to the ground. Myoclonic seizures are an important component of juvenile myoclonic epilepsy, described below. Many of the myoclonic seizure disorders of early childhood, which are often difficult to treat, are also difficult to classify, while myoclonic seizures at all ages can be the presentation of certain metabolic and degenerative diseases.[2] Tonic seizures vary from minor stiffening with tonic upgaze, so that only the whites of the eyes are visible, and neck extension, possibly with respiratory arrest, to generalised rigidity and loss of posture, likened to a felled tree. Atonic seizures also vary from head nods to abrupt falls, typically into a sitting position or forwards, with facial injury. Both atonic and tonic seizures can be primary generalised, as in Lennox-Gastaut syndrome, or secondarily generalised from focal seizures. Drop attacks, therefore, can be due to any of these, as well as brain stem ischaemia, complicated migraine, and cataplexy.

## Unclassifiable seizures

The commonest diagnostic difficulty is the lack of a detailed description of the event, especially its onset, but this can be helped by video recording, in hospital or at home, possibly using a video camcorder lent by the clinician.[3] Interictal EEGs are another source of diagnostic error: in two series of normal children, spike foci were present in 1.9% and 2.4%, while generalised spike and wave occurred spontaneously in 1.2 % and increased with drowsiness or in response to photic stimulation to 8%.[11,12] Since less than 1% of children have epilepsy, interictal EEG changes must occur in children without epilepsy and are, therefore, not specific. In one of these studies, only 7 of the 131 children with EEG abnormalities went on to develop seizures on follow up.[11] By contrast, some epilepsies, especially focal, can be unaccompanied by any change on the surface EEG, due perhaps to a deep origin or to lack of activity during the 20 minute recording. Data are not available for children, but one group who repeated awake EEG recordings in adults with epilepsy found 15% were always normal, 50% intermittently abnormal and only 33% repeatedly abnormal.[13] Focal and other discharges are more easily elicited during sleep, with an 80% sensitivity.[13] The sensitivity of the EEG can also be increased by other techniques such as hyperventilation, intermittent photic stimulation, sleep deprivation or background suppression by intravenous diazepam. Even ictal recordings may not be helpful, especially when there is a deep seated focus, which may not show any changes at the surface or may only show non specific change such as rhythmic slow or attenuation of EEG activity.[2]

### Precipitated seizures

Seizures due to 'primary' syndromes can be precipitated by non specific events including fever, stress, fatigue, sleep deprivation, alcohol, or excitement. Thus breakthrough seizures due to these stimuli do not mean that control is poor and do not necessarily indicate a need to change drug treatment. Seizures may also be provoked by video games in people with several different epilepsy syndromes, where photic or pattern related stimuli result in partial or generalised seizures.[14]

## NEWLY RECOGNISED SEIZURE DISORDERS AND NEWLY RECOGNISED FEATURES OF KNOWN SEIZURE DISORDERS

During the 1980s there were concerted efforts to classify seizure disorders into syndromes, with the aims of allowing more accurate prognosis and treatment for patients and, eventually, understanding their causes. The 1989 ILAE syndromic classification (Table 9.2) is derived from this work.[15] Seizure types, age of onset, clinical, psychometric and other features, and the evolution of the condition all contribute to diagnosis. The major divisions are between focal and generalised epilepsies, and between idiopathic, symptomatic, i.e. lesional, and cryptogenic, i.e. suspected lesional origins. The term 'benign' only means that the seizure disorder usually remits spontaneously, irrespective of treatment. This can cause confusion, since some 'benign' epilepsies can still cause intractable seizures and can have a poor neurological and developmental prognosis.

As with any attempt to bring order to such a large variety of conditions, there are faults, such as its complexity with the inclusion of many rare syndromes, illogicalities (for example infantile spasms and Lennox-Gastaut syndrome are classified as symptomatic/cryptogenic generalised epilepsies but in fact can be of focal or generalised origin and can be idiopathic or lesional), and difficulties in defining some disorders, such as the myoclonic disorders of early childhood. New syndromes are being defined, such as benign infantile

**Table 9.2** Summary of the 1989 International League against Epilepsy classification of epilepsies and epilepsy syndromes

| | | | |
|---|---|---|---|
| *1* | *Localisation related (focal, local, partial) epilepsies and syndromes* | | |
| | 1.1 | Idiopathic | Benign childhood epilepsy with centrotemporal spikes<br>Childhood epilepsy with occipital paroxysms<br>Primary reading epilepsy |
| | 1.2 | Symptomatic | Chronic progressive epilepsia partialis (Kojewnikow's)<br>Syndromes characterised by seizures with specific modes of precipitation<br>Temporal lobe epilepsies<br>Frontal lobe epilepsies<br>Parietal lobe epilepsies<br>Occipital lobe epilepsies |
| | 1.3 | Cryptogenic | |
| *2* | *Generalised epilepsies and syndromes* | | |
| | 2.1 | Idiopathic | Benign neonatal familial convulsions<br>Benign neonatal convulsions<br>Benign myoclonic epilepsy in infancy<br>Childhood absence epilepsy (pyknolepsy)<br>Juvenile absence epilepsy<br>Juvenile myoclonic epilepsy<br>Epilepsy with GTCS on awakening<br>Other generalised idiopathic epilepsies not defined above<br>Epilepsies with seizures precipitated by specific modes of activation |
| | 2.2 | Cryptogenic or symptomatic | West syndrome (Infantile spasms)<br>Lennox-Gastaut syndrome<br>Epilepsy with myoclonic astatic seizures<br>Epilepsy with myoclonic absences |
| | 2.3 | Symptomatic | |
| | 2.3.1 | Non-specific etiology | Early myoclonic encephalopathy<br>Early infantile epileptic encephalopathy<br>Other symptomatic generalised epilepsies not defined above |
| | 2.3.2 | Specific syndromes* | |
| *3* | *Epilepsies and syndromes undetermined whether focal or generalised* | | |
| | 3.1 | With both generalised and focal features | Neonatal seizures<br>Severe myoclonic epilepsy in infancy<br>Epilepsy with continuous spike waves during slow sleep<br>Landau-Kleffner syndrome<br>Other undetermined epilepsies |
| | 3.2 | Without unequivocal generalised or focal features | |
| *4* | *Special syndromes* | | |
| | 4.1 | Situation related seizures | Febrile convulsions<br>Isolated seizures or isolated status epilepticus<br>Secondary to acute metabolic or toxic event |

Idiopathic: no known cause; symptomatic: known, often lesional, cause; cryptogenic: suspected but unproven symptomatic cause; benign: disorder with a high chance of spontaneous remission.
*Those conditions where seizures are a major or presenting feature, e.g. neurodegenerative disease, Angelman syndrome.

convulsions,[16] absences with eyelid myoclonus[17] and autosomal dominant frontal lobe seizures.[18] As the clinical and EEG features of many epilepsies evolve over months or years, early diagnosis can be imprecise. These and other difficulties mean that 35–43% of epilepsies in children and adults fall into special categories.[19,20]

## Localisation related syndromes (partial or focal origin)

At least half of all childhood seizures are of focal origin. The focus can be anywhere in the cortex, but more commonly the frontal or temporal lobes than parietal or occipital. It seems logical that clinical and EEG phenomena should allow localisation to precise cortical areas, as in the 1989 classification, which for example distinguishes seven different frontal syndromes,[15] but in practice this is overambitious: many patients have symptoms overlapping two or more areas, and in some the lesion of origin can be elsewhere, even on the opposite side.[20]

### *Idiopathic focal epilepsies: benign centrotemporal (Rolandic) seizures*

Benign centrotemporal or Rolandic seizures account for 24% of all seizure disorders beginning between 5 and 14 years.[21] Characteristically, seizures mainly occur in the early hours of the morning, begin with an odd sensation on one side of the mouth or throat followed by unilateral contractions of the face, oropharynx (causing odd noises) and arm, with inability to speak and drooling, and may become generalised. The presentation can be with nocturnal generalised tonic-clonic seizures, because the onset is not witnessed. There are typical interictal EEG spikes or spike waves over the centrotemporal regions. In spite of their benign long-term outcome, up to 20% can be resistant to treatment. Most patients only have rare attacks and 21% only have one.[22] Many children with typical EEG changes never have a reported attack. Symptoms usually only last a few years and almost all remit spontaneously by the early teens, although the EEG changes may persist for some years. Although the cause is unknown, there is a genetic contribution.

There are rarer idiopathic focal epilepsies. In benign occipital epilepsy, seizures with visual and other focal phenomena, migraine-like headaches and vomiting are associated with continuous high amplitude spike-wave activity over one or both occipital lobes on eye closure. In benign epilepsy with evoked parietal spikes, high voltage parietal EEG spikes evoked by tapping the foot, a feature present in 1% of normal children, are followed in some by version seizures. In atypical benign partial seizures, seizures reminiscent of benign centrotemporal epilepsy begin in early childhood and are followed by clusters of atonic seizures, possibly with generalised tonic-clonic seizures, absences, or partial motor seizures, more suggestive of Lennox-Gastaut syndrome, which are highly resistant to treatment and are associated with a very abnormal EEG during the clusters. All these still remit during childhood or adolescence.

*Lesional (symptomatic or cryptogenic)*

As well as mesial temporal sclerosis – whose origin is still controversial (see below, febrile fits) – the pathological causes of symptomatic localisation-related epilepsies include malformations, such as focal polymicrogyria; neuronal migration defects encompassing focal pachygyria, cortical dysplasia and heterotopia (nests of neurones in the white matter); hamartomas and tumours, including the recently defined DNET (dysembryoplastic neuroepithelial tumour, a benign slow growing neuroglial lesion), and several rarer conditions, such as chronic inflammation. Whether the epilepsy is 'symptomatic' or 'cryptogenic' depends on the investigation used: 25% of children with normal CT scans in one series had abnormalities on MRI.[23] While ideally every child with lesional epilepsy should have an MRI scan to define their pathology, in practice access to MRI is still limited and the results do not often affect management. MRI is only essential for focal epilepsies that are resistant to treatment, because such patients are worth considering for surgery or may have a tumour.

*Frontal lobe seizures*

Frontal seizures are increasingly recognised, especially in children, although some have been obvious for many years, such as focal motor clonic jerks with a Todd's palsy, or version of the head and eyes. More complex motor behaviour, such as dystonic posturing, particularly at night, or bilateral motor seizures without loss of consciousness can be mistaken for parasomnias or pseudoseizures. Autonomic phenomena can occur, suggesting involvement of the opercular area, where the frontal and temporal lobes touch: hence a gastric aura can be frontal or temporal. Secondary generalisation is common. Brief complex partial seizures of frontal origin can also be frequent, especially in the evening, and often have an abrupt beginning and end, without postictal confusion. The EEG distinguishes most but not all from generalised absences. Frontal foci can be too deep to be detected by a routine surface EEG, but the clinical features captured on video are a helpful diagnostic tool. There is little data on the outcome, but the chances of natural remission seem lower and the response to treatment, including surgery, less certain than in temporal lobe seizures.

*Treatment of localisation related epilepsies*

As therapy has no effect on the natural history of benign epilepsies, some authorities suggest that not all patients need prophylactic treatment, thus avoiding the risk of side effects. If required, both carbamazepine and valproate seem equally effective and to have an equal risk of side effects, but data are limited.[6]

In lesional epilepsies, it is our impression that carbamazepine may have an advantage over valproate, although this has only been demonstrated in adults.[24] Newer antiepileptic drugs, such as vigabatrin and lamotrigine, are effective second line add-on drugs, but neither can be recommended as first line agents in children until long-term safety data are available. Both are relatively nontoxic. Early indications are that lamotrigine causes less neurotoxicity than carbamazepine. Vigabatrin seems particularly effective in children with tuberose sclerosis, but behaviour problems can occur. Gabapentin is currently under trial but anecdotal reports also suggest it may be useful as an add-on agent. Phenytoin is now often considered a third line agent because of its side effects. The natural history suggests that once seizure control has been achieved for 2 years, a trial of drug withdrawal is justified. If seizures recur, a further trial of withdrawal at a later stage may still be worthwhile, although many will relapse.[25]

Surgery is worth considering for intractable seizures and is probably underused. In carefully selected patients, temporal lobe resection can result in up to 90% becoming seizure free or being substantially improved, although the initial response may decline after 5–10 years.[26] The only long-term study of 'temporal lobe' seizures, unfortunately undertaken before the benign Rolandic type was defined, suggests a third of children may spontaneously remit by 15 years of age,[27] so the timing of surgery should not be too early unless there is a good reason, such as a defined lesion or adverse effects on a child's development due to their seizure disorder. Less successful outcomes are seen after focal extra-temporal resections, but even so up to 60% may have similar benefits. Hemispherectomy is still very effective in some severe epilepsies and newer techniques, such as multiple subpial transections, are being evaluated.

## Generalised seizures

Idiopathic generalised seizures often have a major genetic component. The expression of both idiopathic and symptomatic seizures depends on cerebral maturity. An example is the possibility of a patient's epilepsy evolving with age from early infantile epileptic encephalopathy (Ohtahara syndrome) to infantile spasms and then to Lennox-Gastaut syndrome.

### *Absence epilepsies*

Absences occur in several disorders with different prognoses. Classic childhood absence epilepsy remains well defined, with typical clinical and EEG features. An early onset, before the age of 2 years, is now recognised.[28] Failure to induce absences in an untreated child by hyperventilation is generally considered to exclude the diagnosis. The prognosis in childhood absence epilepsy is not quite as benign as originally thought, in that while 50% remit by 13 years, 75% by 18 and nearly 100% by 30, up to 40% will develop generalised tonic-clonic seizures in their teens and the risk of doing so is inversely related to the age of onset. Typical absences starting in the teen years (juvenile absence epilepsy) are less frequent, less sensitive to hyperventilation, and have a poorer prognosis. There is controversy over whether juvenile absence epilepsy is just childhood absence epilepsy with a later onset or a separate syndrome. The risk of later generalised tonic-clonic seizures is also increased by the presence of photosensitivity and the absence of slow posterior rhythms on the EEG.[7] Valproate and ethosuximide are drugs of first choice, but lamotrigine may also be effective. In view of the natural history, drug treatment should be continued until the early teens in most children.

Myoclonic absence epilepsy associates typical absences, with characteristic EEG findings, with marked myoclonic jerks. Seizures are resistant to treatment, persist into late childhood and the intellectual outcome is poor. Treatment has relied on valproate and ethosuximide in combination, although recently lamotrigine has been shown to be effective.[29] Absences with eyelid myoclonus, where the eyes deviate upwards with marked myoclonic fluttering of the eyelids and photosensitivity is often present, are also less responsive to therapy and may persist into adulthood.[17] Juvenile myoclonic epilepsy can also present with childhood absences, but has a very different prognosis from childhood absence epilepsy.

### *Juvenile myoclonic epilepsy*

Juvenile myoclonic epilepsy is a well defined syndrome, causing 4–11% of childhood and adult epilepsies overall, and a higher percentage of idiopathic generalised seizures. Onset can be with absences, at a mean age of 10 years, but as young as 5 years.[30] In teenage years, the commonest presentation is with generalised tonic-clonic seizures in the early morning. Single or multiple myoclonic jerks of the arms after waking, typically causing spilling or dropping of objects ('cup of tea epilepsy'), are characteristic, but often will not be revealed except by direct questioning. The EEG shows generalised spike– or polyspike– wave and up to 40% are photosensitive. Sleep deprivation both provokes attacks and can be used before EEG recordings to increase their sensitivity. This syndrome appears lifelong. If treatment is stopped, 92% relapse within 2 years.[31] Late nights, alcohol, exam stress, and strobe disco lights are all precipitants that should ideally be avoided, often unrealistic advice in this age group! Because of the prognosis and the age of onset, many patients choose to continue treatment to retain a driving licence. There is a strong familial component, with up to 25% of relatives affected by other generalised seizure syndromes and an as yet unproved link to the HLA locus on chromosome 6. Seizures are usually well controlled by valproate; phenytoin and phenobarbitone have been recommended and the effect of lamotrigine is being assessed. Carbamazepine is ineffective and may even worsen seizures – illustrating that treatment should be tailored to syndromes, and that routine prescription of carbamazepine to all patients presenting with generalised tonic-clonic seizures is inadvisable.

*Infantile spasms*

Despite the 1989 classification, infantile spasms are probably best looked upon as a separate seizure type that is not restricted to infancy.[32] Typically, there are both myoclonic (the initial lightening posture change) and tonic (spasm) components. Classically the upper body flexes, with flexion or extension of the legs, but extensor and asymmetric spasms also occur and are more suggestive of a symptomatic cause. Partial seizures occurred in 40% of patients who had 24-hour EEG monitoring and again suggest a lesional cause with a poor outcome; sometimes a series of spasms follows a partial onset.[33] Subtle variants, including upward deviation or adduction of the eyes, grimacing and yawning can also represent seizures. Spasms particularly appear on falling asleep and waking. Hypsarrhythmia is only present in 66% of routine EEGs. Ideally, EEG should include both a sleeping and an awake study: episodes can be captured on awakening, hypsarrhythmia patterns often change in sleep and in some hypsarrhythmia only appears in sleep. The absence of sleep spindles is an ominous feature. Symptomatic spasms are suggested by 'atypical hypsarrhythmia' or focal features: the latter can be revealed at the end of a recording after suppression of hypsarrhythmia by intravenous diazepam.

With improved imaging, an increasing number of causes are being described: structural abnormalities form the largest group, including malformations (e.g. Aicardi syndrome), neuronal migration defects (e.g. laminar heterotopia), tuberous sclerosis and other lesions (e.g. post infarct). Metabolic, chromosomal (Down syndrome) and acquired injuries, e.g. post asphyxial, form the bulk of the remainder. The PEHO syndrome, comprising Progressive encephalopathy with Edema, Hypsarrhythmia and Optic atrophy, is a recent addition.[34] All are associated with a poor outlook for seizure control and for developmental progress. A small number of patients with refractory spasms and normal MRI scans have focal changes on PET (positron emission tomography) scans, representing areas of cortical dysplasia, and their seizures may respond to surgery, though any possible benefit on development is unknown.[35]

A better prognosis has always been recognised in the idiopathic group, but some suggest that this is a subgroup best identified by the reappearance of hypsarrhythmia between each spasm during a cluster, unlike the usual pattern where it is suppressed.[32] Those associated with neurofibromatosis may also do well.[32]

It is, therefore, no longer enough to simply diagnose infantile spasms and start treatment with steroids. All cases should be investigated for a cause. As the outlook in symptomatic cases is poor whatever drug is used, alternative agents without the side effects of steroids seem preferable if effective. Vigabatrin is now often used as a first line treatment of spasms due to tuberous sclerosis and possibly other lesional causes.[2] A Japanese group has found that seizures and hypsarrhythmia stopped within a week of starting oral pyridoxine in doses of 100–400 mg/day in up to 13% of symptomatic and 28% of idiopathic cases.[36] This needs confirmation in other studies, but a trial of pyridoxine seems worthwhile, if only to exclude the rare cases due to pyridoxine dependency. Steroids are still frequently necessary, but the best formulation and dosage regimen is unclear:[2] in symptomatic cases, a short course of oral prednisolone can be effective, followed by high dose valproate and/or benzodiazepines. Longer courses do not seem to have any advantage. The importance of early treatment is also now questioned, especially since the outcome, including sequelae such as autism, depends so much on cause.[2,37]

## Febrile convulsions

The natural history of febrile convulsions has been defined by several epidemiological studies, which have produced two separate but overlapping sets of risk factors, one for further convulsions in subsequent febrile illnesses and the other for the development of later epilepsy. The risk of recurrent febrile convulsions has been quantified at 12% with no risk factors; 50% if the onset is before 16 months, or if a first degree relative has had seizures of any sort, and 75–100% if three or more of the following factors are present: onset before 16 months, first degree relative affected, complex seizures, neurodevelopmental problems and adverse social circumstances.

Neurologically normal children with simple febrile convulsions have a low chance of later epilepsy: only 2.5% have had two or more afebrile seizures by 25 years of age. Complex seizures are risk factors for later epilepsy: prolonged (> 15 minutes), repeated (in the same illness) or focal seizure increases the risk to 7% and all three (present in only 1% of children with febrile convulsions) to 50%.[38,39] Focal febrile convulsions are also associated with an increased risk of late partial seizures.[38,39] Although there is a clear, though rare, association between febrile convulsions and later often refractory partial seizures due to mesial temporal sclerosis, that one causes the other has still not been proved: there are arguments that patients with febrile convulsions are already an abnormal population.[38] While uncertainty persists it seems reasonable to try to prevent prolonged seizures, usually by parents or carers giving rectal diazepam, but there is no evidence that continuous prophylactic antiepileptic therapy affects the long-term outcome.

## KEY POINTS FOR CLINICAL PRACTICE

- Seizures are symptomatic of an underlying disorder which may or may not be epileptic.
- Using the 1981 classification, diagnose the seizure type(s), if possible, as partial (simple or complex), secondary generalised, absence (typical or atypical), myoclonic, tonic, atonic and/or generalised tonic-clonic. Avoid the terms grand mal and petit mal.

- Complex partial seizures and generalised absence seizures can be confused, but most are distinguished by clinical and, particularly, EEG features.
- Tonic seizures are rarely epileptic in normal children and should raise suspicion of syncope or anoxia.
- Generalised tonic-clonic seizures are often secondarily generalised from a partial focus; an aura or a postictal hemiparesis should suggest this possibility.
- Drop attacks may be myoclonic, tonic or atonic seizures, or non-epileptic.
- The EEG helps to classify seizures but is not able to confirm or exclude epilepsy.
- Once seizure types are defined, attempt to diagnose the underlying epilepsy syndrome, using the 1989 classification.
- Benign partial seizures are very common and may not need antiepileptic prophylaxis.
- Not all partial seizures originate from the temporal lobe: frontal lobe seizures are increasingly recognised in children.
- Generalised absence seizures occur in several syndromes with very different prognoses.
- Juvenile myoclonic epilepsy is relatively common and implies a need for lifelong treatment; carbamazepine is contra-indicated.
- Infantile spasms are heterogeneous in aetiology, seizure type and prognosis. Steroids are not always the treatment of first choice.
- Later epilepsy is rare after simple febrile convulsions. The nature of the association with mesial temporal sclerosis is still unclear.
- Tailor the decision to start treatment, the choice of which treatment and when to stop treatment to the epilepsy syndrome.

## REFERENCES

1 Commission on Classification and Terminology of the International League against Epilepsy. Proposal for revised clinical and electroencephalographic classification of epileptic seizures. Epilepsia 1981; 22: 489-501

2 Aicardi J. Epilepsy in Children. New York: Raven Press 2nd edn 1994
3 Stephenson JBP. Fits and faints. Clinics in Developmental Medicine No 109. Oxford: MacKeith Press, 1990
4 Luders HO, Burgess R, Noachtar S. Expanding the International Classification of Seizures to provide localisation information. Neurology 1993; 43: 1650-1655
5 Stefan H. Personal communication, 1994
6 Verity CM, Hosking G, Easter DJ. A multicentre comparative trial of sodium valproate and carbamazepine in paediatric epilepsy. Dev Med Child Neurol 1995; 37: 97-108
7 Loiseau P, Pestre M, Dartigues JF, Commenges D, Barberger-Gateau C, Cohadon S. Long-term prognosis in two forms of childhood epilepsy: typical absence seizures and epilepsy with Rolandic (centrotemporal) EEG foci. Ann Neurol 1983; 13: 642-648
8 Penry JK, Porter RJ, Dreifuss FE. Simultaneous recording of absence seizures with video tape and electroencephalography. A study of 374 seizures in 48 patients. Brain 1975; 98: 427-440
9 Palmini A, Gloor P. The localising value of auras in partial seizures: a prospective and retrospective study. Neurology 1992; 42: 801-808
10 Oller-Daurella L, Oller LF-V. Epilepsy with generalised tonic-clonic seizures in childhood. Does a childhood 'grand mal' syndrome exist? In: Roger J, Bureau M, Dravet Ch, Dreifuss FE, Perret A, Wolf P, eds. Epileptic syndromes in infancy, childhood and adolescence. London: John Libbey, 2nd edn 1992: 161-171
11 Cavazzuti GB, Capella L, Nalin A. Longitudinal study of epileptiform EEG patterns in normal children. Epilepsia 1980; 21: 43-55
12 Eeg-Olofsson O, Petersen I, Sellden U. The development of the electroencephalogram in normal children from the age of 1 through 15 years: paroxysmal activity. Neuropädiatrie 1971; 2: 375-404
13 Binnie CD. Neurophysiological investigation of epilepsy in children. In: Ross EM, Woody RC, eds. Epilepsy. Baillieres Clinical Paediatrics 1994; 2: 585-604
14 Kasteleijn-Nolst Trenite DGA. Video-game epilepsy. Lancet 1994; 344: 1102-1103
15 Commission on Classification and Terminology of the International League against Epilepsy. Proposal for revised classification of epilepsies and epileptic syndromes. Epilepsia 1989; 30: 389-399
16 Lee WL, Low PS, Rajan U. Benign familial infantile epilepsy. J Pediatr 1993; 123: 588-590
17 Panayiotopoulos CP. Fixation off sensitive epilepsy in eyelid myoclonia with absence seizures. Ann Neurol 1987; 22: 87-89
18 Scheffer IE, Bhatia D, Lopes-Cendes I et al. Autosomal dominant frontal lobe epilepsy misdiagnosed as sleep disorder. Lancet 1994; 343: 515-517
19 Furune S, Yasui I, Matsumoto A et al. Classification of epilepsies and epileptic syndromes in young children. Jpn J Psychiatr Neurol 1993; 47: 312-314
20 Manford M, Hart YM, Sander JWAS, Shorvon SD. The National General Practice Study of Epilepsy. The syndromic classification of the International League against Epilepsy applied to epilepsy in a general population. Arch Neurol 1992; 49: 801-808
21 Cavazzuti CB. Epidemiology of different types of epilepsy in school age children in Modena, Italy. Epilepsia 1980; 21: 57-62
22 Loiseau P, Duche B, Cordova S, Dartigues JF, Cohadon S. Prognosis of benign childhood epilepsy with centro-temporal spikes: a follow up study of 168 patients. Epilepsia 1988; 29: 229-235
23 Adams C, Hwang PA, Gilday PL, Armstrong DC, Becker LE, Hoffman HJ. Comparison of SPECT, EEG, CT, MRI and pathology in partial epilepsy. Pediatr Neurol 1992; 8: 97-103
24 Mattson RH, Cramer JA, Collins JF. A comparison of valproate with carbamazepine for the treatment of complex partial seizures and secondarily generalised tonic-clonic seizures in adults. N Engl J Med 1992; 327: 765-771
25 Shinnar S, Berg AT, Moshe SL et al. Discontinuing antiepileptic drugs in children with epilepsy: a prospective study. Ann Neurol 1994; 35: 534-545
26 Engel J. Outcome with respect to epileptic seizures. In: Engel J, ed. Surgical treatment of the epilepsies.New York: Raven Press 1987: 553-571
27 Ounsted C, Lindsay J, Richards P. Temporal lobe epilepsy. A biographical study. London: MacKeith Press 1987
28 Cavazzuti GB, Ferrari F, Galli V, Benatti A. Epilepsy with typical absence seizures with onset in the first year of life. Epilepsia 1989; 30: 802-806

29 Manonmani V, Wallace SJ. Epilepsy with myoclonic absences. Arch Dis Child 1994; 70: 288-290
30 Panayiotopoulos CP, Obeid T, Waheed G. Absences in juvenile myoclonic epilepsy: a clinical and video-electroencephalographic study. Ann Neurol 1989; 25: 391-397
31 Penry JK, Dean JC, Riela AR. Juvenile myoclonic epilepsy: long term response to therapy. Epilepsia 1989; 20 (suppl 4): S19-S23
32 Commission on Pediatric Epilepsy of the International League against Epilepsy. Workshop on infantile spasms. Epilepsia 1992; 33: 195
33 Plouin P, Dulac O, Jalin C, Chiron C. Twenty four hour ambulatory EEG monitoring in infantile spasms. Epilepsia 1993; 34: 686-691
34 Somer M, Sainio K. Epilepsy and the electroencephalogram in progressive encephalopathy with edema, hypsarrhythmia and optic atrophy (the PEHO syndrome). Epilepsia 1993; 34: 727-731
35 Chugani HT, Shields WD, Shewmon DA, Olson DM, Phelps ME, Peacock WJ. Infantile spasms: 1. PET identifies focal cortical dysgenesis in cryptogenic cases for surgical treatment. Ann Neurol 1990; 27: 406-413
36 Ohtahara S, Ohtsuka Y, Yamatogi Y, Oka E, Yoshinaga H, Sato M. Prenatal etiologies of West syndrome. Epilepsia 1993; 34: 716-722
37 Jambaque I, Cusmai R, Curatolo P, Cortesi F, Perrot C, Dulac O. Neuropsychological aspects of tuberous sclerosis in relation to epilepsy and MRI findings. Dev Med Child Neurol 1991; 33: 698-705
38 Annegers JF, Hauser WA, Shirts SB, Kurland LT. Factors prognostic of unprovoked seizures after febrile convulsions. N Engl J Med 1987; 316: 493-498
39 Verity CM, Golding J. Risk of epilepsy after febrile convulsions: a national cohort study. BMJ 1991; 303: 1373-1376

# 10

# Growth and endocrine sequelae following treatment of childhood cancer

*S. M. Shalet*

Over the last three decades there has been a substantial and significant improvement in survival from most forms of childhood cancer.[1,2] For example, the 5-year survival rate for childhood lymphoblastic leukaemia between 1954–1962 was 2% but has risen steadily to reach 61% between 1981–1989 (Table 10.1). Consequently, the number of long-term survivors has increased exponentially such that it has been estimated that, by the year 2000, at least one in a 1000 young adults in the general population will be a survivor of childhood cancer.

The major modalities of treatment are surgery, radiotherapy and cytotoxic chemotherapy. The long-term complications of treatment include growth disturbance, delayed or precocious puberty, induction of endocrine tumours, infertility and a variety of endocrine deficiency states. Virtually all of the endocrine complications described in this review are a consequence of irradiation and/or chemotherapy but, depending on the anatomical site within the body, the tumour itself or surgery may cause endocrine pathophysiology. This review concentrates on endocrine sequelae arising from the treatment of two of the commonest forms of childhood malignancy, brain tumours and acute lymphoblastic leukaemia.

**Table 10.1** Leukaemia, lymphoma and central nervous system tumours. Trends in survival in the north west of England (Blair & Birch, unpublished) by time period of diagnosis

| Diagnosis | 5 year survival rate (%) 1954–62 | 1963-71 | 1972-80 | 1981-89 | Log-rank trend test *P* value |
|---|---|---|---|---|---|
| Acute lymphocytic leukaemia | 2 | 13 | 40 | 61 | < 0.0001 |
| Acute non-lymphocytic leukaemia | 2 | 2 | 16 | 22 | < 0.0001 |
| Hodgkin's disease | 52 | 54 | 83 | 91 | < 0.0001 |
| Non-Hodgkin's lymphoma | 14 | 20 | 35 | 70 | < 0.0001 |
| Ependymoma | 21 | 23 | 22 | 45 | 0.03 |
| Adult astrocytoma | 6 | 15 | 20 | 58 | 0.0001 |
| Juvenile astrocytoma | 64 | 76 | 78 | 92 | 0.01 |
| Medulloblastoma | 24 | 37 | 40 | 51 | 0.001 |

## BRAIN TUMOURS

### Growth impairment

Short stature is a common complication after treatment of brain tumours, such as medulloblastoma, glioma and ependymoma, in childhood. The treatment of these tumours may include neurosurgery, cranial or craniospinal irradiation and chemotherapy. A number of adverse factors may influence the final height achieved by these patients: these include radiation-induced growth hormone deficiency, impaired spinal growth, precocious puberty, chemotherapy, malnutrition and the presence of occult tumour.

### Growth hormone deficiency

Irradiation of the hypothalamic-pituitary axis may produce a range of pituitary hormone deficiencies from isolated growth hormone (GH) deficiency to panhypopituitarism. GH is always the first of the six anterior pituitary hormones to be affected by radiation damage. The degree of pituitary hormonal deficit is related to the radiation dose received by the hypothalamic-pituitary axis, thus after lower radiation doses, isolated GH deficiency ensues, whilst higher doses may produce panhypopituitarism. The greater the radiation dose the earlier GH deficiency will develop after treatment.[3]

There is clear evidence that the hypothalamus is more radiosensitive than the pituitary and, therefore, the primary pathophysiological defect in these children is a disturbance in the neuroregulatory control of GH secretion rather than inadequate GH production from the pituitary.[3]

### Spinal growth

Spinal growth is impaired in those children who have received craniospinal irradiation as part of their treatment[4] and the spinal growth pattern remains unaltered in response to GH therapy. The younger the child at the time of craniospinal irradiation, the greater the loss in growth potential, such that children irradiated at the age of 1 year lose at least 9 cm from their final height.[4] Most of the impairment in spinal growth occurs during puberty, irrespective of the age at which irradiation was administered.

### Precocious puberty

In children irradiated for brain tumours with fields which include a radiation dose to the hypothalamic-pituitary axis in the region of 2500–4700 cGy (1 cGy = 1 rad), the onset of puberty occurs at an early age in both sexes (mean 8.5 years in girls and 9.2 years in boys, plus 0.3 years for every year of age at irradiation[5]). In the context of GH deficiency which, in the isolated idiopathic form, is usually associated with a delay in the onset of puberty, this is abnormal. There is a significant linear association between the age at irradiation and age at onset of puberty in both sexes.[5] At each age of irradiation the estimated age of onset of puberty is approximately 0.7 years earlier in girls than in boys. A similar trend is seen for bone age, which is abnormally early at the time of pubertal onset.

The impact of early puberty in a child with radiation-induced growth failure is to foreshorten the time available for GH therapy. Consequently a number of these children are now treated with a combination of a gonadotrophin releasing hormone (GnRH) analogue, which effectively induces a reversible 'castrate' state medically, and GH therapy. It is relatively easy to halt the progression in pubertal development, but it is too early to analyse the impact of this approach on final height.

### Growth hormone therapy

In children with radiation-induced GH deficiency, GH therapy increases growth velocity and improves final height compared with those who remain untreated. Final height is significantly less than mid-parental height, however, and both spinal irradiation and chemotherapy have a marked effect on growth, which is not overcome with the use of GH replacement therapy in current dosage.[6] In those children who receive craniospinal irradiation, the gain in final height attributable to GH therapy is at the expense of increased skeletal disproportion.

The chances of recurrence of a brain tumour are greatest within 2 years of the primary treatment of the tumour. No evidence exists that GH treatment increases recurrence rates of brain tumours in children with radiation-induced GH deficiency.[7] A reasonable approach, therefore, 2 years after treatment, is to consider the possible need for GH therapy for children with brain tumours treated by standard radiation schedules, including a dose to the hypothalamic-pituitary axis in excess of 3000 cGy. At this time, cytotoxic chemotherapy is completed, the chance of tumour recurrence is low and it has been established that most patients will be GH deficient. In some centres, endocrinologists offer GH therapy routinely at 2 years without recourse to GH tests or evidence of impaired growth. In other centres, endocrinologists insist on biochemical evidence of GH deficiency and a subnormal growth rate.

In practice, our management attempts to match the timing of the introduction of GH therapy with the special circumstances, age, pubertal status and needs of the individual. Early treatment with GH replacement is particularly suitable for the craniospinally-treated child of short parents in whom the growth prognosis is especially poor.

### Thyroid dysfunction

In children receiving craniospinal radiotherapy, the spinal fields of irradiation will necessitate a significant radiation dose reaching the thyroid gland. Subsequent impairment of thyroid function may range from frank hypothyroidism, with an increased serum thyroid stimulating hormone (TSH) concentration and a subnormal serum thyroxine concentration, to subtle disturbance with an increased TSH concentration but normal thyroxine concentration. As expected, there is a significantly increased incidence of thyroid dysfunction after craniospinal irradiation compared with that seen after cranial irradiation. Interestingly, however, there is a significant increase in the incidence of thyroid dysfunction attributable to the adjuvant cytotoxic chemotherapy received by many children treated for brain tumours. Thus both radiation and cytotoxic chemotherapy may damage the thyroid gland.[8, 9]

Obviously, the frankly hypothyroid child requires thyroxine replacement therapy. Similarly, the child with a raised TSH level and a normal thyroxine level should also receive thyroxine replacement. A raised TSH level in a child with an irradiated thyroid gland is of potential carcinogenic importance and, therefore, should be lowered into the normal range. Furthermore, in a child whose growth may be compromised for many reasons, thyroid function should be rendered completely normal.

## Gonadal function

The impact of combination cytotoxic chemotherapy on gonadal function is dependent on the nature and dosage of the drugs received by the child. Drugs that have been shown to cause gonadal damage include the alkylating agents, such as cyclophosphamide, chlorambucil and the nitrosoureas, in addition to procarbazine, vinblastine, cytosine arabinoside and cisplatinum.

It is known that the normal adult testis is extremely sensitive to the effects of external irradiation. However, neither the threshold dose of irradiation required to damage the germinal epithelium in childhood, nor the dose above which irreversible damage occurs, is known. In irradiated girls, the response of the ovary involves a fixed pool of oocytes which once destroyed cannot be replaced. The $LD_{50}$ (the radiation dose causing the death of 50% of cells) for the human oocyte has recently been estimated not to exceed 400 cGy.[10]

The germinal epithelium of the testis is far more vulnerable than the Leydig cells to cytotoxic-induced damage. Thus, in the adolescent boy, puberty is usually completed spontaneously but the testes are pathologically small for the stage of puberty. In girls, fertility prospects are less frequently affected than in boys by cytotoxic-induced damage but if severe ovarian damage has occurred then steroidogenesis as well as fertility is likely to be affected and hormone replacement therapy will be required.

It used to be thought that the prepubertal testis was less vulnerable than the pubertal testis to cytotoxic-induced damage. This has never been confirmed but it is now clear that the testicular germinal epithelium of both prepubertal and pubertal boys may be irreversibly obliterated by gonadotoxic chemotherapy or irradiation.

Both the adjuvant cytotoxic chemotherapy and the spinal fields of irradiation may damage the gonads in children treated for brain tumours. Long-term follow-up in 50 children previously treated for brain tumours with surgery followed by postoperative cranial or craniospinal irradiation and chemotherapy with a nitrosourea, carmustine [BCNU] or lomustine [CCNU], with or without procarbazine has shown that there is a high prevalence of primary gonadal dysfunction.[11,12] Furthermore, from these studies, it is clear that cytotoxic chemotherapy alone is capable of causing gonadal damage.

Both sexes progressed through puberty normally, with consistently raised basal concentrations of follicle-stimulating hormone (FSH) and, occasionally, increased concentrations of luteinizing hormone (LH). The girls achieved menarche at an appropriate age. As adults, most of the boys had inappropriately small testicular volumes, which are likely to be associated with severe oligospermia or azoospermia, and infertility. A sex difference in the reversibility of damage was observed.[11,12] The boys showed no evidence of recovery of germinal epithelial function and no deterioration in Leydig cell function in a follow-up extended to 11 years. In contrast, several girls who had previously been shown to have ovarian damage, have continued with regular menses and normal FSH and oestradiol concentrations. Although it was not known whether these cycles were ovulatory, it is likely that these girls had recovered from the ovarian damage. The prospect of fertility among such girls is good in the early child-bearing years, however, a premature menopause remains a possibility. Many of these children also received spinal irradiation, which results in a scattered irradiation dose to the gonad. In the boys, this results in a small dose to the testis estimated at 46–120 cGy (following a fractionated course of radiotherapy delivering a total dose of 3500 cGy to the whole spine in the Manchester centre). This small radiation dose is likely to contribute to the observed testicular damage. At other centres, individual boys who were treated with craniospinal irradiation but no chemotherapy have developed testicular dysfunction, however, the scattered testicular irradiation dose is unknown.

In girls, the dose of irradiation received by the ovary may show greater variation. In the Manchester centre, a total dose in the range 90–1000 cGy has been estimated to reach the ovaries. The position of the ovaries in relation to the spinal field, and therefore the radiation dose received, can be difficult to estimate as the ovaries are mobile and their position may vary throughout the course of treatment. Nonetheless, the radiation dose received may contribute appreciably to ovarian dysfunction and this may be irreversible.

The scattered dose to the ovary will vary depending on the radiotherapy technique used at different centres. In a large study of gonadal dysfunction following treatment of intracranial tumours, 18 of 42 girls (43%) showed evidence of primary ovarian dysfunction.[13] Seven out of 11 girls who received craniospinal irradiation but no chemotherapy, and 9 out of 14 who had both craniospinal radiotherapy and adjuvant chemotherapy, showed evidence of ovarian dysfunction. The latter results suggest that at that centre,[13] spinal irradiation was the dominant gonadotoxic treatment. Hence, the individual contributions of spinal irradiation and cytotoxic chemotherapy to ovarian damage following the treatment of intracranial tumours will vary depending on the radiotherapy techniques used and the nature of the adjuvant chemotherapy.

## ACUTE LYMPHOBLASTIC LEUKAEMIA

### Growth

Traditionally, children with acute lymphoblastic leukaemia have been treated with combination chemotherapy and cranial irradiation as CNS prophylaxis. Before 1981, most children received a cranial irradiation dose of 2100–2500 cGy. After 1981, the standard prophylactic dose of cranial irradiation was reduced to 1800 cGy and the current UK protocol does not include routine cranial irradiation as prophylaxis.

It is now almost universally agreed that both the above doses of cranial irradiation are capable of adversely affecting GH secretion. It is also believed that, in children who have received either dose of cranial irradiation, there is significant standing height loss and reduced final height.[14] Interpretation of the exact contribution of GH insufficiency to the growth disturbance is complicated by the clear evidence that chemotherapy itself may affect growth adversely.[15–17]

Recent studies have shown that despite not receiving spinal irradiation, not only is final height reduced but marked disproportion is present in 23% (shorter back than legs) of long-term survivors.[14] GH deficiency per se does not cause skeletal disproportion, however, and it is possible that the disproportion is related to chemotherapy. The spine contains large numbers of epiphyses and if chemotherapy has a direct effect on the epiphysial growth plate it seems likely that this might result in greater loss in sitting height than leg length.

The clinical dilemma is how to identify the few children who should receive GH therapy. In the presence of biochemical evidence of GH deficiency those children who are below the tenth centile or whose growth rate is persistently poor after completion of cytotoxic chemotherapy should be considered for a therapeutic trial of GH. It should be understood however that this is an arbitrary definition of GH requirement.

### Obesity

In addition to the reduced stature at final height, body composition is altered in young adult survivors of acute lymphoblastic leukaemia in childhood. Defining obesity as a body mass index (BMI) greater than the 85th centile of the normal population, 23 out of 51 boys (45%) and 30 out of 63 girls (47%) were obese at final height.[18] There was no correlation between any of the auxological parameters of growth and BMI. Thus, approximately 50% of survivors of acute lymphoblastic leukaemia become obese young adults regardless of sex.[18] The obesity does not appear to be due to GH deficiency or early puberty.

## Reproductive axis

Unlike the situation in children irradiated for brain tumours in whom early puberty may occur with equal frequency in either sex, girls but not boys irradiated prophylactically for acute lymphoblastic leukaemia are more likely to undergo puberty early.[19, 20] The probable explanation for sexual dichotomy is the cranial radiation dose. The dose of cranial irradiation employed in the treatment of acute lymphoblastic leukaemia ranged between 1800–2400 cGy compared with the higher irradiation dose of 2500–4700 cGy used to treat childhood brain tumours. The exact reason for the greater vulnerability of the female brain to radiation-induced early puberty is unknown but then idiopathic central precocious puberty is a phenomenon seen almost entirely in girls.

## Combination chemotherapy and the testis

Lendon et al[21] studied testicular histology in 44 boys treated with combination chemotherapy for acute lymphoblastic leukaemia. Based on a count of at least 100 cross-sections of tubules per biopsy, the tubular fertility index (TFI) was calculated as the percentage of seminiferous tubules containing identifiable spermatogonia. The mean TFI in the 44 biopsies was 50% of that in age-matched controls and 18 of the biopsies showed a severely depressed TFI of 40% or less. Previous chemotherapy with cyclophosphamide or cytosine arabinoside (total dose > $1 g/m^2$) depressed the TFI, whereas with increasing time after completion of chemotherapy the TFI improved.

Testicular function was studied in the 44 boys participating in the testicular histology study.[22] Normal Leydig cell function, as assessed by the testosterone response to human chorionic gonadotrophin (HCG), was observed with abnormalities of FSH secretion, consistent with germ cell damage, in the pubertal boys. In this study, all the boys achieved normal adult secondary sex characteristics subsequently and had a serum testosterone concentration within the normal adult range consistent with normal Leydig cell function.[22]

Supportive evidence of germ cell damage in 25 leukaemic boys was seen following chemotherapy with a more intensive schedule that consisted of ten cytotoxic agents including cyclophosphamide and cytosine arabinoside, given for three or four years. In 24 testicular biopsies assessed at the time of completion of chemotherapy, there was an absence of germ cells in 13 and in the remaining 11, the germ cells were markedly depleted.[23]

To assess the reversibility of documented germ cell damage after chemotherapy for ALL in childhood, our group has studied testicular function in 37 male long-term survivors.[24] This study was conducted at two separate time points; initially a wedge testicular biopsy was performed at or near completion of chemotherapy to assess the incidence of occult testicular relapse. The TFI was calculated as described earlier, and subsequently, at a median time of 10.7 years after stopping chemotherapy, the patients were reassessed by clinical examination, measurement of gonadotrophins and testosterone levels and, in 19, by semen analysis. The median TFI for all 37 biopsies was 74% and at reassessment six men had evidence of severe damage to the germinal epithelium. Five of these men had azoospermia and one, who did not provide semen for analysis, had a reduced mean testicular volume and a raised basal FSH level consistent with severe germ cell damage.[24]

Of 11 males who had a TFI less than 50% at testicular biopsy, five recovered normal germ cell function at a median of 10.1 years after completing chemotherapy. 23 of the 26 males who had a TFI greater than 50%, showed completely normal testicular function when reassessed subsequently, and in the remaining three men the results were inconclusive. Clearly, with increasing time after completion of treatment, germ cell function can improve so that normal fertility may be a possibility for some patients who have sustained damage to the germinal epithelium.[24] Nonetheless, the long-term prognosis for fertility may remain poor for at least 10 years in those most severely affected.

## Combined chemotherapy and the ovary

Ovarian damage following combination chemotherapy for acute lymphoblastic leukaemia has been reported only rarely. In contrast, morphological studies have shown that the ovaries from girls treated for acute lymphoblastic leukaemia between one and 12 years of age and studied 1 week to 4 years after diagnosis, demonstrated inhibition of follicular development.[25] The girls, who had received chemotherapy for only a short period of time, had normal ovaries with ample follicular growth and many small non-growing follicles. This implied that cytotoxic drugs rather than the disease itself had disrupted ovarian morphology.[25]

To evaluate ovarian function and pregnancy outcome after treatment of acute lymphoblastic leukaemia, Green et al[26] reported 27 pregnancies in 12 out of 39 women who had been treated for ALL during childhood or adolescence. There were four spontaneous abortions, one stillbirth, and 22 liveborn infants. Two of the liveborn infants had congenital anomalies (one heart murmur; one epidermal naevus) and none of the children (ages 1 month to 10 years) had developed childhood cancer.[26]

Two studies emphasise that the prevalence of ovarian dysfunction partly reflects the length of follow-up. Quigley et al[23] described a high incidence of ovarian damage in 20 girls treated with a rather intensive schedule consisting of ten cytotoxic drugs, including cyclophosphamide and cytosine arabinoside, given for 3 or 4 years. Basal and peak FSH levels after administration of GnRH were significantly higher in both the prepubertal and pubertal girls than in the comparable control groups. Despite clear evidence of primary ovarian damage, none of the girls had a delay in reaching puberty and, indeed as pointed out earlier, puberty occurred rather earlier than in normal contemporaries.[23]

A more long-term study of ovarian function in 40 women, who had remained in first remission following combination chemotherapy for childhood leukaemia over 10 years earlier, showed encouraging results.[27] All achieved adult sexual development and 37 had regular menses. Ten patients had 14 live births and evidence of ovulation was obtained in a further 11 patients. Four showed biochemical evidence of ovarian damage, three of whom received craniospinal irradiation and one cyclophosphamide. Thus, the long-term outlook for ovarian function is good for the majority of childhood acute lymphoblastic leukaemia survivors.[27] A premature menopause, however, remains a possibility if significant follicular depletion has occurred at the time of cytotoxic treatment.

### Testicular irradiation

Brauner et al[28] studied 12 boys with acute lymphoblastic leukaemia who had received direct testicular irradiation (2400 Gy in 12 fractions over 18 days) between 10 months and 8.5 years earlier for a testicular relapse (in nine) and as testicular prophylaxis (in three). Leydig cell dysfunction, manifested by a low or absent testosterone response to HCG, or an increased basal level of plasma LH or both, was present in 10 of the 12 boys. Similar findings were reported by Leiper et al,[29] who studied 11 prepubertal boys who had received 2400 cGy in 10–12 fractions over 14–16 days.

Subsequently it has been shown that severe Leydig cell damage is present fairly soon after irradiation, often within the first year, and that there is no evidence of Leydig cell recovery up to 5 years after irradiation.[30]

A more recent study has examined the effect of 'intermediate' doses of testicular irradiation on Leydig cell function in boys treated for acute lymphoblastic leukaemia.[31] Fifteen boys were studied, twelve received 1200 cGy 'prophylactic' testicular irradiation in six 200 cGy fractions over 8 days, and the other three were treated for overt testicular relapse with 2400 cGy (in two patients) and 1500 cGy (in one patient). The seven patients old enough to provide semen for analysis were azoospermic. Eleven of the 12 patients who received 1200 cGy, as well as the patient who received 1500 cGy, had normal pubertal development for their age, with an appropriate basal testosterone level and response to HCG.[31]

All boys who have received direct testicular irradiation for acute lymphoblastic leukaemia will require a biochemical assessment of testicular function. In the presence of results that indicate Leydig cell failure, if there are no signs of puberty by 13–14 years of age or if there is failure to progress through puberty, then androgen replacement therapy should be initiated.

## BONE MARROW TRANSPLANTATION

Increasing numbers of children with haematological malignancy undergo bone marrow transplant (BMT). Marrow transplant preparative regimens are designed to suppress the immune system and to eradicate the underlying haematological disorder or malignancy. Commonly used regimens have included high dose cyclophosphamide given alone or in combination with total body irradiation or total lymphoid irradiation; more recently the combination of high dose busulphan with cyclophosphamide has been used.

In the survivors, there is a high risk of thyroid, pituitary and gonadal dysfunction; in children, growth is often adversely affected. The relative risk of these adverse events is influenced by the underlying pathological condition, previous treatment for that condition, the use of total body irradiation and the irradiation schedule, and the nature and quantity of the cytotoxic drugs used in the BMT preparative regimen.[32]

## Growth

Total body irradiation has a profound adverse impact upon growth. Potential mechanisms include radiation-induced hypothyroidism, growth hormone deficiency and skeletal dysplasia. Additional adverse factors include the pre-transplant chemotherapy and graft versus host disease. The radiation-induced skeletal dysplasia is associated with poorer growth if the total body irradiation is administered in a single fraction rather than multiple fractions.

In recent years, the combination of busulphan plus cyclophosphamide has been used increasingly, especially in nonlymphocytic leukaemias, lymphomas and thalassaemia, as an alternative to total body irradiation-containing preparative BMT regimens. Disappointingly, however, there is no difference in the impairment of growth rates over the first two post-transplant years in patients treated with busulphan/cyclophosphamide and those treated with cyclophosphamide/total body irradiation.[33]

## Thyroid

As described in the brain tumour section, irradiation to the thyroid region may induce thyroid dysfunction. After a total body irradiation dose of 1000–1200 cGy, the typical biochemical finding is a mildly elevated basal serum TSH level and a normal serum thyroxine concentration. Frank biochemical hypothyroidism with a more elevated TSH level and low thyroxine concentration is less common.

The incidence of thyroid dysfunction following fractionated total body irradiation (15–16%) appears significantly less than that following single dose total body irradiation (46-48%) however, the long-term natural history of the irradiation-induced thyroid dysfunction is unknown and thus the timing of the peak incidence of biochemical thyroid abnormalities has not been established for different total body irradiation schedules.

The other major complication arising from irradiation to the thyroid gland is the development of thyroid tumours, benign and malignant. The latency period between irradiation and the clinical presentation of the thyroid tumour may be up to 30 years. In the largest reported series of children undergoing total body irradiation and BMT, two out of 116 children were found to have thyroid papillary carcinoma 4 and 8 years, respectively, after transplantation.[34]

### Ovarian function

The $LD_{50}$ for the human oocyte has been estimated to be less than 400 cGy.[10] Therefore, it is not surprising that a high prevalence of primary ovarian failure is found after total body irradiation (dose 900–1575 cGy) and cyclophosphamide preparative treatment for a BMT.[32] In view of the age dependency of cytotoxic-induced damage, it might be predicted that the prospects of preserving ovarian function following conditioning regimens for BMT would be greater in girls rather than adult women. There is some suggestion that this is the case, in that amongst 14 girls, who received cyclophosphamide and total body irradiation before BMT performed between 3 and 14 years earlier, four showed recovery of ovarian function, including one who became pregnant and had an elective abortion.[35] The prospects of successful pregnancy may, however, be less good. In a young girl, the uterus and the uterine blood flow are vulnerable to radiation-induced damage,[36] leading subsequently in adult life to a greatly increased risk of miscarriage and low birth weight babies.[37, 38] The increased risk of an adverse fertility outcome was established with a radiation dose of 3000 cGy in childhood but the extent of the risk associated with a total body irradiation dose of 1000–1500 cGy in childhood remains to be established.

### Testicular function

In boys receiving total body irradiation (dose 1000 cGy) prior to BMT, severe damage is inflicted on the germinal epithelium of the testes. During and after completion of puberty, the testes are pathologically small and the serum FSH level markedly elevated. Recovery of spermatogenesis has not yet been observed and is unlikely. Marked changes in Leydig cell function may occur with time, however. Initially the testosterone response to HCG may be greatly impaired in prepubertal life, but the boys of pubertal age, who received total body irradiation but no other testicular irradiation, however, entered or progressed through puberty spontaneously.[39] This implies that 'recovery' of Leydig cell function must occur for spontaneous puberty to ensue. The clinical implication is that the HCG test may prove unreliable in determining the need for exogenous testosterone for induction of puberty, which should therefore depend on clinical judgement.

## CONCLUSIONS

It is clear that several of the endocrine sequelae arising from treatment with radiotherapy and/or chemotherapy are complicated in terms of mechanism of injury, diagnosis and management. The problem is further compounded by the fact that the same child may be affected by more than one complication. For instance, the child treated for a medulloblastoma may grow poorly, develop hypothyroidism, then precocious puberty. Subsequent endocrine management with growth hormone, thyroxine and a GnRH analogue will improve the prognosis for these endocrine complications. Once childhood is completed, however, the young adult is likely to be troubled by the metabolic sequelae of GH deficiency, infertility and possibly, many years later, a thyroid tumour. Surveillance of these patients must, therefore, be lifelong!

Only two, albeit two of the commonest, childhood cancers, have been considered in this review. The clinical approach to the detection of these endocrine sequelae is based on a knowledge of the radiation fields and/or chemotherapy received by the individual child. Thus did the child receive any irradiation to the head, neck, gonads, uterus or any part of the spine? Is the cytotoxic chemotherapy known to be gonadotoxic or could it affect growth?

The management of children with cancer varies in different regions of the UK. In a number of centres the children are totally cared for by specialists but in other centres the management is shared between the local paediatrician and the regional specialist. In the latter situation, the local paediatrician can contribute to the long-term surveillance for endocrine complications by sticking to certain guidelines.

## KEY POINTS FOR CLINICAL PRACTICE

- Regular measurements of standing height and weight are important in all children treated for malignancy. The values should be plotted on UK growth charts. Any significant deviation from usual centile position needs explanation and/or specialist advice. Increasing obesity needs to be tackled early with appropriate advice about diet and exercise.

- In any child who has received irradiation to a part of or the whole spine, sitting height measurements are mandatory. Sitting height and leg length measurements should be plotted on standard UK charts and any significant disproportion noted.

- Following cranial irradiation, pubertal staging should be performed regularly, however young the child. In all other children aged 9 years or older, regular pubertal staging should be performed.

- Palpation of the thyroid gland and thyroid function tests should be performed annually if the child has received neck, craniospinal or total body irradiation.

- Do not hesitate to seek specialist advice if a child with malignancy (past or present) develops an endocrine problem. Often a telephone call will suffice. An unexplained deterioration in growth, precocious puberty, disturbed thyroid function, or a thyroid swelling all require early specialist advice.

## REFERENCES


1 Birch JM, Marsden HB, Morris-Jones PH, Pearson D, Blair V. Improvements in survival from childhood cancer: results of a population based survey over 30 years. BMJ 1988; 296: 1372-1376
2 Stiller CA. Population based survival rates for childhood cancer in Britain, 1980–91. BMJ 1994; 309: 1612-1616
3 Shalet SM. Radiation and pituitary function. N Eng J Med 1993; 328: 131-133
4 Shalet SM, Gibson, B, Swindell R, Pearson D. Effect of spinal irradiation on growth. Arch Dis Child 1987; 62: 461-464
5 Ogilvy-Stuart AL, Clayton PE, Shalet SM. Cranial irradiation and early puberty. J Clin Endocrinol Metab 1994; 78: 1282-1286
6 Ogilvy-Stuart AL, Shalet SM. Growth and puberty after growth hormone therapy following irradiation for brain tumours. Arch Dis Child 1995; in press
7 Ogilvy-Stuart AL, Ryder WDJ, Gattamaneni HR, Clayton PE, Shalet SM. Growth hormone and tumour recurrence. BMJ 1992; 304: 1601-1605
8 Livesey EA, Brook CGD. Thyroid dysfunction after radiotherapy and chemotherapy of brain tumours. Arch Dis Child 1989; 64: 593-595
9 Ogilvy-Stuart AL, Shalet SM, Gattamaneni HR. Thyroid function after treatment of brain tumours in childhood. J Pediatr 1991; 119: 733-737
10 Wallace WHB, Shalet SM, Hendry JH, Morris-Jones PH, Gattamaneni HR. Ovarian failure following abdominal irradiation in childhood: the radiosensitivity of the human oocyte. Br J Radiol 1989; 62: 995-998
11 Clayton PE, Shalet SM, Price DA, Campbell RHA. Testicular damage after chemotherapy for childhood brain tumors. J Pediatr 1988; 112: 922-926
12 Clayton PE, Shalet SM, Price DA, Morris-Jones PH. Ovarian function following chemotherapy for childhood brain tumours. Med Pediatr Oncol 1989; 17: 92-96
13 Livesey EA, Brook CGD. Gonadal dysfunction after treatment of intracranial tumours. Arch Dis Child 1988; 63: 495-500
14 Davies HA, Didcock E, Didi M, Ogilvy-Stuart AL, Wales JKH, Shalet SM. Disproportionate short stature after cranial irradiation and combination chemotherapy for leukaemia. Arch Dis Child 1994; 70: 472-475
15 Kirk JA, Raghupathy P, Stevens MM et al. Growth failure and growth hormone deficiency after treatment for acute lymphoblastic leukaemia. Lancet 1987; I: 190-193
16 Clayton PE, Shalet SM, Morris-Jones PH, Price DA. Growth in children treated for acute lymphoblastic leukaemia. Lancet 1988; I: 460-462
17 Sklar C, Mertens A, Walter A et al. Final height after treatment for childhood acute lymphoblastic leukaemia: comparison of no cranial irradiation with 1800 and 2400 cGy cranial irradiation. J Pediatr 1993; 123: 59-64
18 Didi M, Didcock E, Davies HA, Ogilvy-Stuart AL, Wales JKH, Shalet SM. High incidence of obesity in adult survivors of leukaemia in childhood. J Pediatr 1995: In press
19 Leiper AD, Stanhope R, Kitching P, Chessels JM. Precocious and premature puberty associated with the treatment of acute lymphoblastic leukaemia. Arch Dis Child 1987; 62: 1107-1112
20 Moell C, Garwicz S, Westgren U et al. Disturbed pubertal growth in girls treated for acute lymphoblastic leukaemia. Paediatr Haematol/Oncol 1987; 4: 1-5
21 Lendon M, Hann IM, Palmer ML et al. Testicular histology after combination chemotherapy in childhood for acute lymphoblastic leukaemia. Lancet 1978; II: 439-441
22 Shalet SM, Hann IM, Lendon M, Morris-Jones PH, Beardwell CG. Testicular function after combination chemotherapy in childhood for acute lymphoblastic leukaemia. Arch Dis Child 1981; 56: 275-278
23 Quigley C, Cowell C, Jimenez M et al. Normal or early development of puberty despite gonadal damage in children treated for acute lymphoblastic leukaemia. N Engl J Med 1989; 321: 143-151
24 Wallace WHB, Shalet SM, Lendon M, Morris-Jones PH. Male fertility in long-term survivors of childhood acute lymphoblastic leukaemia. Int J Androl 1991; 14: 312-319
25 Himmelstein-Braw R, Peters H, Faber M. Morphological study of the ovaries of leukaemic children. Br J Cancer 1978; 38: 82-87
26 Green DM, Hall B, Zevon A. Pregnancy outcome after treatment for acute lymphoblastic leukaemia during childhood or adolescence. Cancer 1989; 64: 2335-2339

27 Wallace WHB, Shalet SM, Tetlow LJ, Morris-Jones PH. Ovarian function following the treatment of childhood acute lymphoblastic leukaemia. Med Pediatr Oncol 1993; 21: 333-339
28 Brauner R, Czernichow P, Cramer P et al. Leydig cell function in children after direct testicular irradiation for acute lymphoblastic leukaemia. N Engl J Med 1993; 309: 25-28
29 Leiper AD, Grant DB, Chessels JM. The effect of testicular irradiation on Leydig cell function in prepubertal boys with acute lymphoblastic leukaemia. Arch Dis Child 1983; 58: 906-910
30 Shalet SM, Horner A, Ahmed SR, Morris-Jones PH. Leydig cell damage after testicular irradiation for lymphoblastic leukaemia. Med Pediatr Oncol 1985; 13: 65-68
31 Castillo LA, Craft AW, Kernahan J, Evans RG, Aynsley-Green A. Gonadal function after 12 Gy testicular irradiation in childhood acute lymphoblastic leukaemia. Med Pediatr Oncol 1990; 18: 185-189
32 Shalet SM, Didi M, Ogilvy-Stuart AL, Schulga J, Donaldson MDC. Growth and endocrine function after bone marrow transplantation. Clin Endocrinol 1995; 42: 333-339
33 Wingard JR, Plotnick LP, Freemer CS et al. Growth in children after bone marrow transplantation: busulphan plus cyclophosphamide versus cyclophosphamide plus total body irradiation. Blood 1992; 79: 1068-1073
34 Sanders JE, Buckner CD, Sullivan KM et al. Growth and development in children after bone marrow transplantation. Hormone Res 1988; 30: 92-97
35 Sanders JE, Pritchard S, Mahoney P et al. Growth and development following marrow transplantation for leukaemia. Blood 1986; 68: 1129-1135
36 Critchley HOD, Wallace WHB, Shalet SM, Mamtora H, Higginson J, Anderson DC. Abdominal irradiation in childhood; the potential for pregnancy. Br J Obstet Gynaecol 1992; 99: 392-394
37 Li FP, Gimbrere K, Gelber RD et al. Outcome of pregnancy in survivors of Wilms' tumour. JAMA 1987; 257: 216-219
38 Wallace WHB, Shalet SM, Crowne EC et al. Ovarian failure following abdominal irradiation in childhood: natural history and prognosis. Clin Oncol 1989; 1: 75-79
39 Ogilvy-Stuart AL, El-Abiary W, Gibson B, Stevens RF, Donaldson MDC, Shalet SM. Gonadal function after fraction after fractionated total body irradiation. 1995: Submitted

11

# Vitamin A deficiency: a paediatric priority in the tropics

*K. P. West Jr*

Vitamin A is an essential nutrient required for normal reproduction, embryogenesis, vision, growth, hematopoiesis, immune competence and, ultimately, survival. Experimental vitamin A depletion in animals leads to widespread epithelial metaplasia and keratinization, depressed growth and late-stage weight loss, ocular changes, reproductive failure, depressed immunity, weakened resistance to infection and death.[1,2] The key to most of these functions is the role of vitamin A (and, more broadly, retinoids) in regulating gene expression (via nuclear receptors) and cell differentiation, conceivably in every cell in the body. The role of vitamin A in the visual cycle has long been understood. Although the global food supply of vitamin A is generally adequate,[3] marked inequities in availability and dietary intake (in relation to need) exist by region, social class and age. Thus, in many developing countries, where vast numbers of children (and their mothers) are poorly nourished, vitamin A deficiency is the leading cause of paediatric blindness (due to corneal xerophthalmia) and a major, underlying cause of early childhood death (due to infection).[3]

An estimated 5–10 million children develop xerophthalmia each year, of whom a quarter to a half-million suffer corneal disease, half of whom go blind.[3] However, xerophthalmia represents only the 'tip of the iceberg': systemic (and largely 'subclinical') vitamin A deficiency affects an estimated 125 million pre-school children in the world and, because of its impact on infection, is responsible for an estimated 1.2 to 2.5 million child deaths each year.[4] Additionally, maternal vitamin A deficiency appears to be widespread, with potential consequences for reproductive health and fetal and infant survival, particularly in HIV-infected third-world populations.[5] These sobering figures have made the prevention of vitamin A deficiency an urgent, international health priority to reach stated health goals by the year 2000 and beyond.[6]

This review attempts to: (a) provide the salient clinical, biochemical, immunological and epidemiological features and health consequences of vitamin A deficiency; and (b) update the practising paediatrician and health provider in the tropics on approaches to assessment, treatment and prevention.

## ASSESSMENT OF VITAMIN A STATUS

Prolonged, low dietary intake of vitamin A (preformed and as provitamin A carotenoids) precedes uncomplicated vitamin A deficiency. Dietary assessment, in principle, should detect chronic inadequacies of intake before vitamin A status deteriorates and, thus, serve as the earliest indicator of vitamin A deficiency. For methodologic reasons this is rarely the case. A major role for dietary assessment is to identify food-related behavior and specific foods lacking in the diet that may be causing vitamin A deficiency in individuals and communities to provide a basis for diet counselling and broader food-based, preventive initiatives.

Indicators of vitamin A status essentially reflect tissue concentrations of retinol (in blood, breast milk, tear, liver, total body) or the biological roles in which vitamin A is known to be involved (e.g. retinal function and epithelial differentiation). Plasma (or serum) concentration of retinol continues to be the biochemical standard for assessing vitamin A status, despite considerable laboratory variability, and difficulty in interpreting individual values between 20 μg/dl and 40 μg/dl (0.70–1.40 μmol/l) (due to homeostatic control)[7] and in the presence of acute infection and severe malnutrition which can depress plasma retinol levels.[3] Still, marginal-to-deficient status can safely be inferred when an individual serum retinol is below 20 μg/dl (0.70 μmol/l).[7] Frequency distributions of serum retinol provide a common basis to determine the vitamin A status of populations, especially when expressed as the percent of individuals with below this cut-off (Table 11.1).[7,8] Distributions of serum retinol in populations also reliably respond to effective vitamin A interventions.[7]

Conjunctival impression cytology is a non-invasive technique that assesses vitamin A status by detecting early losses of vitamin A-dependent, mucus-secreting goblet cells and early (pre-xerophthalmic) metaplasia of the epithelium.[7] Surface cells are harvested from the infero-temporal quadrant of the conjunctiva with a small strip or disk of filter paper, that is stained, mounted and examined under a light microscope. It is primarily intended for evaluating the vitamin A status of communities (vs individuals), generating prevalence estimates that are comparable to those obtained by serum retinol determination, and are usually 5–10 times higher than rates of xerophthalmia (reflecting 'subclinical' vitamin A deficiency). While useful for static measurement, the response of conjunctival impression cytology to vitamin A treatment and intervention is variable.[7]

Other measured, biochemical and functional indicators of vitamin A status are either primarily investigational (i.e. relative dose response that estimates hepatic retinol adequacy from two phlebotomies, and stable isotopic dilution that measures body pools of retinol) or show promise but remain to be adequately tested (a single-blood draw modification of the relative dose response, breast milk and tear retinol concentrations, and indicators of retinal function: vision restoration time and pupillary threshold-based dark adaptometry, both following bleaching of the retina with light).[7]

A clinical classification system, developed by the World Health Organization

(WHO), provides a global standard for the diagnosis of xerophthalmia and a basis for determining its public health significance (Table 11.1).[8] It is organized around the roles of vitamin A (a) in the visual cycle of retinal photoreceptors and (b) in maintaining normal epithelial surfaces of the conjunctiva and cornea. The classification reflects a continuum of severity of ocular manifestations (and systemic vitamin A depletion) that include night blindness, conjunctival xerosis with Bitot's spots, corneal xerosis, corneal ulceration and keratomalacia, and corneal scarring.[3,8,9] The consequences of ocular disease are discussed below.

## HEALTH CONSEQUENCES

The effects of vitamin A deficiency on child health can be both subtle (undermining resistance to infection) and dramatic (precipitation of corneal xerophthalmia or death from an acute infection, such as measles, preconditioned by chronic vitamin A deficiency).

### Xerophthalmia

Xerophthalmia is the most common, specific, clinical manifestation of vitamin A deficiency that a practitioner will encounter. Xerophthalmia appears to be a public health problem, based on WHO minimum criteria (Table 11.1), in approximately 40 developing countries,[8] located primarily in the peri-equatorial regions of the world (Fig. 11.1).

#### *Night blindness*

Night blindness is the earliest ocular and behavioral manifestation of xerophthalmia. Vitamin A (11-*cis* retinal) is required for rod (and cone) vision via its participation as a chromophore in the 'visual cycle'. Rod photoreceptors, located in the outer-segment of the retina, contain the visual pigment rhodopsin. Upon being stimulated by light, rhodopsin is 'bleached', causing

**Table 11.1** Criteria for assessing the public health significance of xerophthalmia and vitamin A deficiency among children less than 6 years of age

| Criterion | Minimum prevalence (%) |
|---|---|
| Clinical | |
| Night blindness | 1.0 |
| Bitot's spot | 0.5 |
| Corneal xerosis and/or ulceration/keratomalacia | 0.01 |
| Xerophthalmia-related corneal scars | 0.05 |
| Biochemical | |
| Serum retinol (vitamin A) less than 0.35 μmol/l (10 μg/dl) | 5.0 |

From Sommer[8] with permission (WHO)

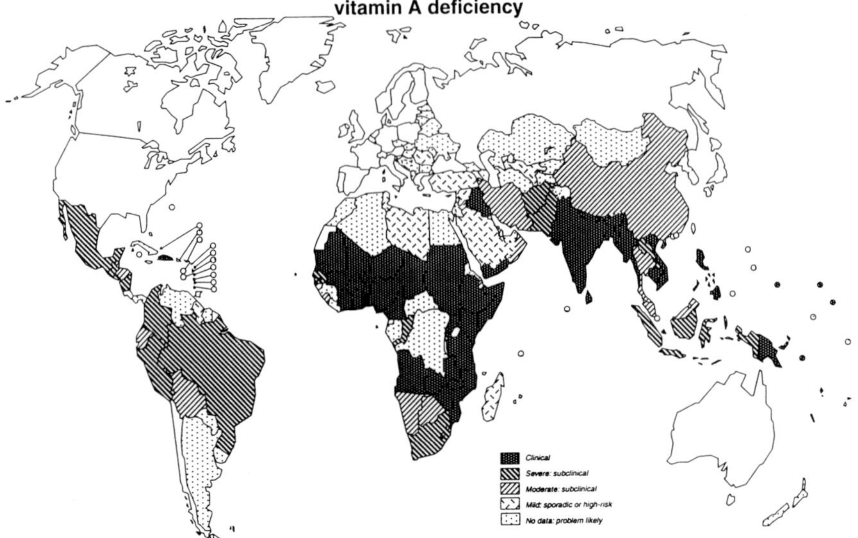


**Fig. 11.1** Global map of vitamin A deficiency as a public health problem (with permission, WHO, March 1995). The designations employed and the presentation of material on the map do not imply the expression of any opinion whatsoever on the part of the World Health Organisation concerning the legal status of any country, territory, city or area or of its authorities, or concerning the delimitation of its frontiers or boundaries. Dotted lines represent approximate border lines for which there may not yet be full agreement.

11-*cis* to isomerize to all-*trans* retinal which, in turn, is released from the opsin molecule. This initiates an electrochemical signal to be carried to the brain where visual images are constructed.[3] In vitamin A deficiency, the threshold for stimulating rods is raised, compromising a subject's ability to see (and function) under dim light.

A reliable, parental history of night blindness can be elicited for children over one year of age using a carefully defined, local term that often translates into 'twilight blindness' or 'chicken eyes'. Chickens lack rods in their retinas and are immobile at night; mothers note the similarity in how their children and chickens behave between dusk and dawn and draw their own 'diagnosis'. Children with a history of night blindness tend to have lower serum retinol levels,[3,9] as well as a higher risk of diarrhoea, respiratory infection[10] and mortality[11] compared to children without night blindness. The condition generally disappears within 24–48 hours after oral treatment with high-potency vitamin A.

Where vitamin A deficiency is endemic, marginally nourished women may also frequently become night blind late in pregnancy and during early lactation,[12] apparently associated with increased demands on vitamin A nutrition imposed by feto-placental utilization. The natural history,

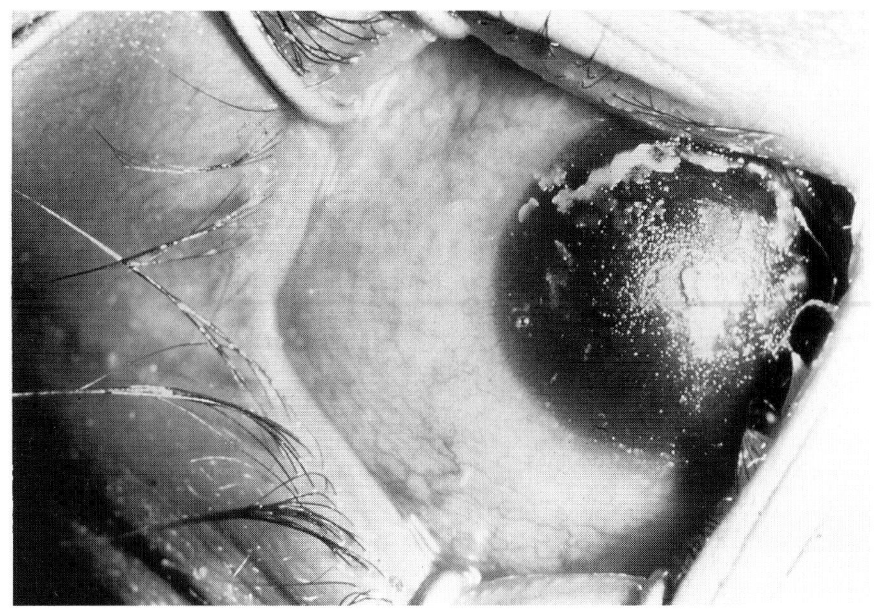

**Fig. 11.2** Corneal xerosis. Note the dry, pebbly appearance of the corneal surface (photograph by Prof. Alfred Sommer;[8] with permission, WHO).

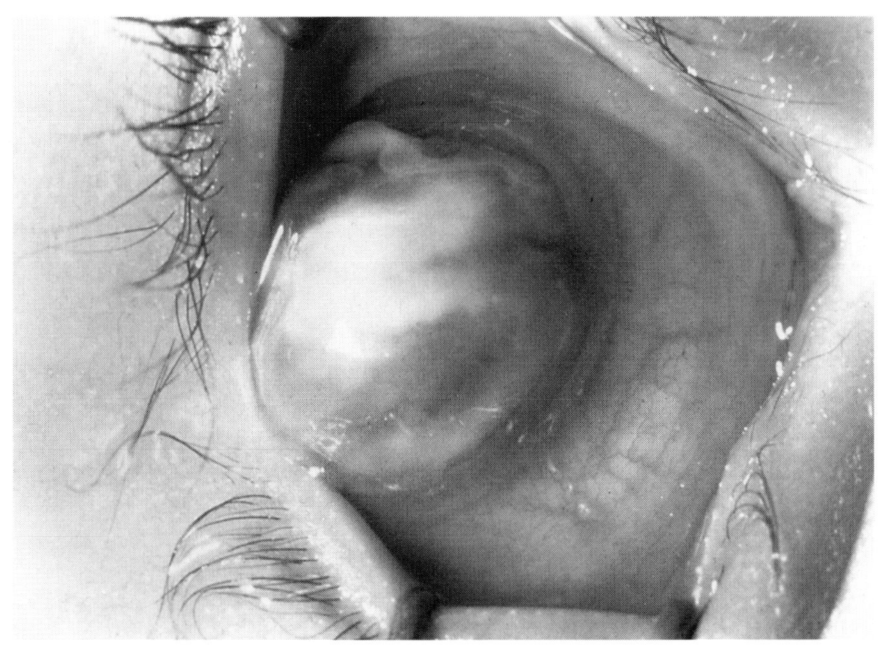

**Fig. 11.3** Keratomalacia (photograph by Prof. Alfred Sommer; [8] with permission, WHO).

epidemiology and health consequences to the fetus and mother associated with maternal night blindness are presently under investigation in Nepal (P. Christian et al, personal communication, 1995).

*Bitot's spots*

During vitamin A deficiency, the normal, columnar epithelium of the conjunctiva undergoes squamous metaplasia, causing a loss of mucus-secreting goblet cells and stratified changes in the epithelium; with advancing deficiency superficial layers of keratinized cells form, leaving the ocular surface dry (xerotic), 'unwettable' by tears and lustreless.[8] Conjunctival xerosis is best observed on oblique illumination with a torch. Mild xerosis is difficult to standardize and is little used to diagnose xerophthalmia. In more advanced deficiency, large, visible squames of sloughed-off keratinized cells and saprophytic bacilli collect on the conjunctival surface forming a 'Bitot's spot' (named after a prominent 19th century French ophthalmologist): Bitot's spots are clinically distinct, nearly always forming temporal to the limbus, and are bilateral. Nasal involvement reflects more advanced deficiency. Bitot's spots may be 'bubbly', 'foamy' or 'cheesy' in appearance and vary in size and shape (classic lesions are 'triangular').[8] Uncomplicated, Bitot's spots that respond to vitamin A rarely progress to corneal disease (though a superficial punctate keratopathy may be visible by light microscopy[3,9]). Still, the presence of vitamin-A responsive Bitot's spots suggests a level of moderate, systemic vitamin A depletion (e.g. low serum retinol and liver stores), possibly indicative of more widespread epithelial metaplasia (as seen in vitamin A-depleted animals[1] and severely deficient children at autopsy[13]), a greater risk of frank, corneal disease in the event of a precipitating illness, early immune impairment,[14] and an increased risk of morbidity[10] and mortality.[11]

Bitot's spots observed in older, school-aged children are more likely to be 'non-responsive' to vitamin A treatment; these children also tend to have normal serum retinol levels.[9,15] Histologically, the underlying keratinization and goblet cell losses are more localized than seen in vitamin A-responsive X1B.[9]

*Corneal xerosis and ulceration or keratomalacia*

As noted above, superficial corneal changes may occur in mild xerophthalmia (night blindness and Bitot's spots). Clinically apparent corneal xerosis, however, represents a more serious, frank keratinization of the corneal epithelium often with stromal oedema.[3] The cornea develops a dry, pebbly, thickened and hazy appearance; the lesions are typically bilateral (Fig. 11.2). Corneal xerosis responds to vitamin A therapy within 2–5 days, with the cornea becoming clear within 2 weeks.[8]

Without vitamin A treatment, the xerotic cornea can rapidly deteriorate, forming sharply demarcated ulcers (corneal ulceration) that can perforate the cornea.[8] Perforations may be plugged with iris, thereby preserving the integrity of the eye. Following high-potency vitamin A therapy, shallow ulcers heal with little scarring, whereas perforated ulcers form leukomas or (if plugged with iris) adherent leukomas.[8] Without treatment the lesion may progress to a full-thickness softening and necrosis of corneal stroma (keratomalacia); the lesions appear grey or yellowish, may or may not protrude from the corneal surface, and often involve the entire cornea (Fig. 11.3). A usual lack of inflammatory infiltrate suggests a metabolic defect giving rise to the lesion. On treatment with vitamin A, necrotic tissue sloughs off leaving a descemetocele, a protruding, (healed) staphyloma or a shrunken, phthisical eye if the ocular contents have been lost. In each case, the eye is blind.[8]

Young (1–4 years), frail and wasted children with a recent history of severe infectious illness (such as diarrhoea or measles) are at highest risk of corneal xerophthalmia. The condition is a medical emergency, requiring immediate large-dose vitamin A and other supportive therapy to save further ocular destruction and the child's life;[8] in-hospital case fatality rates are generally 5–25%.[9]

*Corneal scarring*

Corneal scarring due to xerophthalmia may range from a small nebula, leukoma or adherent leukoma (when the iris is attached to the scarred tissue) where the content and shape of the globe have been largely retained (i.e. due to corneal ulceration) to the more severe, blinding sequelae of staphyloma and phthisis. Close examination of the shape and location of the scar and a careful history (e.g. ruling out trauma, ocular infection, etc.) is always required to determine whether xerophthalmia was the likely cause of a corneal scar. A history of severe infection (such as measles) and wasting malnutrition around the time the lesion appeared supports a diagnosis of vitamin A deficiency in a young child in the absence of a history of traditional medicine use or trauma.[8]

## Childhood mortality and morbidity

Due to its rarity, severe xerophthalmia explains only a small proportion of child mortality attributed to vitamin A deficiency.

A relationship between milder xerophthalmia (night blindness and Bitot's spots) and increased child mortality was first reported by Sommer and colleagues in Indonesia more than a decade ago.[11] Among a group of ~4000 pre-school-aged children examined quarterly for 18 months, the risk of mortality rose in a dose-response manner with the severity of eye signs. Children with night blindness were 3 times more likely to die over a 3 month interval than children with normal eyes; having Bitot's spots was associated with a 6-fold higher risk and having both conditions (night blindness and Bitot's spots) held a 9-fold higher risk of death compared to non-xerophthalmic children. This study suggested that 15–20% of all early childhood deaths (beyond infancy) was associated with clinically evident vitamin A deficiency.[11] Causes of death were not ascertained, but surviving children with mild xerophthalmia were 2–3 times more likely to develop diarrhoeal or a respiratory infection by the next examination compared to non-xerophthalmic children.[10] Numerous studies over the past decade have reported higher risks of persistent diarrhoea or dysentery, respiratory infections, severe measles and otitis media associated with both mild xerophthalmia and subclinical vitamin A deficiency (defined biochemically or histologically).[3]

The observational study in West Java was followed by a randomized community trial in Aceh Province, North Sumatra where pre-school-aged children in half of 450 enrolled villages (~30 000 children) received semi-annually a large dose of vitamin A (200 000 IU for 1–5 years; a half-dose < 12 months). Children in control villages received no vitamin A supplement, although children with xerophthalmia were treated in both groups. After a year, mortality declined by 34% in the vitamin A-supplemented villages[16] (or twice that hypothesized by preventing xerophthalmia alone), raising the possibility that subclinical vitamin A deficiency could also increase the risk of child death.

Since then, six of seven additional community trials carried out in Indonesia, India, Nepal, Ghana and the Sudan have reported reductions of 6% to 54% in pre-school child (6–72 months) mortality with vitamin A supplementation, delivered as a periodic large dose, a small weekly dose, or via a fortified food item (monosodium glutamate) (reviewed in[3,17]). Meta-analyses (combining the estimates from these studies) suggest the expected reduction in mortality following a vitamin A intervention to be 23–34%.[6,17] The actual impact of a program will vary by population, the existing mix of health and nutrition services in an area, and by the evaluation design.[17] Mortality attributed to measles and diarrhoea or dysentery appear to be especially effected. Surprisingly, deaths due to apparent acute, lower respiratory infection have not been reduced by vitamin A.[3]

Morbidity trials carried out to date support the mortality findings: improved vitamin A nutrition appears to reduce the severity of potentially fatal infections rather than the incidence or duration of trivial illnesses. In Ghana, the incidence of sick-child visits to local clinics and hospital admissions (proxies for increasingly severe morbidity) significantly decreased (by 12% and 38%, respectively) among vitamin A-supplemented compared to control children, consistent with the 19% reduction that was observed in mortality.[18] In the plains (terai) of Nepal, where a 30% overall reduction in mortality occurred among vitamin A-supplemented children,[19] ~50% reductions in mortality were observed in children who had persistent (> 7 days) dysentery, diarrhoea and high fever during the week before dosing (K.P. West et al, unpublished data, 1995). In Brazil, prior dosing with vitamin A was associated with milder episodes (lower stool frequencies) among children who subsequently developed diarrhoea,[20] although vitamin A therapy may not noticeably effect the outcome of an ongoing episode of diarrhoea.[21] In contrast, few studies have observed a measurable benefit of vitamin A on the occurrence or severity of acute lower respiratory infections,[3,17] an observation that remains unexplained.

Measles is a potentially highly fatal disease in many developing countries

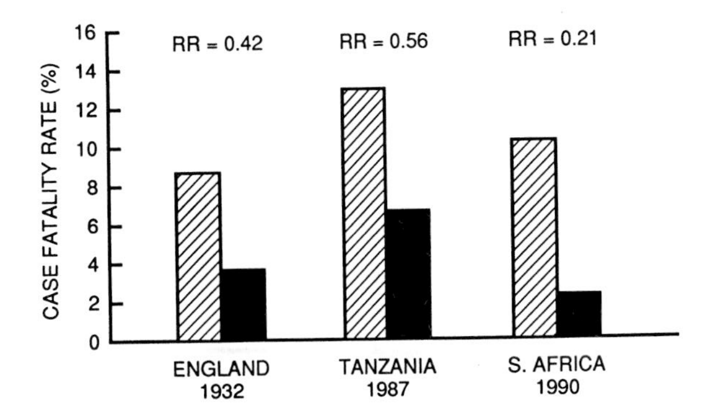


**Fig. 11.4** Impact of vitamin A therapy on measles case fatality in England,[22] Tanzania[23] and South Africa.[24] Hatched bars, untreated; solid bars, vitamin A-treated, RR= relative risk (with permission, Marcel Dekker, Inc.).

that is responsive to vitamin A therapy (200, 000 IU on admission and day 2[22,23]). Concurrent vitamin A supplementation can essentially cut measles case-fatality by half or more,[22–24] (Fig. 11.4) markedly reduce the severity of complications, enhance immune capacity and responsiveness, accelerate recovery[25] and, as a result, lessen demand for hospitalization and intensive care.[26]

*Mechanisms of resistance to infection*

Effects of vitamin A on susceptibility to infection are likely mediated by the vitamin's role in regulating epithelial and immune effector cell differentiation, function and integrity. Vitamin A-depleted animals show diffuse squamous metaplasia, keratinization, and/or losses of mucus-secreting goblet and ciliated cells throughout the respiratory, gastrointestinal and genito-urinary tracts and glandular ducts.[1,2,14] Although data in humans are sparse, autopsy studies in the 1930s reported widespread epidermoid metaplasia in severely vitamin A-deficient, wasted children.[13] These epithelial alterations occur independently of infection; however, such changes may increase the risk of pathogen colonization, invasion and infection. Vitamin A-deficient children exhibit increased bacterial adherence to nasopharyngeal epithelial cells (vs vitamin A-sufficient children)[27] revealing an abnormality that could reflect compromised, local 'offences' (i.e. mucus and enzyme secretions, ciliation and other mechanisms that attack and clear pathogens)[3], in this case, of the respiratory epithelium.[27]

Vitamin A also appears to effect lymphopoiesis and immune effector cell lineage, maturation, expression and trafficking.[3,14] Vitamin A-deficient children exhibit decreased CD4-to-CD8 T cell ratios as well as other abnormalities in T cell subsets that indicate disturbed cellular and T cell-dependent humoral immune function.[2,14] These abnormalities appear responsive to vitamin A repletion. For example, previously vitamin A-deficient children enhance their primary and secondary IgG antibody responses to tetanus toxoid antigen and increase their numbers of circulating CD4 T cells within a few weeks after receiving vitamin A.[14] Among children with severe measles, vitamin A treatment enhances specific IgG antibody levels and the numbers of circulating lymphocytes.[25] Generally, impairment and enhancement of innate, T cell-dependent and antibody-mediated immunity by vitamin A depletion and repletion, respectively, are supported by an extensive experimental animal literature[2, 14] , including Ross in Sommer.[3]

A synergism between vitamin A deficiency and infection also contributes to make matters worse. While children with mild xerophthalmia are more prone to infection,[10] children who acquire infection are also more likely to become vitamin A-deficient.[3,28] There can be several reasons for this: during acute infection dietary vitamin A intake and absorption may be poorer, hepatic mobilization may be impaired (as part of the acute phase response to infection), tissue utilization of retinol may increase and urinary excretion may increase many-fold.[14] By decreasing available vitamin A, these actions, in turn, may further compromise innate and acquired resistance to infection.[2,14]

## KEY EPIDEMIOLOGIC FEATURES

Epidemiologic patterns have emerged that may be helpful in understanding the causality of vitamin A deficiency and identifying and initiating preventive measures in communities.

### Age and gender

The prevalence (risk) of xerophthalmia rises with age through the pre-school years, typically affecting 1–2% of toddlers (1–2 years) and 3–6% of older children (3–6 years). In South Asia, the prevalence continues to increase in the school-age years, though more older children tend to have non-responsive Bitot's spots.[3] Boys tend to be at higher risk of mild xerophthalmia than girls (although corneal disease strikes the two sexes equally).[9] Genetic or diet-and-environmental influences may underlie the gender difference.[3]

### Clustering

Xerophthalmia clusters by geographic areas that often correspond to poverty-stricken populations. High-risk (case-dense) provinces have been identified in most countries where the problem exists.[3] Children in villages where at least one other child has xerophthalmia are roughly twice as likely to have xerophthalmia than children in villages where no prior cases have been reported.[29] The risk concentrates even more within families. Siblings of cases are 7–13 times more likely to have (or develop) xerophthalmia than children from households without a previous case.[29] Shared poverty (by local standards) and dietary constraints appear to underlie higher risks within villages and households.[3,30]

Vitamin A deficiency may also exhibit seasonality; for example, in South Asia prevalence rates of xerophthalmia and mortality tend to be highest in the late-dry and early-monsoon months (April–July).[31] Vitamin A stores may be low and demands high during these months which follow a typical seasonal growth spurt (a few months earlier) and correspond with the 'measles' and early diarrhoea seasons in some areas.[3,31]

Irrespective of causes, locational and seasonal clustering can influence xerophthalmia treatment and vitamin A deficiency prevention decisions. For example, preventive efforts could target highest-risk groups and aim to coordinate vitamin A prophylaxis to reduce seasonal peaks in deficiency.

### Breast feeding and the household diet

Breast feeding appears to protect infants and children from xerophthalmia through the first 3–4 years of life in rural cultures of Asia[9,32] and Africa.[33] The association appears to be dose-responsive: that is, the more frequent the breast feeding the stronger the protective effect.[32] However, the protective effect of breast milk primarily relates to clinical disease since vitamin A supplementation can dramatically reduce mortality from late infancy onward, [3,17] at ages when most children in traditional cultures are still breast feeding. The protection of breast feeding, however, is as much a statement about the inadequacy of a young child's weaning diet as it is about the nutritional (and perhaps extended) benefit of breast milk. In cultures where breast feeding uniformly ceases earlier (i.e. first half of the second year), the risk of xerophthalmia rises 2–5-fold when the weaning diet is routinely lacking vitamin A-rich foods.[30] Dietary studies repeatedly show that (partially and fully weaned) children with xerophthalmia tend to consume foods rich in vitamin A (egg, liver, cheese, milk) and provitamin A-carotenoid rich foods (dark green leaves, yellow and orange fruits and vegetables) less frequently than children without xerophthalmia.[3,30] Not surprisingly, the insufficient diet continues long after the therapeutic effects of vitamin A supplementation have waned, [3] indicating that dietary inadequacy afflicts families over extended periods of time. This may partly explain the high incidence of night blindness in young, pregnant and lactating mothers.[12]

## TREATMENT

Children with any stage of xerophthalmia should be treated with vitamin A according to WHO guidelines (Table 11.2): 200 000 IU vitamin A orally on presentation, the following day and, whenever possible, 1–4 weeks later (infants 6–12 months receive a half-dose and infants < 6 months one-quarter the dose, following the same schedule).[8] Broad-spectrum antibiotic therapy can reduce the risk of secondary infection in children with corneal involvement. Concurrent infections and worm infestation should also be treated with appropriate antibiotics and antihelminthics, respectively; [8] patients with diarrhoea should receive oral rehydration therapy.

**Table 11.2** Treatment schedule for xerophthalmia[8]

| Timing | Dosage[a] |
|---|---|
| Immediately upon diagnosis[b] | 110 mg retinyl palmitate or 66 mg retinyl acetate (200 000 IU) by mouth |
| Next day | 110 mg retinyl palmitate or 66 mg retinyl acetate (200 000 IU) by mouth) |
| Within 1–4 weeks; whenever clinical deterioration occurs; every 2–4 weeks in the presence of persistent kwashiorkor | 110 mg retinyl palmitate or 66 mg retinyl acetate (200 000 IU) by mouth |

[a]Children 6–11 months of age should receive only half the dose shown in this table, and children less than 6 months one-quarter of the dose.
[b]Intramuscular injection of 55 mg water-miscible retinyl palmitate (100 000 IU) is substituted in rare instances when children with severe stomatitis cannot swallow, in cases of persistent vomiting, or if severe malabsorption (as in cystic fibrosis) prevents an adequate response.

Siblings of a case are also at high risk of being vitamin A deficient; while treating the case, consideration should be given to dose these children prophylactically i.e., every 4-6 months. The mother or guardian should be advised to feed properly prepared vitamin A-rich foods (either preformed or provitamin A) to her children to prevent recurrent (in the patient) or initial (in siblings) xerophthalmia and reduce their risk of severe infection. Children should consume any one of the following to meet their daily vitamin A requirements:[8] ~1/2 cup of cooked, dark green leaves, ~1/4 of a cooked, medium-sized carrot, ~2 tablespoons of yellow sweet potato or ripe papaya, half of a ripe mango, or other equivalent deep orange or yellow vegetable or fruit. Food sources of preformed vitamin A are very expensive and often unavailable; nonetheless, mothers should be encouraged to feed their recovered children (and their siblings), perhaps on at least a weekly basis, any of the following, highly protective foods: a cooked egg, 15–30 g of cooked liver, 15–30 g of cheese, or 4–6 oz of milk.

In addition, children with persistent diarrhoea, dysentery or acute respiratory infection, especially in the presence of wasting malnutrition, should be treated with a single 200 000 IU oral dose of vitamin A (repeat doses can be safely given as frequently as every 4 months). Children with severe, protein-energy malnutrition, cases of measles in areas of known vitamin A deficiency or severe, complicated cases of measles irrespective of where they occur, should be given a full treatment regimen of vitamin A (Table 11.2). Dietary counselling should be given whether or not the child has xerophthalmia.[8]

## PREVENTION

The goal of prevention is to insure an adequate vitamin A intake and status of high-risk groups. Three complementary approaches can help achieve this goal: (a) dietary diversification; (b) food fortification with vitamin A; and (c) periodic supplementation of high-risk groups with high-potency vitamin A.[3]

## Dietary diversification

Vitamin A deficiency prevention has a rational dietary solution: increase the intake of local food sources of both preformed retinyl esters and provitamin A carotenoids to levels that at least exceed minimal requirements and, preferably approach recommended daily intakes. The Food and Agriculture Organization of the United Nations has set these levels (termed 'basal' and 'safe') at 200 μg and 450 μg retinol equivalents per day, respectively, for healthy, pre-school-aged children (1–6 years) (reviewed in[3]). These levels can largely be achieved in children by consuming vitamin A-rich foods in amounts specified under 'Treatment'.

Achieving lasting dietary change requires a thorough knowledge of existing food beliefs, dietary habits (in health and disease) and seasonal and geographic food availability that influence vitamin A intake. Efforts to reallocate (often existing) vitamin A-rich foods to children within the household should be a main message. Families with and without xerophthalmic children often differ more in the frequency with which vitamin A-rich foods (papaya/mango, dark green leaves, egg) are fed to their children than in the availability of such foods in the household (with normals being fed these foods more often).[3,9] Where non-availability and price are a concern, home, school and community gardening (combined with nutrition education) may help to increase the supply of food and vitamin A intakes of vulnerable groups (directly or indirectly through economic exchange). It is always important to emphasize periodic intakes of foods containing preformed vitamin A to assure improved status.[3]

## Food fortification

Fortification of food items with vitamin A can be highly effective in improving vitamin A status, although most developing countries have limited experience with this strategy. Successful food fortification requires a relatively centrally processed, technically fortifiable food ('vehicle') that is routinely consumed by vulnerable groups (i.e. children and women in poorer strata of society) within a known range of intake (in the general population, for safety reasons). It also requires a commitment from government and industry, advocacy in the community and a financing plan that can sustain the program.[3] In Guatemala, a national sugar fortification program in the late 1970s elevated and sustained higher serum retinol, iron and ferritin levels in preschool children and breast milk retinol levels in lactating women.[34] Economic hardship and civil strife halted the program in the early 1980s, followed by a marked deterioration in vitamin A status of children. Once the program restarted in 1988, there was an impressive rebound in childhood serum retinol levels.[35]

In the Philippines and Indonesia monosodium glutamate is widely consumed as a flavour-enhancer. Pilot projects have shown fortification of monosodium glutamate to improve vitamin A status,[36,37] decrease xerophthalmia,[36,38] raise haemoglobin levels and decrease mortality of pre-school-aged children.[38] Breast milk retinol concentrations have also risen.[37]. However, technical problems have arisen in maintaining the acceptability of vitamin A-fortified monosodium glutamate during normal, tropical storage conditions, delaying further progress on this product (for the time-being).

Other vitamin A-fortified products that reach the rural and urban poor are increasingly being tested. Fortification of food with vitamin A will likely increase in countries where markets are semi-developed and food processing capabilities are in place. In poorer countries, food aid commodities are increasingly being fortified with micronutrients, including vitamin A.

## Supplementation

Periodic distribution of an oral, high-potency vitamin A supplement is currently the most direct and widely adopted way to improve vitamin A status, prevent xerophthalmia and reduce associated mortality in pre-school children 6 months of age and older.[3,16,17,19] Supplements are normally supplied to countries through UNICEF (~125 million in 1993 alone) as small, gelatinous capsules containing 200 000 IU vitamin A at an approximate (at-port) cost of ~US$0.02.[39] In India, an oily syrup with vitamin A (100 000 IU/ml) is manufactured, bottled and distributed in-country.

Three delivery schemes are used, each representing increasingly wider coverage (program sensitivity).[39] 'Medical' delivery is the most restrictive (specific) and least expensive approach by supplying a limited number of capsules and training to health workers to treat children with xerophthalmia and other high-risk conditions, using the WHO treatment guidelines discussed earlier.

A second, 'targeted' approach involves saturating health and other delivery services to provide high-potency supplements to children whenever possible; that is, during sick and growth monitoring visits, vaccination campaigns, community health and family planning and horticultural extension visits, and so on. This method reaches a larger proportion of potentially high-risk children at low (marginal) cost since it 'piggy backs' vitamin A onto existing health and other delivery services; however, distribution may be difficult to coordinate and coverage is often irregular.

The 'universal' approach represents purposeful, community-based distribution of vitamin A to all target-aged children on a periodic basis, usually every 6 months and (increasingly) organized as coordinated, national or regional campaigns. Distribution may be more frequent (e.g. every 3 months) in refugee settings.[40] Health or volunteer workers are provided supplements and mobilized to dose children with vitamin A in their home. Distribution requires a great deal of coordination, motivation, continuous funding and community involvement, making universal delivery difficult to sustain in the 'long run'. Universal supplementation should reach 65% or more of targeted children to effectively reduce xerophthalmia;[39] mortality rates have been cut by 20–30% when coverage has been ~85% or higher.[3,16,19,39] On the other hand, coverage that is too low (e.g. < 25%) may be useless in reducing either xerophthalmia or mortality.[3,39]

## KEY POINTS FOR CLINICAL PRACTICE

- Vitamin A (through diet or supplements) can prevent xerophthalmia and nutritional blindness, reduce the severity of an infectious illness and dramatically lower the risk of mortality in a young child.

- Treat cases of xerophthalmia (night blindness, Bitot's spots, corneal xerosis, keratomalacia) with 200 000 IU oral vitamin A; give a second dose the next day and a third dose 1–4 weeks later (when possible). Infants 6-11 months old receive a half-dose; < 6 months a quarter. Treat infection and provide appropriate dietary counselling.

- Children with severe measles or wasting malnutrition should receive a full treatment course of vitamin A; also dose one time (as noted above, by age) any child presenting with recurrent diarrhoea or dysentery, pneumonia or febrile illness where vitamin deficiency is endemic.

- A child with xerophthalmia represents a 'window to the family', now and over time: consider supplementing siblings with vitamin A and initiate dietary counselling with follow-up.

- Consider periodic, 'universal' distribution of high-potency vitamin A supplements in communities where xerophthalmia occurs or where protein-energy malnutrition and infectious diseases are common.

## REFERE9NCES

1 Wolbach SB, Howe PR. Tissue changes following deprivation of fat-soluble A vitamin. J Exp Med 1925; 42: 753-777
2 Ross AC. Vitamin A status: relationship to immunity and the antibody response. PSEBM 1992; 200: 303-320
3 Sommer A, West Jr KP. Vitamin A Deficiency: Health, Survival and Vision. New York, NY: Oxford University Press 1995: In press
4 Humphrey JH, West Jr KP, Sommer A. Vitamin A deficiency and attributable mortality among under-5-year-olds. Bull WHO 1992; 70: 225-232
5 Semba RD, Miotti PG, Chiphangwi JD et al. Maternal vitamin A deficiency and mother-to-child transmission of HIV-1. Lancet 1994; 343: 1593-1597
6 West Jr KP (Rapporteur). Bellagio meeting on vitamin A deficiency and childhood mortality. Proceedings of Public Health Significance of Vitamin A Deficiency and Its Control, Bellagio Study and Conference Center of the Rockefeller Foundation. New York, NY: Helen Keller International 1992
7 A brief guide to current methods of assessing vitamin A status. A report of the International Vitamin A Consultative Group (IVACG). Washington, DC: The Nutrition Foundation, Inc. 1993
8 Sommer A. Vitamin A Deficiency and its Consequences: Field Guide to Their Detection and Control. 3rd edn. Geneva, Switzerland: World Health Organization 1995

9 Sommer A. Nutritional Blindness: Xerophthalmia and Keratomalacia. New York, NY: Oxford University Press 1982
10 Sommer A, Katz J, Tarwotjo I. Increased risk of respiratory disease and diarrhea in children with preexisting mild vitamin A deficiency. Am J Clin Nutr 1984; 40: 1090-1095
11 Sommer A, Hussaini G, Tarwotjo I, Susanto D. Increased mortality in children with mild vitamin A deficiency. Lancet 1983; 2: 585-588
12 Katz J, Khatry SK, West Jr KP et al. Night blindness during pregnancy and lactation in rural Nepal. J Nutr 1995: In press
13 Blackfan KD, Wolbach SB. Vitamin A deficiency in infants. A clinical and pathological study. J Pediatr 1933; 3: 679-706
14 Semba RD. Vitamin A, immunity, and infection. Clin Infect Dis 1994; 19: 489-499
15 Sovani I, Humphrey JH, Kuntinalibronto DR, Natadisastra G, Muhilal, Tielsch JM. Response of Bitot's spots to a single oral 100 000- or 200 000-IU dose of vitamin A. Am J Ophthalmol 1994; 118: 792-796
16 Sommer A, Tarwotjo I, Djunaedi E et al, Aceh Study Group. Impact of vitamin A supplementation on childhood mortality: a randomised controlled community trial. Lancet 1986; 1: 1169-1173
17 Beaton GH, Martorell R, Aronson KJ et al. Effectiveness of vitamin A supplementation in the control of young child morbidity and mortality in developing countries. ACC/SCN State of the Art Series Nutrition Policy Discussion Paper No. 13. Geneva, Switzerland: Administrative Committee on Coordination-Subcommittee on Nutrition (ACC/SCN) 1993
18 Ghana VAST Study Team. Vitamin A supplementation in northern Ghana: effects on clinic attendances, hospital admissions, and child mortality. Lancet 1993; 342: 7-12
19 West Jr KP, Pokhrel RP, Katz J et al. Efficacy of vitamin A in reducing preschool child mortality in Nepal. Lancet 1991; 338: 67-71
20 Barreto ML, Santos LMP, Assis AMO et al. Effect of vitamin A supplementation on diarrhoea and acute lower respiratory tract infections in young children in Brazil. Lancet 1994; 344: 228-231
21 Henning B, Stewart K, Zaman K, Alam AN, Brown KH, Black RE. Lack of therapeutic efficacy of vitamin A for non-cholera, watery diarrhoea in Bangladeshi children. Eur J Clin Nutr 1992; 46: 437-443
22 Ellison JB. Intensive vitamin therapy in measles. BMJ 1932; 2: 708-711
23 Barclay AJG, Foster A, Sommer A. Vitamin A supplements and mortality related to measles: a randomised clinical trial. BMJ 1987; 294: 294-296
24 Hussey GD, Klein M. A randomized, controlled trial of vitamin A in children with severe measles. N Engl J Med 1990; 323: 160-164
25 Coutsoudis A, Kiepiela P, Coovadia HM, Broughton M. Vitamin A supplementation enhances specific IgG antibody levels and total lymphocyte numbers while improving morbidity in measles. Pediatr Infect Dis J 1992; 11: 203-209
26 Hussey GD, Klein M. Routine high-dose vitamin A therapy for children hospitalized with measles. J Trop Pediatr 1993; 39: 342-345
27 Chandra RK. Increased bacterial binding to respiratory epithelial cells in vitamin A deficiency. BMJ 1988; 297: 834-835
28 Campos FACS, Flores H, Underwood BA. Effect of an infection on vitamin A status of children as measured by the relative dose response (RDR). Am J Clin Nutr 1987; 46: 91-94
29 Katz J, Zeger SL, West KP Jr, Tielsch JM, Sommer A. Clustering of xerophthalmia within households and villages. Int J Epidemiol 1993; 22: 709-715
30 Mele L, West Jr KP, Kusdiono et al, Aceh Study Group. Nutritional and household risk factors for xerophthalmia in Aceh, Indonesia: a case-control study. Am J Clin Nutr 1991; 53: 1460-1465
31 Sinha DP, Bang FB. Seasonal variation in signs of vitamin-A deficiency in rural West Bengal children. Lancet 1973; 2: 228-231
32 Khatry SK, West Jr KP, Katz J et al. Epidemiology of xerophthalmia in Nepal: a pattern of household poverty, childhood illness and mortality. Arch Ophthalmol 1995; 113: 425-429
33 West Jr KP, Chirambo M, Katz J, Sommer A, Malawi Survey Group. Breast-feeding, weaning patterns, and the risk of xerophthalmia in Southern Malawi. Am J Clin Nutr 1986; 44: 690-697

34 Arroyave G, Aguilar JR, Flores M, Guzman MA. Evaluation of sugar fortification with vitamin A at the national level. Washington, DC: Pan American Health Organization 1979
35 Dary O. Avances en el proceso de fortificacion de azucar con vitamina A en Centro America. Boletin de la Oficina Sanitaria Pan Americana 1994; 117: 529-537
36 Solon FS, Fernandez TL, Latham MC, Popkin BM. An evaluation of strategies to control vitamin A deficiency in the Philippines. Am J Clin Nutr 1979; 32: 1445-1453
37 Muhilal, Murdiana A, Azis I, Saidin S, Jahari AB, Karyadi D. Vitamin A-fortified monosodium glutamate and vitamin A status: a controlled field trial. Am J Clin Nutr 1988; 48: 1265-1270
38 Muhilal, Permaesih D, Idjradinata YR, Muherdiyantiningsih, Karyadi D. Vitamin A-fortified monosodium glutamate and health, growth, and survival of children: a controlled field trial. Am J Clin Nutr 1988; 48: 1271-1276
39 West Jr KP, Sommer A. Delivery of Oral Doses of Vitamin A to Prevent Vitamin A Deficiency and Nutritional Blindness. A State-of-the-Art Review. Rome, Italy: United Nations Administrative Committee on Coordination-Subcommittee on Nutrition 1987
40 Nieburg P, Waldman RJ, Leavell R, Sommer A, DeMaeyer EM. Vitamin A supplementation for refugees and famine victims. Bull WHO 1988; 66: 689-697

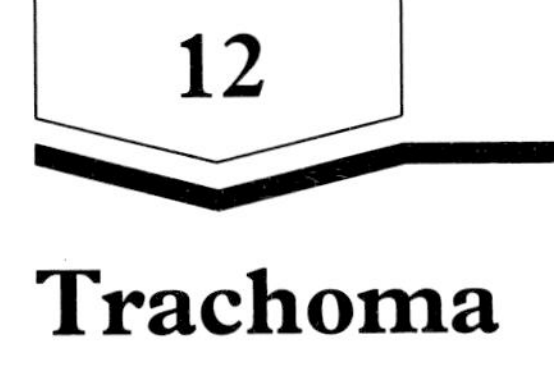

# Trachoma

*S. West L. Bobo*

Trachoma, an ocular infection caused by *Chlamydia trachomatis*, is the leading infectious cause of blindness worldwide. An ancient disease, trachoma is the derivation of a Greek word for 'rough', or 'swelling'.[1] The features of trachoma were described in the Eber's Papyrus.[1] Early descriptions of treatment for trachoma bespoke of its ubiquitous distribution in the 19th and early 20th centuries. In Greece, xysis, the removal of follicles with forceps followed by an application with a copper stick, was proposed. Other treatment regimens included applying leeches to eyebrows, evacuation of the bowel, and topical applications of perchloride, or mercury, to which the disease was described as 'very unresponsive' in a travellers' guide to Africa. Interestingly, early descriptions of the disease included a discussion of possible preventive or public health strategies.[2] In 1920, Elliot recommended avoiding hand/eye transmission, and practising fly control.[3] Trachoma has largely disappeared from North America and Europe, the disappearance occurring well in advance of any pharmaceutical intervention. It continues to be hyperendemic in many areas of Africa, the Middle East, and Asia. Despite considerable advances in understanding the epidemiology of this disease, blindness from trachoma remains a significant public health problem.

## ETIOLOGY

Trachoma is caused by repeated reinfection with *C. trachomatis*, an obligate intracellular bacterium. The chlamydiae have characteristics of both viruses and bacteria, and are given a place in their own order, Chlamydiales. Within the family and genus are three species, *C. trachomatis*, *C. psittaci* and *C. pneumoniae.* The species are separated into several serotypes. Primary ocular serotypes are A, B, Ba, and C. Genital serovars are typically D to K, and L1 to L3 are the lymphogranuloma venereum serotypes. In newborn infants, ocular infection can occur from passage through an infected birth canal resulting in acute or sub-acute, self-limited follicular conjunctivitis. A single episode of acute conjunctivitis is not considered trachoma because there is virtually no risk of sustained inflammation or the adverse sequelae that characterizes repeated bouts of ocular infection with chlamydia in trachoma endemic areas. The repeated episodes of reinfection occurring in childhood and young adulthood appear to be necessary to produce the potentially blinding complications.

Chlamydiae lack a cell wall but contain both noncompartmentalized DNA and RNA. They lack a cytochrome system and cannot produce ATP. Thus, the host cell ATP is used to transport nutrients essential to the chlamydia across the cell membrane. Infection in the epithelial cells begins with endocytosis of the 350 nm infectious particle, the elementary body. Current efforts are underway to determine if there is a specific chlamydial adhesion mechanism, which may include the major outer membrane protein of chlamydia and a specific cell receptor. Endocytosis is followed by transformation of the elementary bodies into reticulate bodies. Although it is clear that one elementary body gives rise to one reticulate body, electron micrographs indicate that one reticulate body may give rise to several elementary bodies. Reticulate bodies are non-infectious, but are metabolically active, and multiply rapidly over the next 15 hours. Twenty hours post-infection, there appears to be an increased expression of the cysteine-rich 60 kDa outer membrane protein that coincides with the transformation of the reticulate bodies into new elementary bodies prior to release from the infected cell. The reticulate bodies and elementary bodies are enclosed in an inclusion body which can occupy up to 90% of the cell cytoplasm. Usually, rupture of the cell follows and infection of other cells by the elementary body results. Electron micrographic studies have shown that some cells can remain persistently infected with aberrant reticulate body-like structures. Although major outer membrane protein, a major immunodominant protein, and chlamydial heat shock protein are produced by both elementary bodies and reticulate bodies, chlamydial lipopolysaccharide is associated mainly with reticulate bodies.

## LABORATORY STUDIES

The laboratory diagnosis of *C. trachomatis* infection can be made by cytological examination of stained slides, by growing the organism in tissue cultured cells, or by detection of chlamydial antigens or nucleic acids. Serological tests for chlamydial IgG are not helpful for diagnosing current infection. The sensitivity and specificity of any of these methods can be greatly altered by the collection, handling and storage of the samples both by the clinician and the laboratory.

### Sample collection

Since chlamydiae are obligate, intracellular bacteria, an adequate number of epithelial cells should be present. Obvious mucus or pus should be removed from the sampling area and the tarsal conjunctivum should be firmly rubbed with a dacron-tipped swab having a plastic or metal shaft. Wood shafts have been shown to contain toxic chemicals for chlamydia. In our experience for processing ocular samples, at least 100 epithelial cells seen microscopically from an ocular sample indicates adequacy for tissue culture or antigen testing.

### Sample transport and storage

If there will be a delay in transport of samples for tissue culture and antigen methods, it is necessary to provide a cold chain. Although freezer storage is optimal for samples which will be analyzed by DNA amplification, refrigerator or room temperature storage in a transport buffer for a period up to 1 month does not affect the test sensitivity.[4,5]

### Giemsa and iodine staining

In 1907, chlamydial inclusions were first observed in conjunctival scrapings from orang-utans who developed follicular conjunctivitis after being infected with human trachoma samplings.[6] Inclusions seen in direct smears after Giemsa staining appear as roundish large structures containing reddish purple elementary or reticulate bodies. Giemsa staining is fast and economical in addition to providing information on the presence of other bacterial pathogens. However, this method is only moderately sensitive ranging from 22–56%, even if active disease is present.[7,8] Iodine stains the glycogen mass, and the inclusions appear reddish-brown for *C. trachomatis*. The other chlamydial species, which do not contain glycogen, appear clear. Iodine staining is even less sensitive than Giemsa.

### Tissue culture

Currently, samples are commonly cultured on cycloheximide-treated McCoy cells. After 48 hours of incubation, samples may be passaged from the original McCoy cell culture to a second culture of McCoy cells to increase recovery rates. Definitive diagnosis is made by staining the McCoy cells with direct fluorescent antibody to major outer membrane protein and observing for inclusions. One of the major advantages of tissue culture over direct cytological methods is that it is nearly 100% specific. However, if the strict requirements for transport and storage are not maintained, the sensitivity of this method decreases dramatically. Ideally, sensitivity is 90% or greater, but this may fall off depending upon length of storage, conditions of storage and faulty transport. In addition, in a setting of chronic or repeated infection, tissue culture may be negative even in symptomatic individuals.[9,10] It is postulated that certain immune factors could play a role in interfering with uptake of the elementary body into the cell or in maturation of the chlamydiae into infectious elementary bodies.[11]

### Antigen detection

Specific identification of *C. trachomatis* in direct conjunctival smears may be made using direct fluorescent antibody microscopy. The elementary bodies stain bright apple green with species-specific anti-major outer membrane protein fluorescein-tagged antibody.[12] This test is expensive, can be subjective, requires a highly trained observer, and for optimal results, maintenance of a cold chain. A non-microscopic antigen detection test currently in use is the enzyme linked immunosorbant assay (ELISA). One commonly used ELISA is genus specific in that the antibody is directed against all *Chlamydia* spp. lipopolysaccharide. For genital samples, ELISA sensitivity ranges from 62–96% and specificity from 86–99% versus cell culture. Best results occur in evaluations on high risk populations. ELISA assay has not been widely used in trachoma investigations. In a study of trachoma in Gambia, chlamydial glycolipid was detected by an amplified antigen detection system in 25% of active cases versus 18% by culture[13]

## Nucleic acid detection

Labeled DNA probes, which can be used to detect specific nucleotide sequences by hybridization to *C. trachomatis* ribosomal RNA, have not been widely evaluated for ocular samples. For genital samples, these probes are 80–95% specific compared to cell culture, and the sensitivity is only about $10^5$–$10^6$ chlamydial genomes.[14,15]

One of the most promising new tests is that of DNA amplification or the polymerase chain reaction (PCR) and the ligase chain reaction. Conserved areas of one *C. trachomatis* major outer membrane protein genome or of the cryptic plasmid can be amplified $10^6$-fold and the DNA is then detected by various methods. If certain factors are controlled, a quantitative estimate of chlamydial DNA load is possible. A chlamydial PCR was evaluated for determining trachoma prevalence in Tanzania, nasal infection, and to investigate ocular re-infection after vaccine in a cynmologous monkey model.[5,10,16] In the Tanzanian studies, it was found that DNA load directly correlated with clinical severity and that response to topical tetracycline therapy could be monitored. In addition, PCR diagnosed clinically inapparent infection in 70% of those subjects with 1–4 follicles by photographic analysis where direct fluorescent antibody was quite insensitive. Nasal infection was 24% pretreatment and directly correlated to severity of inflammation posttreatment. In the animal study, PCR positivity was related to inflammation in culture negative animals who were re-challenged. In studies on low risk populations, PCR correlates well with traditional detection tests. However, in high risk sexually transmitted disease populations and in trachoma endemic areas, PCR detection of *C. trachomatis* surpasses both culture and antigen detection methods.

## Chlamydia typing

Although chlamydial typing is not a routine test, typing plays a central role in understanding the epidemiology of *C. trachomatis* infection. In addition, typing provides relevant information for planning vaccine usage by documenting the fluctuation of antigenic types in a geographic locale.

Based on nucleotide sequencing of the major outer membrane protein gene

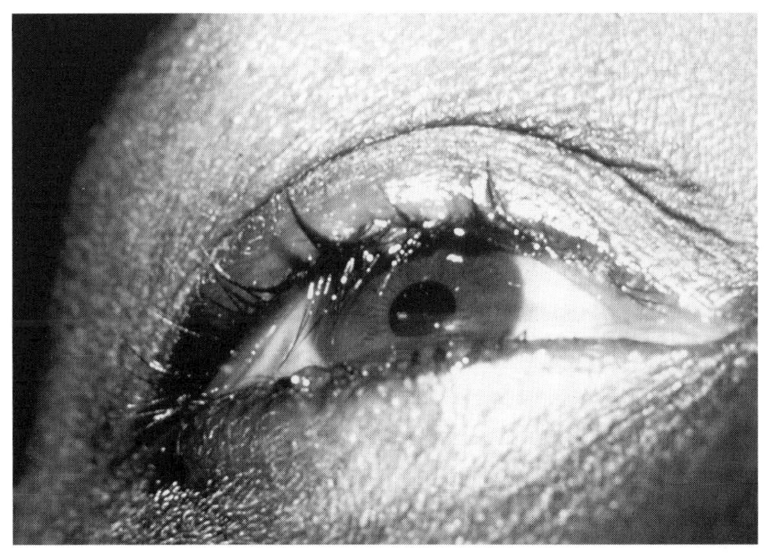

**Fig. 12.1** Patient with trichiasis.

of all the serovars, the major outer membrane protein gene is composed of conserved or species-specific areas and hypervariable or type-specific domains.[17] In addition, in several studies on types isolated from trachoma endemic areas, it was found that for a given serovar, there may exist multiple gene types.[18,19] These observations are important for two reasons. First, immunotyping usually indicates only two trachoma types in a given locale, but gene typing may indicate many more variants. Nucleotide information thus allows a finer evaluation of prevalence, transmission and antigenic variation. Secondly, nucleotide studies of variants can also be linked to analyses of tear or serum antibodies.[20] It is postulated that this antigenic variation could be a mechanism whereby chlamydia escape from immune surveillance would facilitate re-emergence of disease.

For clinicians, the primary emphasis is on use of laboratory studies as an adjunct to diagnosis and treatment. However, the following research areas should be briefly mentioned. There is tremendous activity using a laboratory approach to gain a better understanding of the humoral, mucosal and cellular immune responses to various chlamydial antigens in trachoma. Key questions involve trying to understand why the humoral or local immune response is often not protective, what is the role of cell-mediated factors, and why re-infection leads to blinding sequelae.

## CLINICAL FEATURES

Trachoma is characterized by an acute, inflammatory response to a series of infections throughout childhood, followed by evidence of scarring of the

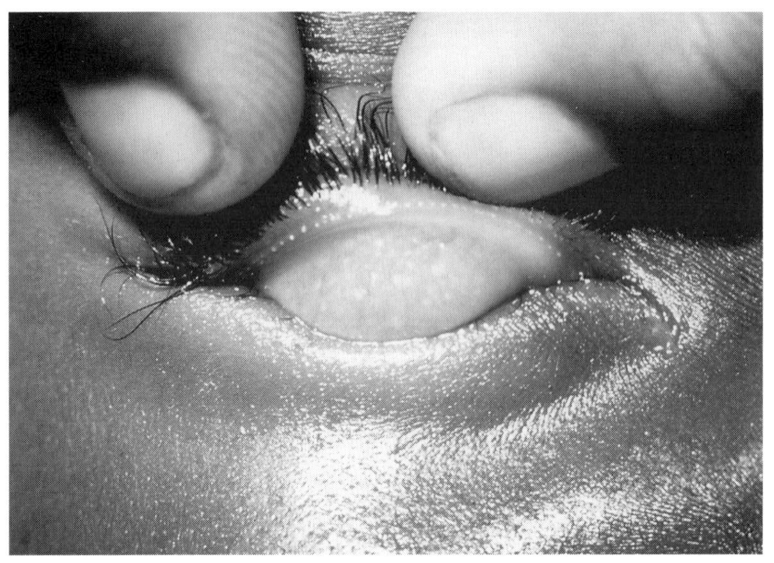

**Fig. 12.2** Follicular trachoma.

sub-conjunctiva. By late childhood and early adulthood, the scarring may be prominent and obscure evidence of active disease. Visual impairment and blindness from corneal scarring most often occur in middle age. Typically, patients with trachoma do not complain of symptoms until the scarring is significant enough to cause trichiasis, or inturned eyelashes (see Fig. 12.1).

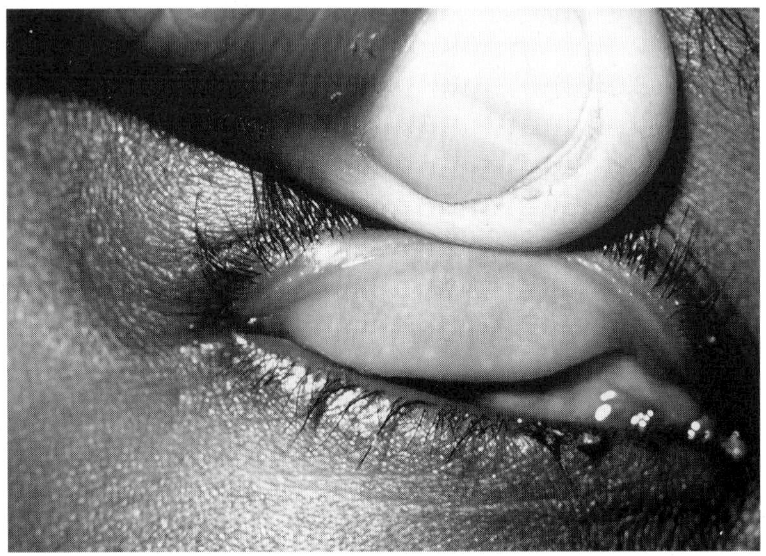

**Fig. 12.3** Patient with papillae and follicles.

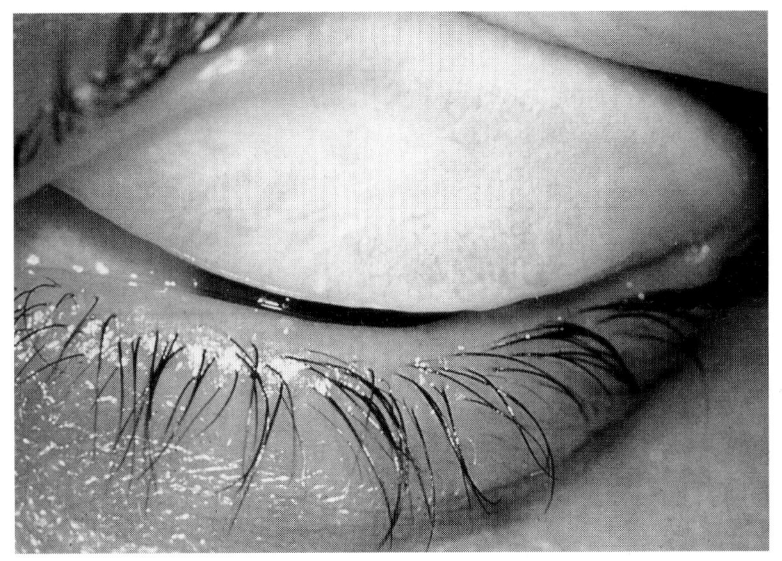

**Fig. 12.4** Patient with extensive scarring.

The community pool of active inflammatory trachoma resides in pre-school children. Children with active trachoma present with follicles and papillae. Follicles are yellow or white round spots occurring in the superior tarsal conjunctiva (see Fig. 12.2). Follicles are avascular lymphoid tissue whose germinal centre contain B lymphocytes surrounded by T cells. Necrosis of the follicle during resolution of the disease may be followed by scarring. In addition to the follicle, signs of trachoma include papillae (Fig. 12.3). The density of these small red dots in the superior tarsal conjunctiva reflects the intensity of inflammation, and are particularly prominent in the presence of a secondary bacterial infection. In hyperendemic trachoma areas, 10% or more of active trachoma cases in children can present as a severe inflammation and thickening of the conjunctiva which obscures the deep tarsal vessels. Follicles are usually present with severe inflammation, but may be difficult to see in the presence of pronounced hyperemia. The presence of pus with severe inflammation usually indicates a bacterial infection. Children with trachoma may have watery eyes and complain, if at all, of a 'gritty' sensation, usually attributable to the follicles.

Corneal changes may also occur during active inflammation, but these signs are not a sensitive indicator of chlamydial infection because they are often absent. Limbal follicles may appear, and new vessels develop producing a corneal pannus. The pannus may extend across the cornea, avoiding the limbal follicles. Once the follicles resolve, depressions remain on the cornea, resulting in the pathognomic sign of trachoma, 'Herbert's pits'.

Herbert's pits, pannus, and scarring of the conjunction are signs of past infection with trachoma. Scars can appear as small, stellate spots, difficult to differentiate from follicles. Severe scarring can result in a 'basket weave' appearance to the conjunctiva (Fig. 12.4). Severe scarring contracts the tarsal plate, rotating the eyelashes inward. When the eye lashes turn in sufficiently to abrade the cornea, a high risk of blindness from corneal scarring and opacification is present. Eyes with trichiasis need appropriate lid surgery to correct the inturned lashes and avoid loss of sight. Trichiasis and corneal opacity are late stages of trachoma and typically appear in adults.

Other conditions can produce a follicular conjunctivitis and should be differentiated from active trachoma. The most common are viral conjunctivitis and vernal catarrh. Viral conjunctivitis presents with follicles, is self-limited, and usually resolves within 2 weeks. Other differential diagnoses include ocular allergies, inclusion conjunctivitis and molluscum contagiosum, which produces a follicular conjunctivitis.

Inclusion conjunctivitis is also caused by *C. trachomatis*, but is usually associated with a genital strain. Neonatal inclusion conjunctivitis occurs after passage through an infected birth canal. Infants present with severe, mucopurulent conjunctivitis, usually within 2 weeks of birth. Silver nitrate is ineffective in preventing chlamydial infection, and infants require systemic antibiotics. Chlamydial inclusion conjunctivitis should be differentiated from gonococcal ophthalmia neonatorum, which is a sight-threatening infection. Ophthalmia neonatorum typically appears within the first 8 days, and the typical Gram-negative intracellular diplococci of *Neisseria gonorrhoeae* can be seen in smears. Penicillin, a cell wall-acting antibiotic, is effective against gonococci, but not against chlamydia, which have no cell wall. Therefore, treatment of mixed infection may require multiple antibiotics. Inclusion conjunctivitis results from an isolated episode of chlamydial infection, whereas repeated episodes of chlamydial infection are the pattern of potentially blinding trachoma.

## TREATMENT

At the outset it should be said that treatment of trachoma requires a community-based approach. Treatment of isolated cases will cure the patient's current infection, but the odds are high that re-infection will occur shortly after treatment in these endemic communities. For many trachoma areas, treatment of the entire community at regular intervals coupled with a public health approach may be the only way to reduce blinding trachoma. This topic is discussed more fully in the next section.

Chlamydia is sensitive to several antibiotics. For neonatal conjunctivitis, recommended treatment is systemic erythromycin 30–50 mg/kg/day for 14 days. Systemic treatment is recommended to reduce the risk of chlamydial pneumonia in newborns who have ocular evidence of chlamydial infection. Development of antibiotic resistance of chlamydia in vivo has not been documented.

Various regimens for treating trachoma with topical antibiotics have been studied. Tetracycline 1% eye ointment or 1% oily tetracycline drops used 1–2 times per day for 4–6 weeks are effective, and tetracycline ointment is relatively inexpensive. Other dosing regimens include use of the ointment 2 times per day for 1–3 weeks, repeated at monthly intervals for 6 months.[21]

There is a new azolide, azithromycin, which is effective against *C. trachomatis*. It has the advantage of requiring only a single dose to be effective due to the high tissue levels and long half-life.[22] Although relatively expensive, it has become the drug of choice for treating chlamydial genital infections. In adults, the dose is 1 g, given once. In Europe, azithromycin can be used in children as young as 6 months for chlamydia infections.

Azithromycin offers the potential for a breakthrough in community-control of trachoma. Studies are currently underway in hyperendemic communities to determine the risk of re-emergent trachoma after mass treatment. Unfortunately, unless a program is developed under which the azithromycin might be given free or subsidized to such communities, it is unlikely to be a practical solution to trachoma control.

## EPIDEMIOLOGY

Trachoma remains the leading infectious cause of blindness worldwide. It is endemic in areas of Africa, Asia, Australia and the Middle East with foci in North and South America. In areas where trachoma has been endemic for a long time, the disease has a characteristic age distribution. Active, inflammatory trachoma is present in children, primarily pre-school children. Prevalence surveys in hyperendemic areas have revealed anywhere from 60–100% of children can have evidence of active disease.[23] Scarring of the conjunctiva can be visible, even at a young age, and identifies those who are at high risk of severe scarring, and possibly trichiasis and entropion.[24]

Rates of active disease decline rapidly after age 10 years, with mothers or caretakers of pre-school children being the primary group of adults with active trachoma.[23] Trichiasis and entropion can occur in young adults, but are typically seen in middle-aged or older adults.

Active trachoma rates may be equal in young boys and girls, or slightly higher in young girls, but scarring, trichiasis, entropion, and corneal opacity preferentially affect women.[23] This is generally thought to be due to the higher likelihood of exposure to constant re-infection experienced by women because of their child care responsibilities.[25] However, one study designed to evaluate the risk of trichiasis in women associated with cumulative years of exposure to child care in a trachoma endemic community did not find any association.[26] Characteristics that predispose women to the blinding sequelae of trachoma need to be further studied.

Several studies have shown that trachoma is hyperendemic in communities characterized by poor sanitation and hygiene, where water is scarce and viewed as a precious resource. Transmission of infection occurs during contact with infected ocular or other secretions. A large fly population contributes to the risk of trachoma, especially severe trachoma, and flies are thought to be physical vectors for chlamydia transmission.[27,28]

Strategies for control of trachoma in endemic communities are now taking a public health approach. Clearly, simply identifying and treating clinically apparent cases is not enough to keep blinding trachoma from these communities. Even the World Health Organization recommendations to treat the entire community have only short-lived benefit; trachoma rates have been shown to fall during and for a few months following mass treatment, but have returned to pretreatment levels within a year. Recent data have shown that children with unclean faces, or who are not washed at least once a day, have an almost 2-fold risk of severe trachoma.[27,29] These children are probably more likely to re-infect themselves and others. Data from a large project in Central Tanzania suggest that mass treatment followed by an intensive campaign to increase face-washing in children results in suppression of rates of severe trachoma for up to a year.[30] Even in areas with water shortage, families can be shown that face-washing requires only a small commitment of water.[31]

Health care professionals working in trachoma endemic communities should consider projects with a community-wide approach to control. These consist of the following components:

1. Identify the magnitude of the trachoma problem. The World Health Organization recommends use of a simple grading scheme for assessment of acute, inflammatory trachoma, scarring, and trichiasis/entropion.[32] Small prevalence surveys, especially among preschool children and middle-aged adults, will provide a picture of high-risk communities.

2. Work with community leaders, women's groups, neighbourhood associations and other community organizations to mobilize a community-based trachoma control program. One component of this must include treatment of existing cases, probably through a mass treatment campaign. However, the community must be aware that prevention through improved hygiene is the only long-term solution to trachoma control.

3. Provide lid surgery for trichiasis/entropion. Effective lid surgery can prevent corneal damage from trichiasis. Safe and effective lid surgery can be carried out by trained eye nurses at minimal cost, and should be part of any community-based strategy.

Trachoma has disappeared in most industrialized countries, and hence has been largely forgotten as a serious public health issue. *C. trachomatis* infection now receives intense attention as a sexually transmitted disease. However, trachoma continues to be a major problem for the communities that often have the fewest resources to take on health issues, and it strikes the most vulnerable members of those communities, children and women. Effective public health measures for trachoma control must re-emerge as priorities for health care professionals responsible for the prevention of blindness in these communities.

## KEY POINTS FOR CLINICAL PRACTICE

- Trachoma is the leading infectious cause of blindness worldwide. It continues to be hyperendemic in many areas of Africa, the Middle East and Asia.
- Trachoma, and acute follicular conjunctivitis of newborns, are caused by an ocular infection with *C. trachomatis*.
- The most sensitive test for the laboratory diagnosis of *C. trachomatis* is use of DNA amplification techniques or PCR detection. Kits are commercially available.
- Where endemic, trachoma is a public health problem, trachoma control necessitates effective treatment and promotion of hygiene measures like face-washing to decrease transmission.
- *C. trachomatis* is sensitive to erythromycin, tetracycline, and the new azolide, azithromycin. Effective treatment of trachoma may require a mass campaign in the community recognizing that young children are the reservoir of infection.

## REFERENCES

1 Duke-Elder SS. Diseases of the outer eye, Part I. System of ophthalmology, Vol. VIII. London: Henry Kempton, 1977: 249-307
2 American Encyclopedia of Ophthalmology, Vol. XVII. Wood CA. Ed. Cleveland Press, 1921: 12887-12892.
3 Elliot RH. Tropical Ophthalmology. London: Oxford University Press, 1920: 300.
4 Taylor HR, Rapoza PA, West S et al. The epidemiology of infection in trachoma. Invest Ophthalmol Vis Sci 1989; 30: 1823-1833
5 Bobo L, Muñoz B, Viscidi R, Quinn T, Mkocha H, West S. Diagnosis of *Chlamydia trachomatis* ocular infection in Tanzania by polymerase chain reaction-enzyme immunoassay. Lancet 1991; 338: 847-850
6 Halberstaester L, von Prowazek S. Uber Zelleinschlusse parasitarer Natur beim Tracho. Arb Gesundheitsa 1907; XXVI: 44-47
7 Rowe DS, Aicardi EZ, Dawson CR, Schachter J. Purulent ocular discharge in neonates. Pediatrics 1979; 63: 628-632
8 Sandstrom KI, Bell TA, Chandler JW et al. Diagnosis of neonatal purulent conjunctivitis caused by *Chlamydia trachomatis* and other organisms. In: Mardh PA, Holmes KK, Oriel JD, Piot P, Schachter J. eds. Chlamydial Infections. Amsterdam: Elsevier 1982: 217-220
9 Viscidi RP, Bobo L, Hook EW, Quinn TC. Transmission of *Chlamydia trachomatis* among sexual partners assessed by polymerase chain reaction. J Infect Dis 1993; 168: 488-492

10 Holland S, Hudson A, Bobo L et al. Demonstration of chlamydial RNA and DNA during a culture-negative state. Infect Immun 1992; 60: 2040-2047
11 Beatty W, Byrne GI, Morrison RP. Morphologic and antigenic characterization of interferon-τ-mediated persistent *Chlamydia trachomatis* infection in vitro. Proc Natl Acad Sci USA 1993; 90: 3998-4002
12 Tam MR, Stamm WE, Handsfield HH et al. Culture-independent diagnosis of *Chlamydia trachomatis* using monoclonal antibodies. N Engl J Med 1984; 310: 1146-1150
13 Mabey DCW, Robertson JN, Ward ME. Detection of *Chlamydia trachomatis* by enzyme immunoassay in patients with trachoma. Lancet 1987; ii: 1491-1492
14 Horn JE, Hammer ML, Falkow S, Quinn TC. Detection of *Chlamydia trachomatis* in tissue culture and cervical scrapings by in situ DNA hybridization. J Infect Dis 1986; 153: 1155-1159
15 Palva A. Nucleic acid spot hybridization for detection of *Chlamydia trachomatis*. FEMS Microbiol Lett 1985; 28: 85-91
16 West S, Muñoz B, Bobo L, Viscidi R, Quinn T. Non-ocular chlamydia infection and risk of ocular reinfection after mass treatment in a trachoma hyperendemic area. Invest Ophthalmol Vis Sci 1994; 34: 3194-3198
17 Yuan Y, Zhang YX, Watkins NG, Caldwell HD. Nucleotide and deduced amino acid sequences for the four variable domains of the major outer membrane proteins of the 15 *Chlamydia trachomatis* serovars. Infect Immun 1989; 57: 1040-1049
18 Dean D, Dawson C, Schachter J, Stephens RS. Comparison of the major outer membrane protein sequence variant regions of B/Ba isolates: a molecular epidemiological approach to *Chlamydia trachomatis* infections. J Infect Dis 1992; 166: 383-392
19 Hayes LJ, Bailey RL, Mabey DCW et al. Genotyping of *Chlamydia trachomatis* from a trachoma-endemic village in the Gambia by a nested polymerase chain reaction: identification of strain variants. J Infect Dis 1992; 666: 1173-1177
20 Jones HM, Schachter J, Stephens RS. Sequence-defined immunoassay for determining serovariant-specific serological responses to *Chlamydia trachomatis* infection. J Infect Dis 1992; 166: 915-919
21 Dawson CR, Jones BR, Tarizzo ML. Guide to Trachoma Control. Geneva: World Health Organization, 1981: 41
22 Martin DH, Mroczkowski TF, Daler ZA et al. Azithromycin for Chlamydial Infectious Study Group. A controlled trial of a single dose of azithromycin for the treatment of chlamydial urethritis and cervicitis. N Engl J Med 1992; 327: 921-925
23 West SK, Muñoz B, Turner VM, Mmbaga BBO, Taylor HR. The epidemiology of trachoma in Central Tanzania. Int J Epidemiol, 1991; 20: 1088-1092
24 Dawson CR, Juster R, Marx R, Daghfous MT, Djerad AB. Limbal disease in trachoma and other ocular chlamydia infections: risk factors for corneal vascularization. Eye 1989; 3: 204-209
25 Congdon N, West S, Vitale S, Ktala S, Mmbaga BBO. Exposure to children and risk of active trachoma in Tanzanian women. Am J Epidemiol 1993; 137: 366-372
26 Turner VM, West SK, Muñoz B et al. Risk factors for trichiasis in women in Kongwa, Tanzania: a case control study. Int J Epidemiol 1993; 22: 341-347
27 West SK, Congdon N, Katala S, Mele L. Facial cleanliness and risk of trachoma in families. Arch Ophthalmol 1991; 109: 855-857
28 Brechner RJ, West S, Lynch M. Trachoma and flies: individual vs environmental risk factors. Arch Ophthalmol 1992; 110: 687-689
29 Taylor HR, West SK, Mmbaga BBO et al. Hygiene factors and increased risk of trachoma in Central Tanzania. Arch Ophthalmol 1989; 107: 1821-1825
30 West S, Muñoz B, Lynch M et al. Impact of face washing on trachoma in Central Tanzania. Lancet 1995; 345: 155-158
31 West S, Lynch M, Turner V et al. Water availability and trachoma. Bull WHO 1989; 67: 71-75
32 Thylefors B, Dawson CR, Jones BR, West SK, Taylor HR. A simple system for the assessment of trachoma and its complications. Bull WHO 1987; 65: 477-483

# 13

# Paediatric literature review – 1994

*T. J. David*

## ALLERGY AND IMMUNOLOGY

### Allergy

Leung DYM. Mechanisms of the human allergic response: clinical implications. Pediatr Clin North Am 1994; 41: 727-743. *Review.*

Munir AKM, Einarsson R, Dreborg SKG. Indirect contact with pets can confound the effect of cleaning procedures for reduction of animal allergen levels in house dust. Pediatr Allergy Immunol 1994; 5: 32-39. *Visits from pet owners confound antigen avoidance procedures.*

### Immunology

Bellanti JA, Kadlec JV, Escobar-Gutiérrez A. Cytokines and the immune response. Pediatr Clin North Am 1994; 41: 597-621. *Review.*

Buckley RH. Breakthroughs in the understanding and therapy of primary immunodeficiency. Pediatr Clin North Am 1994; 41: 665-690. *Review. See also BMJ 1994; 308: 581-585 and Arch Dis Child 1994; 70: 260-263.*

Shirakawa T, Li A, Dubowitz M et al. Association between atopy and variants of the β subunit of the high-affinity immunoglobulin E receptor. Nature Genet 1994; 7: 125-129. *This receptor, subject to maternal modification, may be the atopy-causing locus on chromosome 11q. See also Lancet 1994; 343: 1597-1600. For genetic basis of immunoglobulin-class switching see N Engl J Med 1994; 330: 1008-1009.*

Sullivan KE, Mullen CA, Blaese RM et al. A multi-institutional survey of the Wiskott-Aldrich syndrome. J Pediatr 1994; 125: 876-885. *Only 27% of 154 cases had the classical triad of thrombocytopaenia with small platelets, eczema and recurrent otitis media.*

Walker AM, Kemp AS, Hill DJ et al. Features of transient hypogammaglobulinaemia in infants screened for immunological abnormalities. Arch Dis Child 1994; 70: 183-186. *12 out of 15 had symptoms of either atopic disease or food intolerance and three had gastrointestinal symptoms.*

## CARDIOVASCULAR

Leversha AM, Wilson NJ, Clarkson PM et al. Efficacy and dosage of enalapril in congenital and acquired heart disease. Arch Dis Child 1994; 70: 35-39. *Enalapril was clinically safe and effective, but renal failure was a problem in young infants with left to right shunts.*

Lucas A, Morley R. Does early nutrition in infants born before term programme later blood pressure? BMJ 1994; 309: 304-308. *Data suggest that the long-term rise in blood pressure reported in individuals who had low birth weight at full term is not, as previously speculated, due to poor foetal nutrition or growth as such. See also Arch Dis Child 1994; 70: 536-537.*

Silove ED. Assessment and management of congenital heart disease in the newborn by the district paediatrician. Arch Dis Child 1994; 70: F71-F74. *Review.*

## COMMUNITY

Anonymous. Using medicines in school. Drug Ther Bull 1994; 32: 81-87. *Review.*
Cass HD, Sonksen PM, McConachie HR. Developmental setback in severe visual impairment. Arch Dis Child 1994; 70: 192-196. *Developmental setback in the second or third year occurred in ten (31%) of 32 children who were totally blind.*
Cornelissen P, Bradley L, Fowler S et al. What children see affects how they spell. Dev Med Child Neurol 1994; 36: 716-727. *Unstable binocular control may affect not only how certain children read but also how they spell.*

First LR, Palfrey JS. The infant or young child with developmental delay. N Engl J Med 1994; 330: 478-483. *Review.*

Gandhi KK. Diagnosis and management of nocturnal enuresis. Curr Opin Pediatr 1994; 6: 194-197. *Review.*

Heller DR. Ambulatory paediatrics: stepping out in a new direction? Arch Dis Child 1994; 70: 339-342. *Review.*

Laborde DJ, Weigle KA, Weber DJ et al. The frequency, level, and distribution of fecal contamination in day-care center classrooms. Pediatrics 1994; 94 Suppl: 1008-1011. *Faecal contamination is widespread. See also pp. 987-1008.*

Pocock SJ, Smith M, Baghurst P. Environmental lead and children's intelligence: a systematic review of the epidemiological evidence. N Engl J Med 1994; 309: 1189-1197. *Review. See also Pediatrics 1994; 93: 201-204.*

Wolfe DA, Korsch B. Witnessing domestic violence during childhood and adolescence: implication for pediatric practice. Pediatrics 1994; 94 Suppl: 594-599. *Review.*

Wolke D, Gray P, Meyer R. Excessive infant crying: a controlled study of mothers helping mothers. Pediatrics 1994; 94: 322-332. *Treatment by suitably but briefly trained lay counsellors was an inexpensive and successful treatment. See editorial pp.333-334.*

Zahir M, Bennett S. Review of child development teams. Arch Dis Child 1994; 70: 224-228. *Review.*

## Accidents

Buckley SL. Sports injuries in children. Curr Opin Pediatr 1994; 6: 80-84. *Review. For radiological features see Arch Dis Child 1994; 70: 457-460. For injuries from sports equipment see Arch Pediatr Adolesc Med 1994; 148: 1107-1109.*

Byard RW, Beal S, Bourne AJ. Potentially dangerous sleeping environments and accidental asphyxia in infancy and early childhood. Arch Dis Child 1994; 71: 497-500. *Review of 30 cases of accidental asphyxia in infants and young children who had been left to sleep unattended.*

Chiaviello CT, Christoph RA, Bond GR. Stairway-related injuries in children. Pediatrics 1994; 94: 679-681. *The majority of injuries were minor.*

Gershman KA, Sacks JJ, Wright JC. Which dogs bite? A case-control study of risk factors. Pediatrics 1994; 93: 913-917. *Failure to neuter a dog, and selection of male dogs and certain breeds such as German Shepherd may increase the risk of a dog biting a non household member, who often may be a child.*

Mott A, Evans R, Rolfe K et al. Patterns of injuries to children on public playgrounds. Arch Dis Child 1994; 71: 328-330. *The high fracture rate on modernised bark playgrounds is a problem.*

Nuutinen M, Uhari M, Karvali T et al. Consequences of caustic ingestions in children. Acta Paediatr 1994; 83: 1200-1205. *Report of 98 cases; household vinegar was the most commonly ingested caustic agent.*

Rodgers GC. The role of aversive bittering agents in the prevention of pediatric poisonings. Pediatrics 1994; 93: 68-69. *Review.*

Thomas S, Acton C, Nixon J et al. Effectiveness of bicycle helmets in preventing head injury in children: case-control study. BMJ 1994; 308: 173-176. *Helmets work. See also pp.177, 1521-1522, 1534-1540 and Arch Dis Child 1994; 71: 536-539.*

Yeoh C, Nixon JW, Dickson W et al. Patterns of scald injuries. Arch Dis Child 1994; 71: 156-158. *The best way to reduce scalds would be to reduce the temperature in domestic hot water tanks. For review of burns see Lancet 1994; 343: 216-220.*

## Cerebral palsy

Lingam S, Joester J. Spontaneous fractures in children and adolescents with cerebral palsy. BMJ 1994; 309: 265-266. *Children with cerebral palsy have a tendency to sustain spontaneous fractures. See also Arch Dis Child 1994; 71: 235-238.*

Kuban KCK, Leviton A. Cerebral palsy. N Engl J Med 1994; 330: 188-195. *Review.*

Staiano A, Del Giudice E. Colonic transit and anorectal manometry in children with severe brain damage. Pediatrics 1994; 94: 169-173. *Colonic transit abnormalities in the colon and rectum may explain the constipation seen in severely handicapped children.*

## Child abuse

Adams JA, Harper K, Knudson S et al. Examination findings in legally confirmed child sexual abuse: it's normal to be normal. Pediatrics 1994; 94: 310-317. *Abnormal genital findings were not common in this series of sexually abused girls.*

Toubia N. Female circumcision as a public health issue. N Engl J Med 1994; 331: 712-716. *Review. See also Arch Dis Child 1994; 70: 441-444.*

McClain PW, Sacks JJ, Ewigman BG et al. Geographic patterns of fatal abuse or neglect in children younger than 5 years old, United States, 1979 to 1988. Arch Pediatr Adolesc Med 1994; 148: 82-86. *Understanding the sizable geographic variation in child abuse death rates could lead to effective interventions.*

MacGregor R, Pullar A, Cundall D. Silent at school – elective mutism and abuse. Arch Dis Child 1994; 70: 540-541. *8 of 18 children selectively mute in school had suffered definite or probable abuse compared with only one control.*

Kemp AM, Mott AM, Sibert JR. Accidents and child abuse in bathtub submersions. Arch Dis Child 1994; 70: 435-438. *Out of 44 children who suffered from drowning or near drowning in the bath, there were ten with stories suggestive of abuse.*

Makari GSH, Carroll JE, Burton EM. Hereditary sensory neuropathy manifesting as possible child abuse. Pediatrics 1994; 93: 842-844. *Child abuse was suspected incorrectly in a five year old with burns in whom the mother reported that the child did not seem to feel pain.*

## Immunization

Aickin R, Hill D, Kemp A. Measles immunisation in children with allergy to egg. BMJ 1994; 309: 223-225. *A positive skin prick test to the vaccine did not predict an adverse reaction.*

Baxter DN. Pertussis immunisation of children with histories of neurological problems. BMJ 1994; 309: 1619-1620. *Children with histories of neurological problems can be safely immunised against pertussis. See also Health Trends 1994; 26: 23-24. For immunization myths see pp.1073-1075.*

Bell LM, Lopez NI, Pinto-Martin J et al. Potential impact of linking an emergency department and hospital-affiliated clinics to immunize pre-school-age children. Pediatrics 1994; 93: 99-103. *Routine vaccination in the emergency department would significantly increase immunization percentages.*

Christie CDC, Marx ML, Marchant CD et al. The 1993 epidemic of pertussis in

Cincinnati. Resurgence of disease in a highly immunized population of children. N Engl J Med 1994; 331: 16-21. *The 1993 pertussis epidemic occurred primarily among children who had been appropriately immunised, implying that the whole cell pertussis vaccine failed to give full protection. See also Lancet 1994; 344: 491-492.*

Committee on Infectious Diseases. Update on timing of hepatitis B vaccination for premature infants and for children with lapsed immunization. Pediatrics 1994; 94: 403-404. *Review.*

Gale JL, Thapa PB, Wassilak SGF et al. Risk of serious acute neurological illness after immunization with diphtheria-tetanus-pertussis vaccine. JAMA 1994; 271: 37-41. *No significant increase.*

Grabham T. The new measles campaign. Immunisation should prevent an epidemic predicted by modelling. BMJ 1994; 309: 1102-1103. *Editorial. See also pp. 1161-1162 and Commun Dis Rep CDR Wkly 1994; 4: R141-R155.*

Hall CB, Granoff DM, Gromisch DS et al. Recommended timing of routine measles immunization for children who have recently received immune globulin preparations. Pediatrics 1994; 93: 682-685. *American Academy recommendations.*

Peltola H, Heinonen OP, Valle M et al. The elimination of indigenous measles, mumps, and rubella from Finland by a 12 year, two dose vaccination program. N Engl J Med 1994; 331: 1397-1402. *An immunisation programme using two doses of combined live virus vaccine has eliminated indigenous measles, mumps and rubella from Finland. See editorial pp. 1446-1447.*

Stratton KR, Howe CJ, Johnston RB. Adverse events associated with childhood vaccines other than pertussis and rubella. JAMA 1994; 271: 1602-1605. *Review.*

Watson BA, Starr SE. Varicella vaccine for healthy children. Lancet 1994; 343: 928-929. *Review.*

**Infant feeding**

Cockburn F. Neonatal brain and dietary lipids. Arch Dis Child 1994; 70: F1-F2. *Review.*

Blomquist HK, Jonsbo F, Serenius F et al. Supplementary feeding in the maternity ward shortens the duration of breast feeding. Acta Paediatr 1994; 83: 1122-1126. *Supplementation with formula or donor milk is associated with an increased risk of short duration for breast feeding. For low prevalence of breast feeding in Scotland see BMJ 1994; 308: 824-825.*

Lang S, Lawrence CJ, Orme RL. Cup feeding: an alternative method of infant feeding. Arch Dis Child 1994; 71: 365-369. *Review.*

Lucas A, Morley R, Cole TJ et al. A randomised multicentre study of human milk versus formula and later development in preterm infants. Arch Dis Child 1994; 70: F141-F146. *Donor milk feeding was associated with advantages for later development and may have offset any potentially deleterious effects of its low nutrient content for preterm infants. For neurological outcome see also Lancet 1994; 344: 1319-1322.*

Rudolph CD. Feeding disorders in infants and children. J Pediatr 1994; 125 Suppl: S116-S124. *Review.*

Smith MM, Lifshitz F. Excess fruit juice consumption as a contributing factor in nonorganic failure to thrive. Pediatrics 1994; 93: 438-443. *Large intakes of fruit juices may displace more calorie and nutrient dense foods.*

Kauffman RE, Banner W, Berlin CM et al. The transfer of drugs and other chemicals into human milk. Pediatrics 1994; 93: 137-150. *Review.*

Morton JA. The clinical usefulness of breast milk sodium in the assessment of lactogenesis. Pediatrics 1994; 93: 802-806. *A normal drop in sodium is highly predictive of successful lactation, and a prolonged elevation of sodium signifies impaired lactogenesis with a high risk of failure.*

Varendi H, Porter RH, Winberg J. Does the newborn baby find the nipple by smell? Lancet 1994; 344: 989-990. *When given the choice, newborn infants preferred to feed from an unwashed rather than a washed breast.*

**Sudden infant death syndrome (SIDS)**

Brooks JG, Gilbert RE, Fleming PJ et al. Postnatal growth preceding sudden infant death syndrome. Pediatrics 1994; 94: 456-461. *No difference was found between the postnatal growth of SIDS victims and that of age matched control infants.*

Fleming PJ. Understanding and preventing sudden infant death syndrome. Curr Opin Pediatr 1994; 6: 158-162. *Review. For pulmonary immunopathology see Lancet 1994; 343: 1390-1392. For ethnicity and SIDS see Arch Dis Child 1994; 70: 349-353.*

Fleming PJ, Cooke M, Chantler SM et al. Fire retardants, biocides, plasticisers, and sudden infant deaths. BMJ 1994; 309: 1594-1596. *Review.*

Gilbert R. The changing epidemiology of SIDS. Arch Dis Child 1994; 70: 445-449. *Review For evaluation of government campaign to reduce risk see BMJ 1994; 309: 703-704.*

Mitchell EA, Nelson KP, Thompson JMD et al. Travel and changes in routine do not increase the risk of sudden infant death syndrome. Acta Paediatr 1994; 83: 815-818. *But visits to and by friends or relatives were associated with significantly reduced risk of SIDS, possibly suggesting less social support in SIDS cases.*

Tirosh E, Haddad F, Lanir A et al. Relationship of sweat electrolytes to apparent life-threatening events (ALTE): a case control study. Acta Paediatr

1994; 83: 1268-1271. *A significantly elevated sweat potassium concentration was found in affected cases.*

### Surveillance/screening

Bess FH, Paradise JL. Universal screening for infant hearing impairment: not simple, not risk-free, not necessarily beneficial, and not presently justified. Pediatrics 1994; 94: 330-334. *Review. For distraction testing see Arch Dis Child 1994; 70: 10-13.*

Hammond J, Chinn S, Richardson H et al. Serum total cholesterol and ferritin and blood haemoglobin concentrations in primary schoolchildren. Arch Dis Child 1994; 70: 373-375. *Suggests that an apparently healthy sample of predominantly middle class British children have moderately high levels of iron deficiency, anaemia, and higher than desirable serum cholesterol levels. For unhealthy diets in schoolchildren, see pp. 376-381.*

Jewell G, Reeves B, Saffin K et al. The effectiveness of vision screening by school nurses in secondary school. Arch Dis Child 1994; 70: 14-18. *Vision screening is not the best way to meet the eye/vision needs of secondary schoolchildren.*

## DERMATOLOGY

Harrison SL, MacLennan R, Speare R et al. Sun exposure and melanocytic naevi in young Australian children. Lancet 1994; 344: 1529-1532. *With exposure to intense ultraviolet light, children develop melanocytic naevi early in life and in large numbers.*

Healy E, Simpson N. Acne vulgaris. BMJ 1994; 308: 831-833. *Review.*

Roujeau JC, Stern RS. Severe adverse cutaneous reactions to drugs. N Engl J Med 1994; 331: 1272-1285. *Review.*

## ENDOCRINOLOGY

Donaldson MDC, Thomas PH, Love JG et al. Presentation, acute illness, and learning difficulties in salt wasting 21-hydroxylase deficiency. Arch Dis Child 1994; 70: 214-218. *Report of 63 cases, with a notably high incidence of learning difficulties.*

Donaldson MDC, Chu CE, Cooke A et al. The Prader-Willi syndrome. Arch Dis Child 1994; 70: 58-63. *Review.*

Levine A, Cohen D, Zadik Z. Urinary free cortisol values in children under stress. J Pediatr 1994; 125: 853-857. *Recommendations to increase the dose of steroids to 3–5 times of the baseline in children on steroids during times of stress may be inadequate.*

Lissau I, Sorensen TIA. Parental neglect during childhood and increased risk of obesity in young adulthood. Lancet 1994; 343: 324-327. *Parental neglect is associated with an increased risk of obesity in young adulthood.*

Magiakou MA, Mastorakos G, Oldfield EH et al. Cushing's syndrome in children and adolescents. Presentation, diagnosis and therapy. N Engl J Med 1994; 331: 629-636. *Weight gain and growth retardation are the common clinical characteristics.*

Tillotson SL, Fuggle PW, Smith I et al. Relation between biochemical severity and intelligence in early treated congenital hypothyroidism: a threshold effect. BMJ 1994; 309: 440-445. *There were two distinct groups – those with plasma thyroxine less than 42.8 nmol/l at diagnosis, who showed a global deficit in mean IQ of 10 points, and those with less severe congenital hypothyroidism who showed no deficit. For growth outcome see Arch Dis Child 1994; 70: 464-468.*

Xue-Yi C, Xin-Min J, Zhi-Hong D et al. Timing of vulnerability of the brain to iodine deficiency in endemic cretinism. N Engl J Med 1994; 331: 1739-1744. *Up to the end of the second trimester, iodine treatment protects the fetal brain from the effects of iodine deficiency. Treatment later in pregnancy or after delivery may improve development slightly, but does not improve neurological status. See editorial pp. 1770-1771. For high incidence of goite in Guinea see Lancet 1994; 344: 1675-1678.*

## Diabetes

Atkinson MA, Maclaren NK. The pathogenesis of insulin-dependent diabetes mellitus. N Engl J Med 1994; 331: 1428-1436. *Review.*

Azad K, Parkin JM, Court S et al. Circulating lipids and glycaemic control in insulin dependent diabetic children. Arch Dis Child 1994; 71: 108-113. *Abnormalities in circulating lipids are common in young subjects with diabetes but largely disappear if blood glucose concentrations are reasonably controlled. For autonomic abnormalities and control see pp. 511-515 and for postural vasoconstriction see 70: 22-26.*

Sackey AH, Jefferson IG. Interval between insulin injection and breakfast in diabetes. Arch Dis Child 1994; 71: 248-250. *There should be an interval of about 30 minutes between insulin and breakfast.*

Shield JPH, Baum JD. Prevention of long term complications in diabetes. Arch Dis Child 1994; 70: 258-259. *Review. For extending the honeymoon period see Lancet 1994; 343: 684-685.*

## Growth

Kelnar CJH. Treatment of the short, sexually immature adolescent boy. Arch Dis Child 1994; 71: 285-287. *Review. For constitutional delay see pp. 315-317.*

Khamis HJ, Roche AF. Predicting adult stature without using skeletal age: the

Khamis-Roche method. Pediatrics 1994; 94: 504-507. *A convenient and reliable method in healthy white children.*

Rivkees SA, Danon M, Herrin J. Prednisone dose limitation of growth hormone treatment of steroid-induced growth failure. J Pediatr 1994; 125: 322-325. *When prednisolone dose was greater than 0.35 mg/kg/day, growth hormone did not increase the growth rate.*

Voss LD, Bailey BJR. Equipping the community to measure children's height: the reliability of portable instruments. Arch Dis Child 1994; 70: 469-471. *Inexpensive height measuring equipment, once accurately installed, is no less reliable than the most expensive.*

## ENT

Isaacson G, Rosenfeld RM. Care of the child with tympanostomy tubes: a visual guide for the pediatrician. Pediatrics 1994; 93: 924-929. *Review.*

Klein JO. Lessons from recent studies on the epidemiology of otitis media. Pediatr Infect Dis J 1994; 13: 1031-1034. *Review. For long term sequelae see Pediatr Infect Dis J 1994; 13: 1069-1073.*

Niemela M, Uhari M, Jounio-Ervasti K et al. Lack of specific symptomatology in children with acute otitis media. Pediatr Infect Dis J 1994; 13: 765-768. *Earache, rubbing the ear or feeling of a blocked ear were the most predictive symptoms.*

Otitis Media Guideline Panel. Managing otitis media with effusion in young children. Pediatrics 1994; 94: 766-773. *Review. See also Curr Opin Pediatr 1994; 6: 3-6 and BMJ 1994; 308: 1129-1132.*

Ruuskanen O, Heikkinen T. Viral-bacterial interaction in acute otitis media. Pediatr Infect Dis J 1994; 13: 1047-1049. *Review. For choice of antibiotics, see pp.1050-1057.*

Sáez-Llorens X. Pathogenesis of acute otitis media. Pediatr Infect Dis J 1994; 13: 1035-1038. *Review. For diagnosis and surgical management see pp. 1039-1046 and 1058-1063.*

Shian W-J, Chi C-S. Sudden hearing loss caused by Epstein-Barr virus. Pediatr Infect Dis J 1994; 13: 756-758. *Report of 2 cases.*

## GASTROENTEROLOGY

Bealer JF, Natuzzi ES, Buscher C et al. Nitric oxide synthase is deficient in the aganglionic colon of patients with Hirschsprung's disease. Pediatrics 1994; 93: 647-651. *The aganglionic colon is deficient in NO synthase-containing nerves. This deficiency could prevent smooth muscle relaxation in the aganglionic colon.*

Burn J, Chapman PD, Eastham EJ. Familial adenomatous polyposis. Arch Dis Child 1994; 71: 103-107. *Review.*

Catassi C, Rätsch I-M, Fabini E et al. Coeliac disease in the year 2000: exploring the iceberg. Lancet 1994; 343: 200-204. *Screening of 3351 subjects aged 11–15 years uncovered 11 with coeliac disease, most of whom had no serious symptoms. See editorial pp. 188.*

Ekbom A, Wakefield AJ, Zack M et al. Perinatal measles infection and subsequent Crohn's disease. Lancet 1994; 344: 508-510. *Reports a significant excess of Crohn's disease among persons born during or just after a measles epidemic. For domestic hygiene and risk of Crohn's disease see Lancet 1994; 343: 766-767.*

Fleisher DR. Functional vomiting disorders in infancy: Innocent vomiting, nervous vomiting, and infant rumination syndrome. J Pediatr 1994; 125 Suppl: S84-S94. *Review.*

Friesen CA, Streed CJ, Carney LA et al. Esophagitis and modified Bernstein tests in infants with apparent life-threatening events. Pediatrics 1994; 94: 541-544. *Oesophageal acidification is a cause of apnoea, whether or not there is oesophagitis.*

Gormally S, Drumm B. *Helicobacter pylori* and gastrointestinal symptoms. Arch Dis Child 1994; 70: 165-166. Review. *See also BMJ 1994; 308: 750-753 and 309: 1119-1123.*

Loeing-Baucke V. Constipation in children. Curr Opin Pediatr 1994; 6: 556-561. *Review. For encopresis without constipation see Arch Dis Child 1994; 71: 186-193.*

Rosenthal E, Diamond E, Benderly A et al. Cholestatic pruritus: effect of phototherapy on pruritus and excretion of bile acids in urine. Acta Paediatr 1994; 83: 888-891. *Report of benefit in 7 year old boy.*

Sachar DB. Budesonide for inflammatory bowel disease. N Engl J Med 1994; 331: 873-874. *Review. See pages pp.836-845. For cyclosporin therapy see Arch Dis Child 1994; 71: 243-247.*

Smyth RL, van Velzen D, Smyth AR et al. Strictures of ascending colon in cystic fibrosis and high-strength pancreatic enzymes. Lancet 1994; 343: 85-86. *Report of 5 children with colonic strictures. See also pp.108-110, 1230 and J Pediatr 1994; 125: 587-589.*

Warburton ARE, Jones PH, Bruce J. Zoonotic transmission of giardiasis: a case control study. Commun Dis Rep CDR Wkly 1994; 4: R32-R36. *Strong association between giardiasis and contact with farm animals.*

## GENETICS AND MALFORMATIONS

### Genetics

Gusella JF, MacDonald ME. Huntington's disease and repeating trinucleotides. N Engl J Med 1994; 330: 1450-1451. *The longer the sequence of repeats the earlier of the onset of symptoms. See also pp. 1401-1406. For DNA repeats see 331: 191-193 and for DNA repeats and the Marfan syndrome see pp.148-153.*

Lazaro C, Ravella A, Gaona A et al. Neurofibromatosis type 1 due to germ-line mosaicism in a clinically normal father. N Engl J Med 1994; 331: 1403-1407. *This and another report (see pp. 1408-1415) illustrate the importance of genetic mosaicism in the origins of human genetic disorders. See editorial pp. 1447-1449.*

Malkin D, Friend SH. Screening for cancer susceptibility in children. Curr Opin Pediatr 1994; 6: 46-51. *Review.*

Rosenstein BJ. Genotype-phenotype correlations in cystic fibrosis. Lancet 1994; 343: 746-747. *Review. For carrier screening see BMJ 1994; 308: 1451-1452.*

**Malformations**

Noonan JA. Noonan syndrome: An update and review for the primary pediatrician. Clin Pediatr (Phila ) 1994; 33: 548-555. *Review.*

Seller M, J. Risks in spina bifida. Dev Med Child Neurol 1994; 36: 1021-1025. *Review. For defective folate metabolism see Br J Obstet Gynaecol 1994; 101: 197-202 and Lancet 1994; 343: 307.*

Lie RT, Wilcox AJ, Skjaerven R. A population-based study of the risk of recurrence of birth defects. N Engl J Med 1994; 331: 1-4. *Comment among women whose first infant has a birth defect, the risk of the same defect in the second infant is substantially increased and the risk of a different defect in the second infant is slightly increased. See editorial pp. 48-49.*

HAEMATOLOGY

Armitage JO. Bone marrow transplantation. N Engl J Med 1994; 330: 827-838. *Review.*

Dover GJ, Valle D. Therapy for β-thalassemia – a paradigm for the treatment of genetic disorders. N Engl J Med 1994; 331: 609-610. *Review. For desferrioxamine therapy see 567-572.*

Draper G, McNinch A. Vitamin K for neonates: the controversy. A definitive conclusion is still not possible. BMJ 1994; 308: 867-868. *Review. See also pp. 908-910 and Lancet 1994; 343: 352.*

Hann IM. The use of haemopoietic growth factors in blood disorders. Arch Dis Child 1994; 71: 543-547. *Review.*

Hoyer LW. Hemophilia A. N Engl J Med 1994; 330: 38-47. *Review.*

Lilleyman JS. Intracranial haemorrhage in idiopathic thrombocytopenic purpura. Arch Dis Child 1994; 71: 251-253. *UK survey data suggesting that intracranial haemorrhage occurs in less than one child with ITP in 100, a much lower figure than previously supposed. For treatment with methylprednisolone or immunoglobulin see N Engl J Med 1994; 330: 733-737 and 783-784.*

**Sickle cell disease**

Platt OS. Easing the suffering caused by sickle cell disease. N Engl J Med 1994; 330: 783-784. *Review. For methylprednisolone therapy see pp. 733-737.*

Platt OS, Brambilla DJ, Rosse WF et al. Mortality in sickle cell disease. Life expectancy and risk factors for early death. N Engl J Med 1994; 330: 1639-1644. *50% of patients with sickle cell anaemia survived beyond the fifth decade. A high level of foetal haemoglobin predicted improved survival.*

## INFECTIOUS DISEASE

Barnett ED, Bauchner H, Teele DW et al. Serious bacterial infections in febrile infants and children selected for lumbar puncture. Pediatr Infect Dis J 1994; 13: 950-953. *The decision to perform lumbar puncture identifies children at risk of having not only meningitis but other serious bacterial illnesses.*

Belhorn TH, Lucky AW. Atypical varicella exanthems associated with skin injury. Pediatr Dermatol 1994; 11: 129-132. *The injury to the skin during the incubation period may result in severe localized disease.*

Brown DWG, Ramsay MEB, Richards AF et al. Salivary diagnosis of measles: a study of notified cases in the United Kingdom, 1991–3. BMJ 1994; 308: 1015-1017. *Saliva is a valid alternative to serum for IgM detection. Rubella and parvovirus are responsible for only a minority of incorrectly diagnosed cases of measles in the UK.*

Cantwell MF, Shehab ZM, Costello AM et al. Brief report: congenital tuberculosis. N Engl J Med 1994; 330: 1051-1054. *Report of two cases and review of literature. See also Pediatr Infect Dis J 1994; 13: 738-741. For global challenge of tuberculosis see Lancet 1994; 344: 277-279.*

Chosidow O, Chastang C, Bruce C et al. Controlled study of malathion and d-phenothrin lotions for *Pediculus humanus* var capitis-infested schoolchildren. Lancet 1994; 344: 1724-1727. *After 7 days the success rate of malathion was 95% and of d-phenothrin 39%.*

Enders G, Miller E, Cradock-Watson J et al. Consequences of varicella and herpes zoster in pregnancy: prospective study of 1739 cases. Lancet 1994; 343: 1548-1551. *1373 women who had varicella and 366 who had herpes zoster during the first 36 weeks of gestation were follows up; 9 cases of congenital varicella syndrome were identified, all occurring after maternal varicella during the first 20 weeks of gestation. The highest risk was observed between 13 and 20 weeks' gestation. See also N Engl J Med 1994; 330: 901-905 and 381: 482.*

Friedland IR, McCracken GH. Management of infections caused by antibiotic-resistant *Streptococcus pneumoniae.* N Engl J Med 1994; 331: 377-382. *Review.*

Grayston JT. *Chlamydia pneumoniae* (TWAR) infections in children. Pediatr Infect Dis J 1994; 13: 675-685. *Review.*

Guerina NG, Hsu H-W, Meissner HC et al. Neonatal serologic screening and early treatment for congenital *Toxoplasma gondii* infection. N Engl J Med 1994; 330: 1858-1863. *Routine neonatal screening for toxoplasmosis identifies congenital infections that are subclinical, and early treatment may reduce the severe long-term sequelae.*

Hall CB, Long CE, Schnabel KC et al. Human herpes virus-6 infection in children. A prospective study of complications and reactivation. N Engl J Med 1994; 331: 432-438. *In young children HHV-6 infection is a major cause of visits to the emergency department, febrile seizures, and hospitalization. For clinical features of roseola, see Pediatrics 1994; 93: 104-108.*

Herrera R, Hobar PC, Ginsburg CM. Surgical intervention for the complications of meningococcal-induced purpura fulminans. Pediatr Infect Dis J 1994; 13: 734-737. *Eighteen of 152 patients with meningococcal septicaemia developed purpura fulminans, and 13 of these needed surgery (e.g. skin graft, debridement, amputation). For role of heparin see pp. 867-873.*

Hull HF, Ward NA, Hull BP et al. Paralytic poliomyelitis: seasonal strategies, disappearing disease. Lancet 1994; 343: 1331-1337. *Review.*

Jaskiewicz JA, McCarthy CA, Richardson AC et al. Febrile infants at low risk for serious bacterial infection. An appraisal of the Rochester criteria and implications for management. Pediatrics 1994; 94: 390-396. *Confirms the ability of low risk criteria to identify infants unlikely to have serious bacterial infection. See editorial pp.397-399.*

Kerr-Muir MG. *Toxocara canis* and human health. BMJ 1994; 309: 5-6. *Review.*

Liu H-C, Tsai T-C, Chang P-Y et al. Varicella orchitis: report of two cases and review of the literature. Pediatr Infect Dis J 1994; 13: 748-750. *Resolved without sequelae.*

Mäkelä MJ, Mertsola J, Ruuskanen O. Respiratory syncytial virus infection in children. Curr Opin Pediatr 1994; 6: 17-22. *Review.*

Papenek PJ. Small round structured viruses: airborne transmission and hospital control. Lancet 1994; 343: 1240-1241. *Review.*

Priebe CJ, Nizet V. A 5 year old girl with varicella and acute onset of fever, stridor, and respiratory distress. Curr Opin Pediatr 1994; 6: 36-41. *Acute epiglotitis due to group A streptococcus in a child with chicken-pox.*

Rice P, Simmons K, Carr R et al. Near fatal chickenpox during prednisolone treatment. BMJ 1994; 309: 1069-1070. *Reminder of important hazard of steroid therapy.*

Sawyer SM, Johnson PDR, Hogg GG et al. Successful treatment of epiglottitis with two doses of ceftriaxone. Arch Dis Child 1994; 70: 129-132. *A short course of ceftriaxone is safe and efficacious.*

Weber K, Pfister H-W. Clinical management of Lyme borreliosis. Lancet 1994; 343: 1017-1020. *Review. For basic science of clinical aspects see pp. 1013-1016.*

## AIDS

Anonymous. Features of children perinatally infected with HIV-1 surviving longer than 5 years. Lancet 1994; 343: 191-195. *A substantial number do survive. Severe disease, low CD4 cell numbers, and p24 antigenaemia do not necessarily preclude long term survival.*

Ammann AJ. Human immunodeficiency virus infection/AIDS in children: the next decade. Pediatrics 1994; 93: 930-935. *Review. For evaluation of symptom free children born to infected mothers see J Pediatr 1994; 125: 345-351.*

Anonymous. Prevention and treatment of *Pneumocystis carinii* pneumonia in patients infected with HIV. Drug Ther Bull 1994; 32: 12-15. *Review. See also Arch Dis Child 1994; 70: 241-244 and Lancet 1994; 344: 5-6.*

Blanche S, Mayaux M-J, Rouzioux C et al. Relation of the course of HIV infection in children to the severity of the disease in their mothers at delivery. N Engl J Med 1994; 330: 308-312. *In infants whose HIV infection is maternally acquired, the rate of disease progression varies directly with the severity of the disease in the mother at the time of delivery. See also pp.1905-1906, 331: 1173-1180 and J Pediatr 1994; 125: 345-351.*

Church JA. The diagnostic challenge of the child born 'at risk' for HIV infection. Pediatr Clin North Am 1994; 41: 715-726. *Review. For review of epidemiology of HIV infection see Acta Paediatr 1994; 83 Suppl. 400: 5-14.*

Fowler MG. Pediatric HIV infection: neurologic and neuropsychologic findings. Acta Paediatr 1994; 83 Suppl. 400: 59-62. *Review.*

Italian Register for HIV Infection in Children. Human immunodeficiency virus type 1 infection and breast milk. Acta Paediatr 1994; 83 Suppl. 400: 51-58. *Review. For case of HIV from pooled breast milk see Lancet 1994; 344: 1432.*

Newell ML, Peckham C, Dunn D et al. Natural history of vertically acquired human immunodeficiency virus-1 infection. Pediatrics 1994; 94: 815-819. *Progression not as fast as previously suggested. For neurodevelopmental effects of perinatally acquired HIV infection see pp.883-891.*

Papola P, Alvarez M, Cohen HJ. Developmental and service needs of school-age children with human immunodeficiency virus infection: a descriptive study. Pediatrics 1994; 94: 914-918. *Most of 90 school-age children with perinatally acquired HIV had cognitive defects.*

Spector SA, Gelber RD, McGrath N et al. A controlled trial of intravenous immune globulin for the prevention of serious bacterial infections in children receiving zidovudine for advanced human immunodeficiency virus infection. N Engl J Med 1994; 331: 1181-1187. *Intravenous immune globulin decreases the risk of serious bacterial infections, but only in children who are not receiving co-trimoxazole as prophylaxis. See editorials pp.1222-1225.*

## Gastroenteritis

Guarino A, Canani RB, Russo S et al. Oral immunoglobulins for treatment of acute rotaviral gastroenteritis. Pediatrics 1994; 93: 12-16. *Oral immunoglobulin is associated with a faster recovery.*

Anonymous. Cryptosporidiosis associated with farm visits. Commun Dis Rep CDR Wkly 1994; 4: 73-76. *Children who visit farms with young lambs risk developing cryptosporidiosis.*

Brown KH, Peerson JM, Fontaine O. Use of nonhuman milks in the dietary management of young children with acute diarrhea: a meta-analysis of clinical trials. Pediatrics 1994; 93: 17-27. *Most can be managed with continued feeding of undiluted non-human milk.*

Kelly CP, Pothoulakis C, LaMont JT. *Clostridium difficile* colitis. N Engl J Med 1994; 330: 257-262. *Review. For clinicopathological conference see N Engl J Med 1994; 330: 420-426.*

Saavedra JM, Bauman NA, Oung I et al. Feeding of *Bifidobacterium bifidum* and *Streptococcus thermophilus* to infants in hospital for prevention of diarrhoea and shedding of rotavirus. Lancet 1994; 344: 1046-1050. *Can reduce the incidence of acute diarrhoea and rotavirus shedding.*

## Hepatitis

Alter MJ. Transmission of hepatitis C virus – route, dose, and titer. N Engl J Med 1994; 330: 784-786. *Review. For long-term outcome of infection see Pediatr Infect Dis J 1994; 13: 769-773.*

Anonymous. Prevention and control of hepatitis A. Drug Ther Bull 1994; 32: 9-15. *Review.*

Gregorio GV, Mieli-Vergani G, Mowat AP. Viral hepatitis. Arch Dis Child 1994; 70: 343-348. *Review.*

McIntosh EDG. Molecular biology, pathogenesis, and prevention of hepatitis B virus infection in children. Curr Opin Pediatr 1994; 6: 7-16. *Review.*

Ohto H, Terazawa S, Sasaki N et al. Transmission of hepatitic C virus from mothers to infants. N Engl J Med 1994; 330: 744-750. *HCV is vertically transmitted from mother to infant, and the risk of transmission is correlated with the titre of HCV RNA in the mother.*

**Meningitis**

Bradley JS. Dexamethasone therapy in meningitis: potentially misleading anti-inflammatory effects in central nervous system infections. Pediatr Infect Dis J 1994; 13: 823-826. *Report of 3 cases. For risk of gut bleeding see Lancet 1994; 343: 792.*

Newton RW. Tuberculous meningitis. Arch Dis Child 1994; 70: 364-366. *Review. For review of bacterial meningitis see Curr Opin Pediatr 1994; 6: 29-35.*

Voss L, Lennon D. Epidemiology, management, and prevention of meningococcal infections. Curr Opin Pediatr 1994; 6: 23-28. *Review.*

**Parvovirus**

Brown KE, Hibbs JR, Gallinella G et al. Resistance to parvovirus B19 infection due to lack of virus receptor (erythrocyte P antigen). N Engl J Med 1994; 330: 1192-1196. *People who did not have P antigen, which is the cellular receptor for parvovirus B19, are naturally resistant to infection with this pathogen. For congenital anaemia due to parvovirus see Lancet 1994; 343: 895-896 and for review of parvovirus see BMJ 1994; 308: 149-150.*

Finkel TH, Török TJ, Ferguson PJ et al. Chronic parvovirus B19 infection and systemic necrotising vasculitis: opportunistic infection or aetiological agent?. Lancet 1994; 343: 1255-1258. *Report of 3 patients with parvovirus infection in association with systemic necrotising vasculitis. For parvovirus and Kawasaki disease see Lancet 1994; 343: pp 1260-1261 and 344: pp. 58-59.*

METABOLIC

Barton JS, Hindmarsh PC, Scrimgeour CM et al. Energy expenditure in congenital heart disease. Arch Dis Child 1994; 70: 5-9. *Energy expenditure was increased in congenital heart disease.*

Fleming PJ, Howell T, Clements M et al. Thermal balance and metabolic rate during upper respiratory tract infection in infants. Arch Dis Child 1994; 70: 187-191. *Infants respond to respiratory infection by heat conservation. In the older infants the increase in metabolic rate may result in fever. For determinants of energy expenditure see J Pediatr 1994; 125: 362-367.*

Jackson AA. Urea as a nutrient: bioavailability and role in nitrogen economy. Arch Dis Child 1994; 70: 3-4. *Review.*

Kelly DA. Organ transplantation for inherited metabolic disease. Arch Dis Child 1994; 71: 181-183. *Review.*

Rizzo WB, Roth KS. On 'being led by the nose': rapid detection of inborn errors of metabolism. Arch Pediatr Adolesc Med 1994; 148: 869-872. *Review.*

## MISCELLANEOUS

Cherryman GR. Magnetic resonance imaging in paediatrics. Arch Dis Child 1994; 70: 82-83. *Review.*

Goetting MG. Mastering pediatric cardiopulmonary resuscitation. Pediatr Clin North Am 1994; 41: 1147-1182. *Review.*

Hamilton AB, Zeltzer LK. Visceral pain in infants. J Pediatr 1994; 125 Suppl. S95-S102. *Review.*

Lucas A. Role of nutritional programming in determining adult morbidity. Arch Dis Child 1994; 71: 288-290. *Review.*

Macrae DJ. Paediatric intensive care transport. Arch Dis Child 1994; 71: 175-178. *Review.*

Saper CB, Breder CD. The neurologic basis of fever. N Engl J Med 1994; 330: 1880-1886. *Review. For chemical and glass thermometers see Arch Dis Child 1994; 71: 259-260.*

Staples B, Pharoah POD. Child health statistical review. Arch Dis Child 1994; 71: 548-554. *Review.*

Zideman DA, Bingham R, Beattie T et al. Guidelines for paediatric life support. BMJ 1994; 308: 1349-1355. *Review. For open cardiac massage see Pediatrics 1994; 93: 392-393.*

## NEONATOLOGY

Ahlfors CE. Criteria for exchange transfusion in jaundiced newborns. Pediatrics 1994; 93: 488-494. *The bilirubin/albumin ratio is a simple way of incorporating the serum albumin concentration into exchange transfusion criteria. See also pp.50-53.*

Ahluwalia JS, Morley CJ, Mockridge JNA. Computerised determination of spontaneous inspiratory and expiratory times in premature neonates during intermittent positive pressure ventilation. II: results from 20 babies. Arch Dis Child 1994; 71: F161-F164. *This new technique can distinguish between the effect of the ventilatory and that of spontaneous respiration on the chest wall of preterm infants.*

Beeby PJ, Elliott EJ, Henderson-Smart DJ et al. Predictive value of umbilical artery pH in preterm infants. Arch Dis Child 1994; 71: F93-F96. *Umbilical artery pH is not significantly associated with any outcome, in contrast to a low one minute Apgar (<4) which remained a significant risk factor for neonatal death and cerebral palsy.*

Choonara I. Percutaneous drug absorption and administration. Arch Dis Child 1994; 71: F73-F74. *Review. See also F122-F124.*

Croucher C, Azzopardi D. Compliance with recommendations for giving vitamin K to newborn infants. BMJ 1994; 308: 894-895. *More than 10% of breast fed infants did not receive a second dose of Vitamin K and less than 40% received a third dose. See also Arch Dis Child 1994; 70: 248-251.*

Davies J, Gault D, Buchdahl R. Preventing the scars of neonatal intensive care. Arch Dis Child 1994; 70: F50-F51. *Scarring and the need for plastic surgery were prevented by using subcutaneous hyaluronidase and saline flushing.*

Donn SM. Alternatives to ECMO. Arch Dis Child 1994; 70: F81-F83. *Review.*

Doyal L, Wilsher D. Towards guidelines for withholding and withdrawal of life prolonging treatment in neonatal medicine. Arch Dis Child 1994; 70: F66-F70. *Review. See also 71: F142-F144.*

Evans N. Cardiovascular effects of dexamethasone in the preterm infant. Arch Dis Child 1994; 70: F25-F30. *Myocardial hypertrophy occurs in most treated infants, and in some it is severe.*

Ewer AK, Durbin GM, Morgan MEI et al. Gastric emptying in preterm infants. Arch Dis Child 1994; 71: F24-F27. *Expressed breast milk emptied twice as fast as formula milk.*

Gaffney G, Sellers S, Flavell V et al. Case-control study of intrapartum care, cerebral palsy, and perinatal death. BMJ 1994; 308: 743-750. *Suboptimal care seems to have a role in only a small proportion of all cases of cerebral palsy. See also Arch Dis Child 1994; 70: F195-F200.*

Hall CJ. Perinatal asphyxia in less developed countries. Arch Dis Child 1994; 71: F1-F3. *Review.*

Kao LC, Durand DJ, McCrea RC et al. Randomized trial of long-term diuretic therapy for infants with oxygen-dependent bronchopulmonary dysplasia. J Pediatr 1994; 124: 772-781. *Long-term diuretic therapy in stable infants with oxygen dependent BPD, after extubation, improves pulmonary function but does not decrease the number of days of supplemental oxygen.*

Langbaum M, Eyal FG. A practical and reliable method of measuring blood pressure in the neonate by pulse oximetry. J Pediatr 1994; 125: 591-595. *Measurements of blood pressure in the neonate by pulse oximetry wave form analysis are more accurate than those obtained by the oscillometric method. For poor understanding of oximetry by doctors and nurses see Lancet 1994; 344: 1339-1342.*

Lin C, Chen W, Kang-Wen W. Povidone-iodine in umbilical cord care interferes with neonatal screening for hypothyroidism. Eur J Pediatr 1994; 153: 756-758. *May cause false positive TSH levels.*

McDonnell M, Serra-Serra V, Gaffney G et al. Neonatal outcome after pregnancy complicated by abnormal velocity waveforms in the umbilical artery. Arch Dis Child 1994; 70: F84-F89. *The infant with abnormal velocity waveforms was significantly more growth retarded, had lower platelet counts at birth, and was more likely to become thrombocytopenic in the first week.*

Mehta A. Prevention and management of neonatal hypoglycaemia. Arch Dis Child 1994; 70: F54-F59. *Review. See also pp.F59-F65.*

Ng PC. Systemic fungal infections in neonates. Arch Dis Child 1994; 71: F130-F135. *Review.*

Olsen JH, Hertz H, Blinkenberg K et al. Vitamin K regimens and incidence of childhood cancer in Denmark. BMJ 1994; 308: 895-896. *No association between vitamin K and childhood cancer.*

Paes BA, Modi A, Dunmore R. Changing physicians' behavior using combined strategies and an evidence-based protocol. Arch Pediatr Adolesc Med 1994; 148: 1277-1280. *An evidence-based protocol resulted in a huge reduction of unnecessary investigations.*

Pharoah POD, Stevenson CJ, Cooke RWI et al. Clinical and subclinical deficits at 8 years in a geographically defined cohort of low birthweight infants. Arch Dis Child 1994; 70: 264-270. *Low birth weight children have significant subclinical deficits of cognitive and motor function. For the prevalence of behaviour disorders see pp.271-274.*

Pryds O. Low neonatal cerebral oxygen delivery is associated with brain injury in preterm infants. Acta Paediatr 1994; 83: 1233-1236. *It is unclear whether decreased oxygen delivery is a contributing factor to brain damage or whether it is a marker of existing injury.*

Rautonen J, Mäkelä A, Boyd H et al. CRIB and SNAP: assessing the risk of death for preterm neonates. Lancet 1994; 343: 1272-1273. *Clinical risk index for babies (CRIB) is the most useful score for comparing the performance of neonatal intensive care units. See also pp. 124-125 and pp. 344.*

Rozé J-C, Storme L, Véronique Z et al. Echocardiographic investigation of inhaled nitric oxide in newborn babies with severe hypoxaemia. Lancet 1994; 344: 303-306. *Nitric oxide may improve systemic oxygenation in neonates with severe hypoxaemia. For general reviews of nitric oxide see Lancet 1994; 343: 1199-1206, Br Med J 1994; 309: 453-457 and J Roy Coll Phys Lond 1994; 28: 209-219.*

Rush MG, Shenai JP, Parker RA et al. Intramuscular versus enteral vitamin A supplementation in very low birth weight neonates. J Pediatr 1994; 125: 458-462. *The enteral route is less effective.*

Sahni R, Wung J-T, James LS. Controversies in management of persistent pulmonary hypertension of the newborn. Pediatrics 1994; 94: 307-309. *Review. See also pp. 303-306 and Curr Opin Pediatr 1994; 6: 239-247.*

Saigal S, Feeny D, Furlong W et al. Comparison of the health-related quality of life of extremely low birth weight children and a reference group of children at age eight years. J Pediatr 1994; 125: 418-425. *Use of McMaster quality of life score system to assess long-term burden. See also pp. 411-417.*

Schwartz RM, Luby AM, Scanlon JW et al. Effect of surfactant on morbidity, mortality, and resource use in newborn infants weighing 500 to 1500 g. N Engl J Med 1994; 330: 1476-1480. *The introduction of surfactant has led to decreased mortality and morbidity in very-low-birth-weight infants and to decreased use of resource both for infants who survive and for those who die.*

Sims DG, Heal CA, Bartle SM. Use of adrenaline and atropine in neonatal resuscitation. Arch Dis Child 1994; 70: F3-F10. *The use of these drugs for resuscitation at birth and in the first week of life of extremely preterm infants may be inappropriate.*

Soothill PW. Diagnosis of intrauterine growth retardation and its fetal and perinatal consequences. Acta Paediatr 1994; 83 Suppl. 399: 55-59. *Review.*

Stephenson T, Zuccollo J, Mohajer M. Diagnosis and management of non-immune hydrops in the newborn. Arch Dis Child 1994; 70: F151-F154. *Review.*

Synnott MB, Morse DL, Hall SM. Neonatal meningitis in England and Wales: a review of routine national data. Arch Dis Child 1994; 71: F75-F80. *Review.*

Valaes T, Petmezaki S, Henschke C et al. Control of jaundice in preterm newborns by an inhibitor of bilirubin production: studies with tin-mesoporphyrin. Pediatrics 1994; 93: 1-11. *Tin mesoporphyrin, by inhibiting the production of bilirubin, substantially moderates the development of hyperbilirubinemia in preterm newborns.*

Volpe JJ. Brain injury caused by intraventricular hemorrhage: is indomethacin the silver bullet for prevention? Pediatrics 1994; 93: 673-676. *Review. See also pp. 677-679.*

Whitelaw A, Mutch L, Stewart A et al. Randomised trial of early tapping in neonatal posthaemorrhagic ventricular dilatation: results at 30 months. Arch Dis Child 1994; 70: F129-F136. *Early tapping not recommended on the basis of this data. For infantile hydrocephalus epidemiology see pp. F123-F128.*

Wyatt JS. Noninvasive assessment of cerebral oxidative metabolism in the human newborn. J R Coll Phys Lond 1994; 28: 126-132. *Review.*

## NEPHROLOGY

Buys H, Pead L, Hallett R et al. Suprapubic aspiration under ultrasound guidance in children with fever of undiagnosed cause. BMJ 1994; 308: 690-692. *The use of ultrasound guidance simplifies suprapubic aspiration of urine in babies.*

Dohil R, Roberts E, Verrier Jones K et al. Constipation and reversible urinary tract abnormalities. Arch Dis Child 1994; 70: 56-57. *The bladder residue and upper renal tract dilation after micturition were significantly increased in the group with constipation and improved after treatment.*

Fernandes ET, Reinberg Y, Vernier R et al. Neurogenic bladder dysfunction in children: review of pathophysiology and current management. J Pediatr 1994; 124: 1-7. *Review.*

Hiraoka M, Kasuga K, Hori C et al. Ultrasonic indicators of ureteric reflux in the newborn. Lancet 1994; 343: 519-520. *Ballooning of the renal pelvis during voiding was consistently seen in all five affected renal pelvises.*

Marra G, Barbieri G, Dell'Agnola CA et al. Congenital renal damage associated with primary vesicoureteral reflux detected prenatally in male infants. J Pediatr 1994; 124: 726-730. *Severe primary reflux associated with hydronephrosis usually effects male infants and may be due to abnormal embryological development of the male urethra.*

Moake JL. Haemolytic-uraemic syndrome: basic science. Lancet 1994; 343: 393-397. *Review. For clinical practice see pp. 398-401, and for correspondence see pp. 1042-1043.*

Neuhaus TJ, Fay J, Dillon MJ et al. Alternative treatment to corticosteroids in steroid sensitive idiopathic nephrotic syndrome. Arch Dis Child 1994; 71: 522-526. *52% of 429 children required at least one course of alternative treatment such as cyclophosphamide, levamisole, cyclosporin, chlorambucil, azathioprine or vincristine.*

Pead L, Maskell R. Study of urinary tract infection in children in one health district. BMJ 1994; 309: 631-634. *Urinary tract infection is much commoner in children than widely believed and 1/1000 boys and 1.5/1000 girls had abnormalities of the urinary tract.*

Smellie JM, Poulton A, Prescod NP. Retrospective study of children with renal scarring associated with reflux and urinary infection. BMJ 1994; 308: 1193-1196. *Efforts to reduce the incidence and severity of renal scarring should be directed towards rapid diagnosis and effective early management of urinary tract infection in infancy and childhood. Siblings and offspring of known patients with severe reflux nephropathy should be investigated for reflux.*

Stokland E, Hellström M, Hansson S et al. Reliability of ultrasonography in identification of reflux nephropathy in children. BMJ 1994; 309: 235-239. *The low sensitivity and specificity and poor agreement between observers mean that ultrasonography is not accurate enough to identify those who are at risk of future complications.*

Watson AR. Consensus statement on management and audit potential for steroid responsive nephrotic syndrome. Arch Dis Child 1994; 70: 151-157. *Review.*

Yang L-Y, Chen W-P, Lin C-Y. Lupus nephritis in children – a review of 167 patients. Pediatrics 1994; 94: 335-340. *Data on clinical course, histopathology, and prognosis.*

## NEUROLOGY

Abu-Arefeh I, Russell G. Prevalence of headache and migraine in schoolchildren. BMJ 1994; 309: 765-769. *In a survey of 2165 primary and secondary school children in Aberdeen, the prevalence rate for migraine was 10.6%.*

Bouza H, Dubowitz LMS, Rutherford M et al. Late magnetic resonance imaging and clinical findings in neonates with unilateral lesions on cranial ultrasound. Dev Med Child Neurol 1994; 36: 951-964. *The presence or absence of hemiplegia, or its severity, could not be predicted from either early ultrasound or later MRI appearances.*

Gordon N. Recurrent vomiting in childhood, especially of neurological origin. Dev Med Child Neurol 1994; 36: 463-467. *Review.*

Hrachovy RA, Frost JD, Glaze DG. High-dose, long-duration versus low-dose, short-duration corticotropin therapy for infantile spasms. J Pediatr 1994; 124: 803-806. *No major difference in the effectiveness of these two regimens. See also Dev Med Child Neurol 1994; 36: 863-872.*

Lin J-P, Brown JK, Walsh EG. Physiological maturation of muscles in childhood. Lancet 1994; 343: 1386-1389. *A child's muscles are initially slow to relax, but relaxation doubles in speed up to adult rates by early adolescence.*

Lipton SA, Rosenberg PA. Excitatory amino acids as a final common pathway for neurologic disorders. N Engl J Med 1994; 330: 613-622. *Review.*

Niemann G, Wakat J-P, Krägeloh-Mann I et al. Congenital hemiparesis and periventricular leukomalacia: pathogenetic aspects on magnetic resonance imaging. Dev Med Child Neurol 1994; 36: 943-950. *Review.*

O'Dwyer N, Neilson P, Nash J. Reduction of spasticity in cerebral palsy using feedback of the tonic stretch reflex: A controlled study. Dev Med Child Neurol 1994; 36: 770-786. *Stretch reflex gain was significantly reduced in all test subjects. For role of selective dorsal rhizotomy see pp. 755-769, and for factors associated with inability to walk see pp. 787-795.*

Pääkkö E, Löppönen T, Saukkonen A-L et al. Information value of magnetic resonance imaging in shunted hydrocephalus. Arch Dis Child 1994; 70: 530-535. *MRI is recommended as the primary imaging method for all children with shunted hydrocephalus.*

Pollack IF. Brain tumours in children. N Engl J Med 1994; 331: 1500-1507. *Review.*

Rao JN. Botulinum toxin in the cerebral palsies. BMJ 1994; 309: 1526-1528. *Review.*

Raphael J-C, Chevret S, Chastang C et al. Randomised trial of preventive nasal ventilation in Duchenne muscular dystrophy. Lancet 1994; 343: 1600-1604. *Ventilation did not improve respiratory handicap and reduced survival.*

Rosenbloom L. Dyskinetic cerebral palsy and birth asphyxia. Dev Med Child Neurol 1994; 36: 285-289. *The pattern of birth asphyxia which precedes the development of spastic quadriplegia is different from that which precedes dyskinetic cerebral palsy.*

**Epilepsy**

Hewertson J, Poets CF, Samuels MP et al. Epileptic seizure-induced hypoxemia in infants with apparent life-threatening events. Pediatrics 1994; 94: 148-156. *Epileptic seizures in infants can manifest as apnoea and severe hypoxaemia despite a normal EEG between events.*

Kalayci O, Coskun T, Tokatli A et al. Infantile spasms as the initial symptom of biotinidase deficiency. J Pediatr 1994; 124: 103-104. *Infants with infantile spasms should be examined carefully for hallmarks of biotinidase deficiency, such as alopecia and seborrheic dermatitis.*

Scheffer IE, Bhatia K, P., Lopes-Cendes I et al. Autosomal dominant frontal epilepsy misdiagnosed as sleep disorder. Lancet 1994; 343: 515-518. *Clusters of brief motor attacks occurring in sleep, with onset in childhood, was often misdiagnosed as night terrors, nightmares, hysteria, or paroxysmal nocturnal dystonia.*

Sheth RD, Bodensteiner JB. Effective utilization of home-video recordings for the evaluation of paroxysmal events in pediatrics. Clin Pediatr (Phila ) 1994; 33: 578-582. *Useful practical advice.*

Sturniolo MG, Galletti F. Idiopathic epilepsy and school achievement. Arch Dis Child 1994; 70: 424-428. *Under achievement occurred in 61%.*

Tennison M, Greenwood R, Lewis D et al. Discontinuing antiepileptic drugs in children with epilepsy. A comparison of a six-week and a nine-month taper period. N Engl J Med 1994; 330: 1407-1410. *There was no difference.*

ORTHOPAEDICS

Aronsson DD, Goldberg MJ, Kling TF et al. Developmental dysplasia of the hip. Pediatrics 1994; 94: 201-208. *Developmental dysplasia replaces the term congenital hip dislocation. For role of ultrasound in diagnosis see Arch Dis Child 1994; 70: 362-363. For the hip in cerebral palsy see Dev Med Child Neurol 1995; 37: 3-18.*

Hamanishi C, Tanaka S. Turned head – adducted hip – truncal curvature syndrome. Arch Dis Child 1994; 70: 515-519. *A report of 108 neonates and infants who showed this clinical triad.*

Hughes LO, Aronson J. Skeletal infections in children. Curr Opin Pediatr 1994; 6: 90-93. *Review. For value of CRP, ESR and white cell count see Pediatrics 1994; 93: 59-62.*

Kilmartin TE, Barrington RL, Wallace WA. A controlled prospective trial of a foot orthosis for juvenile hallux valgus. J Bone Joint Surg 1994; 76: 210-214. *Biomechanical orthoses should not be used to treat juvenile hallux valgus.*

Lonstein JE. Adolescent idiopathic scoliosis. Lancet 1994; 344: 1407-1412. *Review.*

## PSYCHIATRY

Friedman RC, Downey JI. Homosexuality. N Engl J Med 1994; 331: 923-930. *Review.*

Jones P, Rodgers B, Murray R et al. Child developmental risk factors for adult schizophrenia in the British 1946 birth cohort. Lancet 1994; 344: 1398-1402. *The origins of schizophrenia may be found in early life.*

Krener P. Factitious disorders and the psychosomatic continuum in children. Curr Opin Pediatr 1994; 6: 418-422. *Review.*

Stores G. Investigation of sleep disorders including home monitoring. Arch Dis Child 1994; 71: 184-185. *Review.*

## RESPIRATORY

Brabin B, Smith M, Milligan P et al. Respiratory morbidity in Merseyside schoolchildren exposed to coal dust and air pollution. Arch Dis Child 1994; 70: 305-312. *Increased prevalence of respiratory symptoms in children exposed to coal dust.*

Couriel JM. Passive smoking and the health of children. Thorax 1994; 49: 731-734. *Review. See also BMJ 1994; 308: 384-389.*

Henderson AJW. Bronchoalveolar lavage. Arch Dis Child 1994; 70: 167-169. *Review.*

Klassen TP, Feldman ME, Watters LK et al. Nebulized budesonide for children with mild-to-moderate croup. N Engl J Med 1994; 331: 285-289. *A single 2 mg dose of nebulised budesonide was associated with clinical improvement in children with mild to moderate croup. See editorial pp. 322-323.*

Lund-Olsen I, Lundbäck A, Gnarpe J et al. Prevalence of specific antibodies to *Chlamydia pneumoniae* in children with acute respiratory infections. Acta Paediatr 1994; 83: 1143-1145. *Antibodies were found in 2/42 children under 10 years and in 17/33 of those aged 13–15 years.*

Margolis PA, Ferkol TW, Marsocci S et al. Accuracy of the clinical examination in detecting hypoxemia in infants with respiratory illness. J Pediatr 1994; 124: 552-560. *Auscultatory findings contributed little. Five clinical findings accounted for almost all the accuracy: attentiveness, consolability, respiratory effort, colour, and movement.*

Nikolaizik WH, Warner JO. Aetiology of chronic suppurative lung disease.

Arch Dis Child 1994; 70: 141-142. *A report of 41 patients; six had congenital malformations, seven had primary ciliary dyskinesia, 11 had immunological abnormalities and two had bronchiectasis due to aspiration.*

Ring JC, Stidham GL. Novel therapies for acute respiratory failure. Pediatr Clin North Am 1994; 41: 1325-1363. *Review.*

Samuels MP, Poets CF, Southall DP. Abnormal hypoxemia after life-threatening events in infants born before term. J Pediatr 1994; 125: 441-446. *Recognition and treatment of baseline hypoxaemia may reduce the risk of further events. For noninvasive monitoring see Pediatrics 1994; 93: 737-746.*

## Asthma

Agertoft L, Pendersen S. Influence of spacer device on drug delivery to young children with asthma. Arch Dis Child 1994; 71: 217-220. *Spacer volume does not seem to be so important for children aged 10–25 months as long as spacers with a volume lower than 750 ml are used.*

Anderson HR, Butland BK, Strachan DP. Trends in prevalence and severity of childhood asthma. BMJ 1994; 308: 1600-1604. *Documents a small increase in the prevalence of wheezy children and a greater increase in persistent wheezing, but severe attacks of chronic disability have fallen. See also pp. 1584-1586, 1591-1600.*

Austin JB, Russell G, Adam MG et al. Prevalence of asthma and wheeze in the Highlands of Scotland. Arch Dis Child 1994; 71: 211-216. *Results do not support the hypothesis that asthma is more common in urban than rural areas, and do not support an association between atmospheric pollution and the prevalence of asthma. See also BMJ 1994; 309: 619-620.*

Bergman DA, Cooley JR, Hilman BC et al. Practice parameter: the office management of acute exacerbations of asthma in children. Pediatrics 1994; 93: 119-122. *Recommendations for management out of hospital of acute exacerbations of asthma.*

Connett GJ, Warde C, Wooler E et al. Prednisolone and salbutamol in the hospital treatment of acute asthma. Arch Dis Child 1994; 70: 170-173. *Routine steroid treatment for asthma admissions can facilitate the safe discharge of an increased number of children within a short period of treatment.*

DeNicola LK, Monem GF, Gayle MO et al. Treatment of critical status asthmaticus in children. Pediatr Clin North Am 1994; 41: 1293-1324. *Review.*

Dukes MNG, Holgate ST, Pauwels RA. Report of an international workshop on risk and safety of asthma therapy. Clin Exp Allergy 1994; 24: 160-165. *Review.*

Helms PJ. Wheezing infants. Clin Exp Allergy 1994; 24: 97-99. *Review. For lack of benefit from cromoglycate see Arch Dis Child 1994; 71: 331-334.*

Gustafsson PA, Björkstén B, Kjellman N-IM. Family dysfunction in asthma: a prospective study of illness development. J Pediatr 1994; 125: 493-498. *Dysfunctional family interaction seems to be the result rather than the cause of the asthma.*

Kikuchi Y, Okabe S, Tamura G et al. Chemosensitivity and perception of dyspnea in patients with a history of near-fatal asthma. N Engl J Med 1994; 330: 1329-1334. *Reduced chemosensitivity to hypoxia and blunted perception of dyspnea may predispose patients to fatal asthma attacks. See editorial pp. 1383-1384.*

Korppi M, Kuikka L, Reijonen T et al. Bronchial asthma and hyperreactivity after early childhood bronchiolitis or pneumonia: an 8-year follow-up study. Arch Pediatr Adolesc Med 1994; 148: 1079-1084. *The risk of asthma and bronchial hyperreactivity were both increased.*

McKenzie SA. Aminophylline in the hospital treatment of children with acute asthma. On the way out. BMJ 1994; 308: 1384. *Review. See also Pediatrics 1994; 93: 205-210 and Lancet 1994; 343: 1006-1008.*

Oswald H, Phelan PD, Lanigan A et al. Outcome of childhood asthma in mid-adult life. BMJ 1994; 309: 95-96. *Many children do not grow out of asthma, and the more troublesome their asthma is, the less likely they are to do so. See also pp. 72-73 and 90-93.*

Seaton A, Godden DJ, Brown K. Increase in asthma: a more toxic environment or a more susceptible population? Thorax 1994; 49: 171-174. *Changes in diet (less fruit and fresh fish) may be a more likely explanation for the increase in asthma than changes in air pollution or house dust mites.*

Sly PD, Cahill P, Willet K et al. Accuracy of mini peak flow meters in indicating changes in lung function in children with asthma. BMJ 1994; 308: 572-574. *The values obtained should be interpreted cautiously. See editorial pp. 548-549. For symptom based outcome measures see BMJ 1994; 309: 1065-1068.*

Taylor MRH. Asthma: audit of peak flow rate guidelines for admission and discharge. Arch Dis Child 1994; 70: 432-434. *PEFR can help to reduce unnecessary admission. (Guidelines: above 60% of expected, admission unnecessary; 40–60% – consider admission, less than 40%, admission necessary).*

**Cystic fibrosis**

Fuchs HJ, Borowitz DS, Christiansen DH et al. Effect of aerosolized recombinant human DNase on exacerbations of respiratory symptoms and on pulmonary function in patients with cystic fibrosis. N Engl J Med 1994; 331: 637-642. *DNase reduced but did not eliminate exacerbation to respiratory symptoms, resulted in slight improvement in pulmonary function, and was well tolerated. See editorial pp. 672-673.*

Hanukoglu A, Bistritzer T, Rakover Y et al. Pseudohypoaldosteronism with increased sweat and saliva electrolyte values and frequent lower respiratory tract infections mimicking cystic fibrosis. J Pediatr 1994; 125: 752-755. *Four patients with severe hypoaldosteronism had frequently recurring lower respiratory tract infections and persistently elevated sweat electrolyte values.*

Harris CE, Wilmott W. Inhalation-based therapies in the treatment of cystic fibrosis. Curr Opin Pediatr 1994; 6: 234-238. *Review.*

Hung JCC, Hambleton G, Super M. Evaluation of two commercial jet nebulisers and three compressors for the nebulisation of antibiotics. Arch Dis Child 1994; 71: 335-338. *In terms of aerosol droplet size, nebulisation time, and aerosol output, there is a considerable difference between different jet nebulisers and compressors. Even with the best combination, only around 50% of the nominal dose was released as a respirable aerosol.*

Konstan MW, Stern RC, Doershuk CF. Efficacy of the flutter device for airway mucus clearance in patients with cystic fibrosis. J Pediatr 1994; 124: 689-693. *In a small sample, the flutter device was more effective than conventional techniques in clearing mucus from the airways.*

Lipuma JJ, Marks-Austin KA, Holsclaw Jr DS et al. Inapparent transmission of *Pseudomonas (Burkholderia) cepacia* among patients with cystic fibrosis. Pediatr Infect Dis J 1994; 13: 716-719. *Pulmonary colonization may not be detected for as long as 2 years after acquisition. For cross-infection see Pediatr Pulmonol 1994; 18: 108-113, J Pediatr 1994; 124: 694-702 and Arch Pediatr Adolesc Med 1994; 148: 805-812.*

Ramsey BW, Boat TF. Outcome measures for clinical trials in cystic fibrosis. J Pediatr 1994; 124: 177-192. Review.

Weaver LT, Green MR, Nicholson K et al. Prognosis in cystic fibrosis treated with continuous flucloxacillin from the neonatal period. Arch Dis Child 1994; 70: 84-89. *Continuous prophylactic flucloxacillin from early diagnosis is associated with improved clinical progress during the first two years of life.*

## RHEUMATOLOGY

Sponseller PD. Back pain in children. Curr Opin Pediatr 1994; 6: 99-103. *Review.*

## SURGERY

Chwals WJ. The metabolic response to surgery in neonates. Curr Opin Pediatr 1994; 6: 334-340. *Review.*

Dollery CM, Sullivan ID, Bauraind O et al. Thrombosis and embolism in long-term central venous access for parenteral nutrition. Lancet 1994; 344:

1043-1045. *In 34 children and adolescents with gut failure who received parenteral nutrition major thrombosis and/or embolism was identified in 12 patients, and 4 died as a consequence.*

Eason JD, McDonnell M, Clark G. Male ritual circumcision resulting in acute renal failure. BMJ 1994; 309: 660-661. *Tight bandaging after ritual circumcision may cause urinary obstruction and acute renal failure. For ureteral obstruction after appendicitis see Lancet 1994; 344: 99-100.*

Lund DP, Murphy EU. Management of perforated appendicitis in children: a decade of aggressive treatment. J Pediatr Surg 1994; 29: 1130-1134. *Review.*

Seashore JH, Touloukian RJ. Midgut volvulus. An ever-present threat. Arch Pediatr Adolesc Med 1994; 148: 43-46. *Neonates with a short history of bile stained vomiting are most likely to have midgut volvulus complicating malrotation.*

## THERAPEUTICS

Anonymous. Treating moderate and severe pain in infants. Drug Ther Bull 1994; 32: 21-24. *Review. For pain management in intensive care see Pediatr Clin N Am 1994; 41: 1183-1199 and for pain, trauma and memory see Curr Opin Pediatr 1994; 6: 411-417.*

Bauchner H, Vinci R, May A. Teaching parents how to comfort their children during common medical procedures. Arch Dis Child 1994; 70: 548-550. *Review. For distraction techniques see Pediatrics 1994; 93: 384-388 and 797-801.*

Como JA, Dismukes WE. Oral azole drugs as systemic antifungal therapy. N Engl J Med 1994; 330: 263-272. *Review.*

Coté CJ. Sedation protocols – why so many variations. Pediatrics 1994; 94: 281-283. *Review.*

Everard ML, Evans M, Milner AD. Is tapping jet nebulisers worthwhile? Arch Dis Child 1994; 70: 538-539. *Tapping a nebuliser causes droplets adhering to the internal walls to fall to the base of the chamber and become available for nebulisation increasing up to a further 40% of drug.*

McClure RJ, Prasad VK, Brocklebank JT. Treatment of hyperkalaemia using intravenous and nebulised salbutamol. Arch Dis Child 1994; 70: 126-128. *Nebulised salbutamol should be the first choice emergency treatment of hyperkalaemia.*

Nunn J, Lowry L, Lowry R. The use of aspirin in children under 12 years old attending a paediatric dentistry department in a dental hospital. Health Trends 1994; 26: 31-32. *Of 129 children under 12, 72 (56%) had taken an analgesic in the previous six months, and 12 (17%) of these had taken aspirin.*

Orlowski JP. Emergency alternatives to intravenous access: intraosseous, intratracheal, sublingual, and other-site drug administration. Pediatr Clin North Am 1994; 41: 1183-1199. *Review.*

Russell G. Inhaled corticosteroid therapy in children: an assessment of the potential for side effects. Thorax 1994; 49: 1185-1188. *Review.*

TROPICAL

Adegbola RA, Falade AG, Sam BE et al. The etiology of pneumonia in malnourished and well-nourished Gambian children. Pediatr Infect Dis J 1994; 13: 975-982. *Report of 159 cases. For hypoxia in pneumonia see BMJ 1994; 308: 119-120.*

Bredow MT, Jackson AA. Community based, effective, low cost approach to the treatment of severe malnutrition in rural Jamaica. Arch Dis Child 1994; 71: 297-303. *Management consisted of carefully delivered dietary advice, antibiotics, antihelminthics, and vitamin supplements.*

Khanum S, Ashworth A, Huttly SRA. Controlled trial of three approaches to the treatment of severe malnutrition. Lancet 1994; 344: 1728-1732. *After one week of in-patient care, at home management of severely malnourished children is a cost effective strategy.*

Morley CJ, Rashiq H, Thomas IRJ et al. Use of Baby Check to assess the severity of illness in babies attending a clinic in the Gambia. J Trop Pediatr 1994; 40: 144-148. *The use of Baby Check could be a valuable tool for the identification of babies that require referral.*

Raymond EG, Tafari N, Troendle JF et al. Development of a practical screening tool to identify preterm, low-birthweight neonates in Ethiopia. Lancet 1994; 344: 524-527. *Neonatal body measurements can be combined into a pragmatic accurate screening tool suitable for clinical use in developing countries.*

Rodrigues MESM, Melo M, Reis FJC et al. Concentration of electrolytes in the sweat of malnourished children. Arch Dis Child 1994; 71: 141-143. *Malnourished children have raised sweat sodium and chloride concentrations when compared with well nourished children, but electrolyte values were not in the cystic fibrosis range.*

Sloan NL, Camacho LWL, Rojas EP et al. Kangaroo mother method: randomised controlled trial of an alternative method of care for stabilised low-birthweight infants. Lancet 1994; 344: 782-785. *Substantially lower incidences of severe illnesses, especially lower respiratory tract infection, was seen with the kangaroo mother method.*

Solomon T, Felix JM, Samuel M et al. Hypoglycaemia in paediatric admissions in Mozambique. Lancet 1994; 343: 149-150. *Hypoglycaemia should be sought in all severely ill children. See also pp. 732-733.*

**Gastroenteritis**

Grange AO, Santosham M, Ayodele AK et al. Evaluation of a maize-cowpea-palm oil diet for the dietary management of Nigerian children with acute, watery diarrhea. Acta Paediatr 1994; 83: 825-832. *Children can safely consume the diet during acute watery diarrhoea without increasing the risk of treatment failure. For hydrolyzed lactalbumin based oral rehydration solution see pp.819-824.*

Maulén-Radován I, Brown KH, Acosta MA et al. Comparison of a rice-based, mixed diet versus a lactose-free, soy-protein isolate formula for young children with acute diarrhea. J Pediatr 1994; 125: 699-706. *The mixed diet resulted in improved clinical outcomes compared with the lactose-free, soy protein isolate formula.*

## Immunization

Pruksakorn S, Currie B, Brandt E et al. Towards a vaccine for rheumatic fever: identification of a conserved target epitope on M protein of group A streptococci. Lancet 1994; 344: 639-642. *The highly conserved part of the M protein may be a suitable target for vaccines to prevent streptococcal infections and their sequelae.*

van Niekerk ABW, Vries JB, Baard J et al. Outbreak of paralytic poliomyelitis in Namibia. Lancet 1994; 344: 661-664. *Report of the factors that may have had a role in this outbreak. For details of outbreak in an unvaccinated community in the Netherlands see pp. 665-670, and for editorial see pp. 630-631.*

## Infant feeding

Cohen RJ, Brown KH, Canahuati J et al. Effects of age of introduction of complementary foods on infant breast milk intake, total energy intake, and growth: a randomised intervention study in Honduras. Lancet 1994; 344: 288-293. *Breast fed infants self regulate their total energy intake when other foods are introduced, and there was no advantage in introducing complementary foods before six months in this population.*

Molbak K, Gottschau A, Aaby P et al. Prolonged breast feeding, diarrhoeal disease, and survival of children in Guinea-Bissau. BMJ 1994; 308: 1403-1406. *The benefit of breast feeding is not restricted to infancy.*

## Malaria

Alonso PL, Smith T, Armstrong Schellenberg JRM et al. Randomised trial of efficacy of SPf66 vaccine against *Plasmodium falciparum* malaria in children in southern Tanzania. Lancet 1994; 344: 1175-1181. *SPf66 is safe, immunogenic and reduces the risk of clinical malaria among children exposed to intense Plasmodium falciparum transmission. See editorial pp. 1172-1173.*

Loevinsohn ME. Climatic warming and increased malaria incidence in Rwanda. Lancet 1994; 343: 714-718. *Findings suggest a link between the upsurge of malaria and enhanced transmission resulting from the concurrence of increased temperature and rainfall.*

Newton CRJC, Peshu N, Kendall B et al. Brain swelling and ischaemia in

Kenyans with cerebral malaria. Arch Dis Child 1994; 70: 281-287. *Brain injury and cerebral malaria may be due in part to secondary systemic and intracranial factors as well as to the direct effect of intravascular sequestration.*

## Vitamin A

Bhandari N, Bhan MK, Sazawal S. Impact of massive dose of vitamin A given to preschool children with acute diarrhoea on subsequent respiratory and diarrhoeal morbidity. BMJ 1994; 309: 1404-1407. *Lack of impact on acute lower respiratory tract related mortality after vitamin A supplementation, and a possible reduction in the severity of diarrhoea.*

Barreto ML, Santos LMP, Assis AMO et al. Effect of vitamin A supplementation on diarrhoea and acute lower-respiratory-tract infections in young children in Brazil. Lancet 1994; 344: 228-231. *The reduction in severity of diarrhoea may be the most important factor in the lowering of mortality by vitamin A supplementation.*

Semba RD, Miotti PG, Chiphangwi JD et al. Maternal vitamin A deficiency and mother-to-child transmission of HIV-1. Lancet 1994; 343: 1593-1596. *Maternal vitamin A deficiency contributes to mother-to-child transmission of HIV.*

# Index

* after page numbers refers to papers in the literature review section (Chapter 13)